Aptasensors for Point-of-Care Diagnostics of Cancer

From lab to clinics

Online at: https://doi.org/10.1088/978-0-7503-5012-9

IOP Series in Global Health and Radiation Oncology

Series editor
Wilfred Ngwa
Dana-Farber/Harvard Cancer Center, University of Massachusetts Lowell, Johns Hopkins University, USA

Editor biography
Wilfred Ngwa is the Director of the Global Health Catalyst, a cross-institutional collaboration initiative launched at Harvard to catalyse high impact collaborations in global health. He currently serves as Adjunct Professor at the University of Massachusetts, as Associate Professor of Radiation Oncology at Johns Hopkins University and as ICTU Distinguished Professor of Public Health. He is a chair of the Lancet Oncology Commission for Sub-Saharan Africa, has published three books on global health and serves on the editorial board of a number of journals, including ASCO's *Journal of Global Oncology, Ecancermedicalsciences*, and *Frontiers in Oncology*. He has won many awards from Harvard, the USA National Institutes of Health, and international professional organisations for his innovations and leading work in global health to address disparities in the USA and globally.

Aims and scope
This series includes books in the emerging area of global radiation oncology and its applications in global health. Building on the published book by the series editor entitled *Emerging Models for Global Health in Radiation Oncology*, it will further detail the work being done globally to promote cancer research and awareness, particularly in lower-income countries.

A full list of titles published in this series can be found here: https://iopscience.iop.org/bookListInfo/iop-series-in-cancer-research-for-global-radiation-oncology#series.

Aptasensors for Point-of-Care Diagnostics of Cancer

From lab to clinics

Edited by
Arpana Parihar
CSIR-Advanced Materials and Processes Research Institute (AMPRI), Bhopal, India

Pushpesh Ranjan
CSIR-Advanced Materials and Processes Research Institute (AMPRI), Bhopal, India

Raju Khan
CSIR-Advanced Materials and Processes Research Institute (AMPRI), Bhopal, India

IOP Publishing, Bristol, UK

ISBN 978-0-7503-5012-9 (ebook)
ISBN 978-0-7503-5010-5 (print)
ISBN 978-0-7503-5013-6 (myPrint)
ISBN 978-0-7503-5011-2 (mobi)

DOI 10.1088/978-0-7503-5012-9

Version: 20231201

IOP ebooks

British Library Cataloguing-in-Publication Data: A catalogue record for this book is available from the British Library.

Published by IOP Publishing, wholly owned by The Institute of Physics, London

IOP Publishing, No.2 The Distillery, Glassfields, Avon Street, Bristol, BS2 0GR, UK

US Office: IOP Publishing, Inc., 190 North Independence Mall West, Suite 601, Philadelphia, PA 19106, USA

Dedicated to Almighty, who gave us the strength to complete this work.

Contents

Preface

The global burden of cancer-associated death can be reduced by employing early and cost-effective point-of-care (POC) diagnostics. The early detection and timely management of cancer have proven clinical benefits. The CT-Scan, PET, MRI, and tissue biopsy are conventional gold-standard methods for cancer diagnosis. These techniques are invasive, costly, and need expensive setup and skilled personnel, which makes them out of reach to people belonging to low- and middle-income countries. The high incidence rate with poor prognosis created a huge need for the development of low-cost, highly specific POC devices for disease management in the field of cancer diagnostics. This book aims to present the current state-of-art of aptasensors-based POC devices and addresses its present and future prospects for the diagnosis of cancer biomarkers. The key element in this book will be the current advancement of the POC aptasensors, their working principle, and their wider applicability along with future developments. This book also focuses on the advanced design and fabrication of robust miniaturized lab-on-chip devices with enhanced features. Additionally, the usage of nanostructured materials and their significance in the construction of POC aptasensors will be discussed. From a futuristic point of view, the integration of the POC aptasensors-based sensing platform with the wireless platform (internet of medical things) for intelligent disease management will provide researchers with novel mechanistic insight in a concise and well-framed manner, which can be exploited for the development of novel aptasensors for onsite disease diagnostics. Overall, the perfect amalgamation of multidisciplinary fields such as oncology, nano-biotechnology, chemistry, material science, physics, and the healthcare industry would open new ways in the field of cancer diagnostics. Further, the present book emphasizes the target-specific design and fabrications of aptasensors and their potential applications for cancer biomarkers diagnostics. Aptamers are a good alternative to antibody-based biosensors and are designed to target specific biomarkers associated with cancer; however, the role of aptasensors and transducing techniques, including electrochemical and optical, should be designed carefully so that the captured behavior of target analytes can be measured properly. The advancement of aptasensors may become a milestone in analytical biosensors for the detection of cancer biomarkers from the lab to the medical and clinical platforms. This book supports readers with the current state-of-the-art POC aptasensors-based devices and addressed its present and future prospects for the diagnosis of cancer biomarkers. This book will demonstrate the current advancement of the POC aptasensors diagnostic devices, their working principle, and the historical overview of their utility along with future developments. This book would enable readers with a cutting-edge technological platform on the current understanding of the POC aptasensors devices along with insightful mechanistic findings of this rapidly developing diagnostic technology as an alternative to conventional antibody-based diagnostic modalities. This book is intended to inculcate the state-of-art emerging knowledge and wider diagnostic applications of aptasensors for cancer diagnosis.

This comprehensive work in this book has been compiled into 12 chapters, which would be useful for researchers, scholars, and manufacturers in medical device design, bioengineering, nanobiotechnology, materials science, biomaterials, and biochemistry. Chapters 1 and 2 discuss an overview and a brief history of aptamer-based POC detection from the lab to clinical applications along with a brief explanation and advantages of aptamers in diagnostics systems for disease management. Chapter 3 discusses the aptamer-based biosensor devices and aspects such as the characterization of bio-recognition probes with their respective analytes, immobilization onto electrode surfaces, and the development of anti-fouling surface chemistries. Special attention will be on different types of surface chemistry used for the development of simple, sensitive, and cost-effective aptasensors. Chapter 4 will include the use of aptasensor techniques to detect metastatic cancer cells. Besides, a brief explanation of the immobilization techniques as receptors on the sensor surface along with *in vitro* assays in real-time detection of cancer cells will be presented. Chapter 5 will explain the excellent features of the label-free aptasensors for the sensitive and accurate monitoring of cancer biomarkers. Also, the role of advanced nanomaterials in the construction of aptasensors for POC testing will be discussed. Chapter 6 discusses the synthesis and selection of aptamers specifically against cancer biomarkers and cells. Additionally, the advantages of nanomaterials that improve the affinity of aptamers in comparison to antibodies are discussed. Chapter 7 intends to describe recent advances made in the field of electrochemical aptasensors for the detection of cancer biomarkers such as specific genes, microRNA, proteins, circulating tumor cells, cell lines, and exosomes or exosome-derived biomarkers. Chapter 8 will summarize the recent developments in different approaches belonging to optical aptasensor technologies being widely employed for their simple operation, sensitivity, and early cancer diagnostics. It will also shed some light on the limitations, advantages, and current challenges in clinical diagnostics, and elaborate on some future perspectives. Chapter 9 highlights the recent progress in aptamer-based screening with emphasis on the integration of aptamers with various forms of LOC devices, including microfluidic chips and paper-based microfluidic devices. Chapter 10 summarizes the cutting-edge developments in nanotechnology/nanobiotechnology applications for cancer diagnosis. In addition, the challenges in the translation of nanotechnology-based diagnostic methods into clinical applications are also discussed. Chapter 11 discusses the role of aptamers in the current diagnostic and therapeutic applications and addresses the challenges associated with them. The chapter also sheds light on the implementation of aptamer conjugates for diagnostic purposes and, finally, the therapeutic aptamers under clinical investigation, challenges therein, and their future directions will also be discussed. Chapter 12 aims to discuss the fundamentals and highlight the clinical applications of aptamers-based platforms in cancer diagnosis and treatment in special context to technology developed in labs and transferred to industry/clinics.

With Warm Regards
Arpana Parihar
Pushpesh Ranjan
Raju Khan

Acknowledgments

The editors gratefully appreciate the support from all authors of the respective chapters in this book. Their sincere efforts, quick response, and analytical approach have been highly valued and acknowledged. The editors are grateful to the director of the CSIR-AMPRI, Bhopal, Madhya Pradesh, India, for his wise counsel and guidance. The Department of Science and Technology, Government of India, is gratefully acknowledged for providing fellowship to Dr Arpana Parihar (DST/ WOS- B/HN-4/2021) under the DST-WoS-B Scheme. Dr Raju Khan is thankful to SERB (IPA/2020/000130) for financial support.

Editor biographies

Dr Arpana Parihar

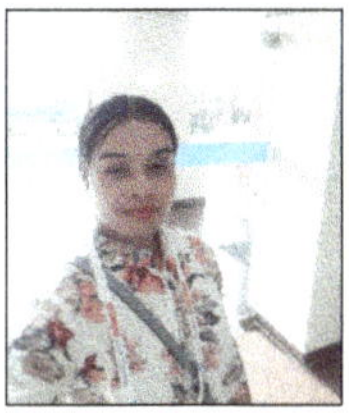

Dr Arpana Parihar is a DST Women Scientist B at CSIR-Advanced Materials and Processes Research Institute (AMPRI), Bhopal, India. She did her PhD at Raja Rammana Centre for Advanced Technology (RRCAT), Indore, and postdoctoral research work at the Centre for Biomedical Engineering (CBME), Indian Institute of Technology (IIT), Delhi. Dr Parihar is awarded prestigious GATE, CSIR-NET, DST-WoS A, and WoS B fellowships. She has more than 8 years of research and teaching experience in the field of disease therapeutics and diagnostics. Her research work in the field of cancer therapeutics and fabrication technologies (micro/nano-fabrication) for bio-devices/bio-medical POCT devices for early diagnosis of cancer and infectious disease gained considerable attention. She has published over 35 articles, 5 edited books, and written 25 book chapters with reputed publishers.

Pushpesh Ranjan

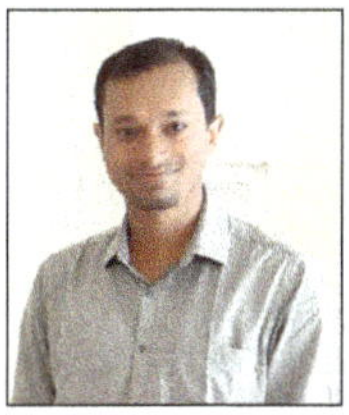

Pushpesh Ranjan is currently pursuing his Doctorate from CSIR-Advanced Materials and Processes Research Institute (AMPRI), Bhopal under the guidance of Dr Raju Khan. He completed his M.Sc. (Chemistry) from Dr Harisingh Gour Central University, Sagar, MP in the year 2017. He qualified as a CSIR-JRF and GATE and joined as a PhD candidate in Chemical Sciences in CSIR-AMPRI, Bhopal in 2018. His research interest lies in the synthesis of hybrid nanocomposites of ionic liquids with graphene materials and the development of a biosensor for the diagnosis of cancer biomarkers. He has published 19 manuscripts in reputed journals and 15 book chapters in IOP, Elsevier, and CRC Taylor and Francis under his research profile.

Dr Raju Khan

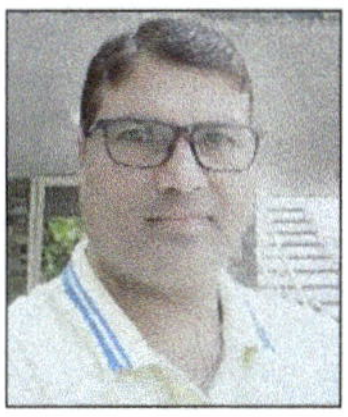

Dr Raju Khan, FRSC is currently working as a Senior Principal Scientist and Professor at CSIR-Advanced Materials and Processes Research Institute (AMPRI), Bhopal, MP, India. He has more than 15 years of experience in electrochemistry exploring electrochemical properties of nanostructure to design and develop efficient biosensor devices for health care monitoring. He has published 95 articles with high citation scores in several renowned scientific journals and 2 patent files filled. Apart from this, he has shown his workmanship by writing 35 book chapters in esteemed publishers like Elsevier, Taylor and Francis, and IOP. He has also shown his proficiency by editing 20 books with various reputed publishers.

List of contributors

Rajesh Ahirwar
Department of Environmental Biochemistry, ICMR-National Institute for Research in Environmental Health, Bhopal Bypass Road, Bhauri, Bhopal 462030, India

Aadil Ashraf
Department of Biotechnology, Pondicherry University, Pondicherry 605014, India

Lal Singh Banjara
Government Indira Gandhi Home Science Girls PG College, Shahdol, Madhya Pradesh 484001, India

Murthy Chavali
Office of the Dean (Research), Dr Vishwanath Karad MIT World Peace University (MIT-WPU), Kothrud, Pune, Maharashtra 411038, India

Rishibha Dixit
Algal Biotechnology Laboratory, Department of PG Studies and Research in Biological Science, Rani Durgavati University, Jabalpur, Madhya Pradesh 482001, India

Supraja Enamala
Sreerama Engineering and MBA College, Karkambadi, Tirupati 517520, India

S M Faheem
School of Lifesciences, Manipal Academy of Higher Education, G04, Dubai International Academic City (DIAC), PO Box, Dubai 345050, UAE

Ali Firoozbakhtian
Nanobiosensors Lab, Department of Life Science Engineering, Faculty of New Sciences and Technologies, University of Tehran, Tehran 1439817435, Iran

Nkurunziza Florien
Department of Biotechnology, Maharishi Markandeshwar University, Mullana, Ambala 134003, India

Sonu Gandhi
DBT-National Institute of Animal Biotechnology (DBT-NIAB), Hyderabad, Telangana 500032, India

Mohammad Reza Ganjali
Center of Excellence in Electrochemistry, School of Chemistry, College of Science, University of Tehran, Tehran 1439817435, Iran

Kritika Gaur
Central Sheep and Wool Research Institute. ICAR- Indian Council of Agricultural Research, Avikanagr, Malpura, Rajasthan, India

Debanjan Ghosh
Department of Biotechnology, Pondicherry University, Pondicherry 605014, India

Javad Gilnezhad
Center of Excellence in Electrochemistry, School of Chemistry, College of Science, University of Tehran, Tehran 1439817435, Iran

Shagun Gupta
Department of Biotechnology, Maharishi Markandeshwar University, Mullana, Ambala 134003, India

Sakshi Hardaha
Department of Biotechnology, Pondicherry University, Pondicherry 605014, India

Morteza Hosseini
Nanobiosensors Lab, Department of Life Science Engineering, Faculty of New Sciences and Technologies, University of Tehran, Tehran 1439817435, Iran

Payal B Joshi
Shefali Research Laboratories, Ambernath, Thane, Maharashtra, India

Deepak Kala
Department of Biotechnology Engineering and Food Technology, Chandigarh University, Mohali 140413, India

Ankur Kaushal
Department of Biotechnology, Maharishi Markandeshwar University, Mullana, Ambala 134003, India

Nabab Khan
CSIR-Institute of Himalayan Bioresource Technology (IHBT), PO Box No. 6, Palampur, Himachal Pradesh 176061, India

Raju Khan
CSIR-Advanced Materials and Processes Research Institute (AMPRI), Hoshangabad Road, Bhopal, Madhya Pradesh 462026, India and Academy of Scientific and Innovative Research (AcSIR), Ghaziabad 201002, India

Enamala Manoj Kumar
Bioserve Biotechnologies (India) Private Limited Unit: D4-7, 1st Floor, Industrial Estate, Moula Ali, Hyderabad, Telangana 500040, India

S Krishnamoorthi
Department of Chemistry, Institute of Science, Banaras Hindu University, Varanasi, Uttar Pradesh 221005, India

Ajay Kumar Meena
Regional Ayurveda Research Institute, Amkho, Gwalior 474009, India

Sayali Mukherjee
Amity Institute of Biotechnology, Amity University, Uttar Pradesh, Lucknow Campus, Lucknow, Uttar Pradesh, India

Soumyadeep Mukherjee
Department of Botany, Banaras Hindu University, Varanasi, Uttar Pradesh 221005, India

Arpana Parihar
CSIR-Advanced Materials and Processes Research Institute (AMPRI), Hoshangabad Road, Bhopal, Madhya Pradesh 462026, India

Pushpesh Ranjan
CSIR-Advanced Materials and Processes Research Institute (AMPRI), Hoshangabad Road, Bhopal, Madhya Pradesh 462026, India and Academy of Scientific and Innovative Research (AcSIR), Ghaziabad 201002, India

Mohd. Abubakar Sadique
CSIR-Advanced Materials and Processes Research Institute (AMPRI), Hoshangabad Road, Bhopal, Madhya Pradesh 462026, India and Academy of Scientific and Innovative Research (AcSIR), Ghaziabad 201002, India

Deepshikha Shahdeo
DBT-National Institute of Animal Biotechnology (DBT-NIAB), Hyderabad-500032, Telangana

Surbhi Sharma
Department of Biotechnology, Maharishi Markandeshwar University, Mullana, Ambala 134003, India

Tanushree Sharma
Amity Institute of Biotechnology, Amity University Uttar Pradesh Lucknow Campus, Lucknow, Uttar Pradesh, India and Molecular and Human Genetics, Banaras Hindu University, Varanasi, Uttar Pradesh 221005, India Uttar Pradesh, India

Rudramani Tiwari
Department of Chemistry, Institute of Science, Banaras Hindu University, Varanasi, Uttar Pradesh 221005, India and Regional Ayurveda Research Institute, Amkho, Gwalior 474009, India

Subhash Chandra Verma
Regional Ayurveda Research Institute, Amkho, Gwalior 474009, India

Shalu Yadav
CSIR-Advanced Materials and Processes Research Institute (AMPRI), Hoshangabad Road, Bhopal, Madhya Pradesh 462026, India and Academy of Scientific and Innovative Research (AcSIR), Ghaziabad 201002, India

Chapter 1

Aptamer-based point-of-care testing: an overview from past to future

Rajesh Ahirwar and Nabab Khan

Aptamers are a widely acknowledged affinity reagent evolved to meet most diagnostic and/or therapeutic applications. These single-stranded short oligonucleotides can be easily modified and tethered onto diverse polymers (plastic, cellulose) and nano- and micro-particles (gold, magnetic, upconverting phosphors) to device diagnostic tools and techniques in various formats. Their competency for use in point-of care (POC) diagnostics meeting the ASSURED criteria (affordable, sensitive, specific, user-friendly, robust, equipment free and deliverable) has been vastly researched. This chapter provides an elementary introduction to the use of aptamers as a molecular recognition element in multiple conventional as well as novel diagnostic platforms used for POC diagnostics. Technological advances in aptamer-based POC diagnostic platforms are also discussed.

1.1 Introduction to aptamers

Aptamers are small non-coding functional oligonucleotides that are artificially raised by combinatorial methodology of *in vitro* selection termed as systematic evolution of ligands by exponential enrichment (SELEX). These tiny oligonucleotides have the capability of selectively binding their targets through an adaptive recognition mechanism, thus achieving the same level of target affinity and specificity as offered by other conventional biorecognition molecules such as antibodies. To date, numerous aptamers have been identified against several targets such as antibiotics [1], amino acids [2], proteins [3], viruses [4], and even whole cell and cellular components [5]. The term 'aptamer' is derived from the combination of a Latin word '*aptus*' which means 'to fit', and a Greek word '*méros*' meaning 'part'. Aptamers are nucleic acid molecules that differ vastly from other major categories of non-coding oligonucleotides (table 1.1).

doi:10.1088/978-0-7503-5012-9ch1

Table 1.1. Key differences among various categories of non-coding oligonucleotides.

Oligonucleotides	Structural form	Major target	Mechanism of action/use
Aptamer	ss RNA or DNA	Metabolites, peptides, proteins	Selective binding; diagnostic and therapeutic applications
Antisense	ss DNA	mRNA	Binds to mRNA and inhibits translation
Decoy nucleic acid	ds DNA	Transcription factor	Traps TF and inhibits transcription
Ribozyme	ss RNA	mRNA	Cut the mRNA and controls expression
siRNA	ds RNA	mRNA	Cuts the mRNA and controls expression
miRNA	ss RNA	mRNA	Binds to mRNA and inhibits translation
anti-miRNA	ss RNA/ DNA	miRNA	Binds to miRNA and inhibits its activity

ss-single stranded, ds-double stranded.

The history of aptamer selection trails back to the 1990s when three independent groups, Tuerk and Gold [6], Ellington and Szostak [7], and Robertson and Joyce [8] materialized the concept of aptamers. To understand the nature of the translational regulation of 43 mRNA by the phage T4 replicase, Craig Tuerk mutated the 8-nucleotide stretch within the regulatory loop of the mRNA. Systematic exposure of the resulting pool of mutated sequences ($4^8 = 65\ 536$) to the T4 replicase resulted in identification of two sequences with similar binding affinity. This experiment for the first time laid the fundamentals of systematic evaluation of ligands by exponential enrichment (SELEX) screening. At the same time, while investigating if the RNA molecules can adapt structures that act as binding pockets for small molecules, Ellington and Szostak utilized a similar strategy to identify a subpopulation of RNA molecules that bind specifically to a variety of organic dyes. This finding also designated the resultant ligands as *aptamers*, to describe their target-fitting characteristic. These experiments established the fundamentals for the discovery of aptamers. In the last two decades, the method of aptamer selection has witnessed many modifications to assist in the identification of target and utility-specific aptamers and rapid screening.

Evolving from these classical experiments, the conventional method of aptamer selection relies on oligonucleotide libraries custom synthesized based on combinatorial chemistry to screen aptamers through the SELEX method. A typical oligonucleotide library has a central randomized region of 30–60 nt, flanked by two fixed regions of 18–22 nt [9]. The fixed regions are needed as priming sequences for amplification during SELEX enrichment. This makes every sequence in an oligonucleotide library to have an average length of 50–80 nucleotides. As the success of a SELEX screening hugely depends on the number and diversity of sequences used, it is very important to synthesize a library of a highly diverse nature. Generally, to obtain a sufficiently diverse oligonucleotide library, the lengths of fixed priming sequences are kept to a minimum, while the random part is kept long, and the synthesis scale is in the micromolar range. However, due to mass limitation (total mass of all the sequences in a library) and the coupling efficiency of oligonucleotide synthesis, the majority of libraries are synthesized at the nanomole scale to give nucleic acid pools of up to 10^{15} individual sequences [10]. Table 1.2 outlines some of the interesting theoretical aspects of a typical DNA/RNA library [11].

Over the past three decades, a large number of aptamers have been screened and tested in multiple diagnostic and therapeutic applications [12]. In particular, aptamers have been raised as substitutes to conventional antibodies (table 1.3) in diagnostics because of their easy and cheap production that also lacks the batch-to-batch variability. They are also easy to chemically modify, and have a better shelf life, stability, and non-immunogenicity [13]. The few of the key advantages of aptamers over antibody counterparts include:

Size: One of the most essential characteristics of the aptamers is their size. Typical size of aptamers (7–15 kDa) is approximately one-tenth the size of an average IgG antibody. Compared to antibodies, the small size of aptamers allows them to easily diffuse in liquid media, and readily penetrate the tissues, along with their faster renal clearance. Nevertheless, modifications such as cholesterol and PEG attachment increases the serum half-life and lowers the rate of renal clearance [14].

Stability: Ability of the aptamers to withstand the denaturation problem (by reversible renaturation) and add additional weightage to their utility in biological applications. Although aptamers do not require protection from proteases, they are susceptible to nuclease degradation. Particularly, the RNA aptamers are more prone to nuclease degradation due to the presence of the 2′-OH on the sugar moiety [15, 16].

Table 1.2. Representation of sequences in the naive pool of a typical DNA/RNA library [11].

Random region (nt)	Number of possible unique sequences ($= 4^{nt}$)	Average representation ofeach unique sequence (synth. scale = 0.1 nmol)	Average representation of each unique sequence (synth. scale = 25 nmol)
5	1.06×10^{3}	5.96×10^{10}	1.56×10^{13}
10	1.06×10^{6}	5.76×10^{7}	1.46×10^{13}
15	1.16×10^{9}	56 000	$1.461 \times {}^{07}$
18	6.96×10^{10}	880	2.26×10^{5}
19	2.76×10^{11}	220	55 000
20	1.16×10^{12}	55	14 000
21	4.46×10^{12}	14	3400
22	1.86×10^{13}	3.4[a]	860
23	7.06×10^{13}	0.86	210
24	2.86×10^{14}	0.21	53
25	1.16×10^{15}	5.36×10^{-2}	13
26	4.56×10^{15}	1.36×10^{-2}	3.3[b]
30[b]	1.26×10^{18}	5.26×10^{-5}	1.36×10^{-2}
40	1.26×10^{24}	5.06×10^{-11}	1.26×10^{-8}
60	1.26×10^{36}	4.56×10^{-23}	1.16×10^{-20}

[a] Beyond diversity limit; some possible sequences are absent.

[b] Beyond synthesizer limit for 1 μmol scale synthesis; some sequences are not produced.

adaptability of the aptamers which assures selective target recognition and binding. Some of the major diagnostic techniques that have shown promising results using aptamer as a molecular recognition element include the enzyme-linked aptamer/oligonucleotide assays, lateral flow assay, nanoparticle-based 'on' and 'off' colorimetric and fluorescence assays, and electrochemical biosensing tools and techniques [21, 22].

1.2 Point-of-care testing

Timely detection of diseases and their causative agents is of utmost importance to derive effective therapeutics and other disease prevention and management strategies. The tools and techniques of clinical diagnosis hold a long history, with only few tests available in the early days that allow disease diagnosis at the patient's bedside. Later, automated technologies allowed centralized clinical laboratories to run large numbers of tests. Sending samples to specialized laboratories and waiting hours to days for results became a common practice. Subsequent advances in biological, material and engineering sciences allowed researchers to come up with tests that can be done anywhere, within or outside laboratories, at home, in a primary, secondary, or tertiary health care facility, in ambulances, at an accident scene, or anywhere but near a patient. Also, these tests provide results quickly so that they can be acted upon without delay. Often referred to as 'self tests' or 'home tests', these tests are now called point-of-care tests (POCTs). Various schools of thought persist defining POCTs; some suggest POCs to be tests that lead to an improved health outcome, others complement them to have such a fast turnaround time that the communication of results to the decision makers is possible within a day. Also, they allow both a health practitioner as well as a layman to easily perform the test and understand the outcome. Broadly, the ASSURED criterion (Affordable, Sensitive, Specific, User-friendly, Robust, Equipment-free, and Deliverable to those who need these tools) is one that is adopted by most to define POCTs.

POCTs have emerged as a useful diagnostic aid that allows early detection, prevention, and easy management of chronic health conditions. POCTs have witnessed huge demand for rapid screening for infectious diseases and critical parameters. For example, POCTs for blood glucose, activated clotting time, oxygen saturation, blood gases and electrolytes, hemoglobin/hematocrit, rapid HIV, thyroid stimulating hormone, human chorionic gonadotropin, creatinine, lipid profile, fecal occult blood, etc, have already made their entry into the clinical market.

1.3 Aptamer-based POCTs

POC testing tools use a variety of affinity molecules/reagents such as enzymes, antibodies, nucleic acids, glycan, and aptamers to assist in selective detection of target molecules/metabolites and subsequent generation of colorimetric, fluorometric or electrochemical signals [23, 24]. While the use of antibodies in diagnostics have been reported over a period of 11 decades, aptamers entered into diagnostic applications for less than 4 decades ago. Notwithstanding, aptamers have many advantages over antibodies. In particular, aptamer-based POC testing tools/methods harness and benefit from the low-cost, easy modification and functionalization capability (on to a variety of molecules, including nanoparticles and fluorophores), high specificity, slow off rates and high stability of aptamers [25]. Aptamer-based POCTs following 'ASSURED' criteria could be fruitful for home, communities, clinics, peripheral laboratories and hospitals-based settings [26].

Aptamer-based assays, such as aptamer-linked immunosorbent assay ALISA)/ enzyme-linked aptamer sorbent assay (ELASA)/enzyme-linked oligonucleotide assay (ELONA), gold nanoparticle-based aggregation assays, nanozyme (peroxidase like nanoparticles)-based assays, dot-blots assays, etc, have been widely reported in the literature [27]. A few of these POCTs have been discussed in detail in the below sections.

1.3.1 Lateral flow assay-based aptamer POCTs

Lateral flow assays (LFAs) are paper-based devices for the detection of target analytes in complex sample mixtures. LFA are performed on paper-based multi-strip (absorbent sample pad, conjugate release pad, detection zone, and wicking pad) devices, as shown in figure 1.2, that carry immobilized antibodies/aptamers and nanoparticles/chromogens, which move unidirectionally through capillary action upon addition of a liquid sample or sample extract on the test strip to produce results within a few minutes [28]. The absorbent pad is often made of cellulose acetate or glass fiber for their inertness towards proteins and other biomolecules. The sample migrates from the sample pad to conjugate release pad that holds the detector particles via electrostatic interaction between the nitrate ester and peptide bond of conjugated antibodies and to keep them functionally stable until the test is performed. Aptamers are conjugated with either AuNPs (red color) or latex microsphores (blue color). Target analytes present within the sample bind with the labeled aptamer and migrate further along the test strip into the detection zone. The detection zone consists of two regions—test and control, to indicate the presence or absence of an analyte in the sample through an appropriate response indicated on the test line. The control region or control line indicates the proper flow of solvent/ liquid through the strip [29].

In a typical aptamer-based LFA, the conjugation pad contains dried detection labels, such as aptamer-modified AuNPs, which migrate upon resuspension towards the test and control zones after addition of the test analyte sample onto the pad (figure 1.2). Aptamer-based LFAs offer an ideal POC testing method for a variety of targets. They can be designed in different formats and using different labels. Often, different detection strategies are employed for a different category of targets. For example, the three most widely used formats of aptamer LFA for proteins or large target molecule detection are sandwich (utilize two aptamers to bind at different sites of the target proteins), competitive (sample target competes with other target molecules integrated in the LFA strips), and adsorption–desorption assay formats. These assays are based on target-induced dissociation or displacement, target induced reassembling of aptamer fragments (split aptamers reassemble come together in the presence of the target), and target induced structure switching

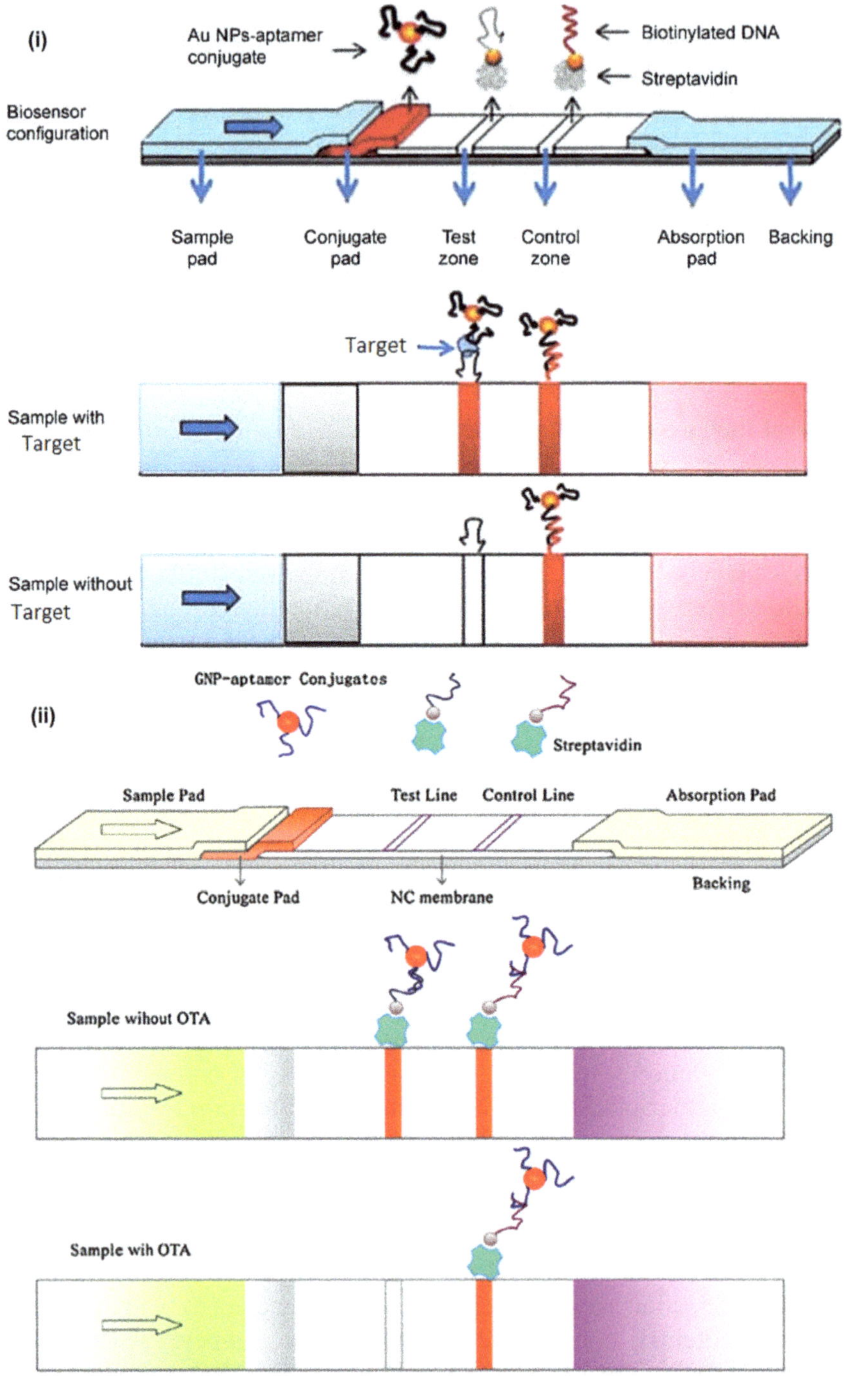

Figure 1.2. Schematic presentation of a sandwich and competitive aptamer-based LFA for (i) thrombin detection. Reproduced with permission from [30]. Copyright (2009) American Chemical Society (ii) Ochratoxin A detection. Reproduced with permission from [32]. Copyright (2011) Elsevier.

(aptamer under conformational change upon binding to their targets). An example of sandwich assay format is adopted by Xu *et al*, in which two aptamers that bind at two different sites of analytes are used (figure 1.2(i)) to detect thrombin protein [30]. The first aptamer (thiolated) is conjugated to AuNPs, and used as a recognition element by drying it on the conjugate pad. The second aptamer (biotinylated) served as a capture probe, which is sprayed on the test line via biotin-streptavidin interaction. Addition of sample solution containing target analyte on the sample pad leads to capillary flows of mixture into the conjugate pad, where the analyte binds to the AuNP-labeled aptamer. The resulting AuNP-aptamer-analyte complex then migrates along the strip towards the nitrocellulose membrane, where the analyte is selectively captured by the second aptamer already present immobilized on the test line, producing a red band in the test zone. Excess/unbound AuNP-aptamer passing the test line is captured through hybridization between the immobilized DNA probes and the primary aptamer in the control zone, producing another red band in the control zone. Presence of two bands indicates a positive result, while only one band (in the control zone) indicates absence of the analyte in samples [30].

A competitive assay format-based aptamer LFA POCT was developed by Wang *et al* in 2011 for the detection of mycotoxins with only one aptamer [32]. The thiolated aptamer polyadenylated at another end is conjugated to AuNPs. A biotin-modified complementary strand termed as DNA probe 1 is immobilized via streptavidin binding onto the test zone. On the other hand, a biotin-modified poly DNA probe 2 is immobilized onto the control line through streptavidin binding. Here, competitive affinity interaction between DNA probe 1 and the target molecule for binding to aptamers forms the basis of detection. In the presence of an analyte, the AuNP-aptamer bound to the analyte, decreasing the effective concentration of AuNP-aptamer for hybridization with DNA probe 1 on the test line and resulting in a weaker intensity of colorimetric signal (figure 1.2(ii)). The unbounded AuNP–apatmer hybridizes with DNA probe 2 on the control line. In this format, the concentration of analyte in the sample is inversely proportional to the intensity of the color signal.

Yet another format, the adsorption–desorption using AuNP as labels, was reported by Ranganathan *et al* in 2020 to detect human epidermal growth factor receptor 2 (HER2) in serum samples [33]. Authors prepared the LFA strip by coating with streptavidin and pullulan mixture at the test line, and a cationic charged polymer named polydiallyldimethylammonium chloride (PDDA) at the control line. Biotinylated HER2 aptamers coated onto AuNPs were used in the assay. In the presence of HER2 in the sample solution, it binds selectively to its aptamer, resulting in the release from AuNPs surface. Applying this solution onto the LFA strip result in the absence of a red signal on the test zone as the aptamer–HER2 complex was bound to the streptavidin on the membrane. The control zone turned red due to non-specific adsorption of anionic AuNPs by the cationic PDDA. In the absence of analyte, the aptamer–AuNP conjugate remained intact, leading to generation of a red signal on the test zone due to aptamer–AuNP binding to the streptavidin. The control zone turned red as before (figure 1.3(i)). Using this approach, the authors were able to detect HER2 with a LOD of 20 nM within approximately 30 min.

Furthermore, different strategies have been reported to increase the assay sensitivity of LFA POCTs to detect low concentrations of analyte. For example, replacing AuNPs with fluorescent labels or using enzymatic reactions to generate a colorimetric signal is one of the most common and popular methods to increase sensitivity. In this regard, enzyme mimetic nanomaterials or nanozymes with intrinsic enzymatic activity are a good option due to their unique properties compared to natural enzymes. Multiple aptamer-based LFA POCTs are reported in the literature to detect various biomarkers, microorganisms, hormones, and antibiotics (table 1.3) [31]. For example, an aptamer-based fluorescence quenching LFA can be devised by using fluorophores and AuNP-aptamer complex. The DNA-probe modified fluorophores when immobilized onto test line binds with AuNP-aptamer complexes through hybridization of the aptamer to the short complementary sequence on the fluorophore, causing quenching of fluorescent signal in the absence of target analyte. In presence of the target, the aptamer-AuNPs binds with the target

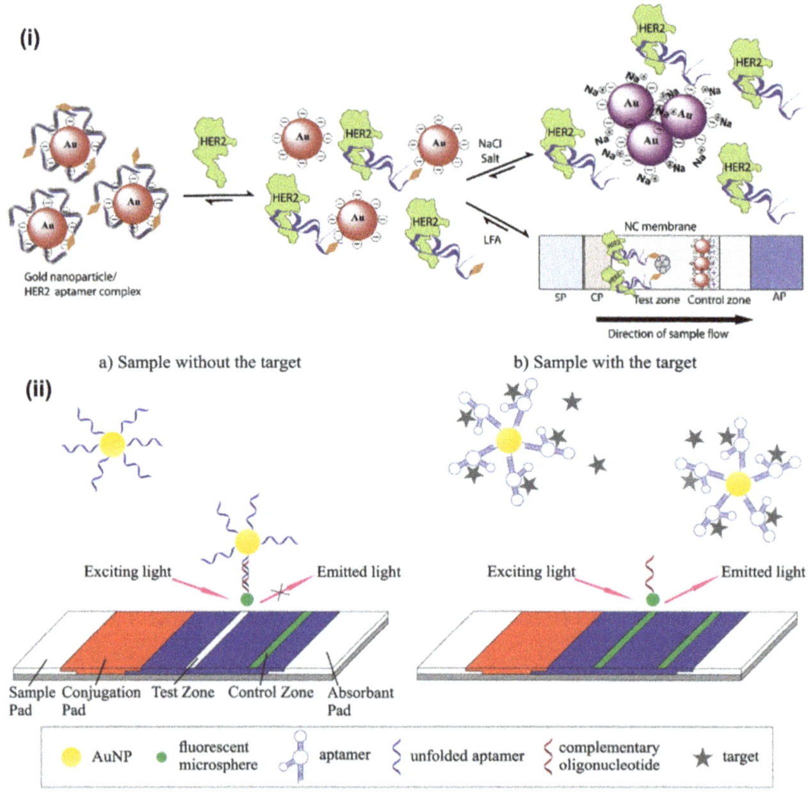

Figure 1.3. Schematic presentation of the principle of (i) adsorption–desorption based LFA. Reproduced with permission from [33]. Copyright (2019) Elsevier. (ii) The aptamer-based fluorescence quenching LFA. Reproduced with permission [34]. Copyright (2018) AIMS Press.

analyte and competes with the complementary sequence in the test zone for binding to aptamers. As less aptamer binds on the test zone, this leads to an increase in the fluorescent signal on the LFA device (figure 1.3(ii)) [34]. A descriptive overview of multiple lateral flow-based POC tests reported for the detection of biomarkers, microorganisms, hormones, and antibodies is provided in table 1.4.

1.3.2 Dot-blot based aptamer POCT

Dot-blotting is a routinely used POCT which is principally similar to aptamer-ELISA (ALISA), except the test is performed on nitrocellulose (NC) or another similar polymer membrane such as polyvinylidene fluoride (PVDF). A typical dot-blot assay involves the immobilization of the target antigen onto an NC or PVDF membrane by direct spotting, and after drying for a few minutes at room temperature, the remaining sites on the membrane are blocked with 1% non-protein blocking reagent, or 5% skim milk, or 5% BSA, or a mixture of 5% casein and 1% non-protein blocking reagents to minimize the non-specific binding of the detection probe. The resulting nitrocellulose membrane immobilized with the target protein is then incubated with the corresponding labelled aptamer diluted in an appropriate binding buffer, followed by signal production via a peroxidase activity reaction (figure 1.4) [35].

Various versions of dot-blots are reported in the literature. For example, Wang *et al* reported in 2013 an aptamer-based dot-blot POCT for the detection of immunoglobulin E [36]. The immobilized IgE on the nitrocellulose membrane was detected through a biotinylated aptamer and avidin-conjugated horseradish to produce a blue-colored insoluble product as a dot on the membrane. Based on a linear response relationship between the spot intensity and the concentration of IgE (intensity of the dots increased with increasing concentration of IgE) over the range of 50 nmol l^{-1} to 1 μmol l^{-1}, authors reported achieving a detection limit of 2.89 nmol l^{-1} for IgE [36]. In another study, Dorraj *et al* reported in 2015 an

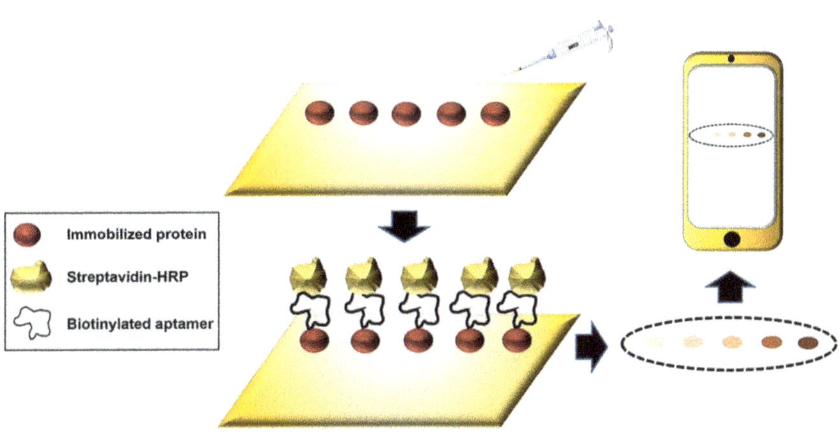

Figure 1.4. Schematic presentation of an aptamer-based dot-blot POCT. Reproduced with permission from [35]. Copyright (2021) Elsevier.

Table 1.4. Aptamer-based lateral flow POCTs for detection of biomarkers, microorganisms, hormones, and antibiotics [31].

Strategy	Analyte	Label	Test line	Control line	LOD	Detection range	Matrix
Conjugation of AuNPs with dopamine duplex aptamer and dissociation of duplex in the presence of target	Dopamine	AuNPs	Streptavidin-biotinylated cDNA3	Streptavidin-biotinylated cDNA1	50 ng ml^{-1}	nr *	Urine
Desorption of biotin-modified aptamer from AuNPs surface in the presence of analyte	HER2	AuNPs	Streptavidin and pullulan mixture	Cationic charged PDDA polymer	20 nM	nr	Human serum
Competitive reaction between CA125 conjugated with AuNPs and unlabeled CA125 for binding to capture probe	CA125	AuNPs nanozyme	CA125 specific aptamer	—	5.21 U ml^{-1}	7.5–200 U ml^{-1}	Human serum
An aptamer-based hook-effect-recognizable three-line LFA	Thrombin	AuNPs	Biotinylated aptamer—poly A tail	Botinylated poly T probe (C-DNA)	0.85 nM	1 nM–100 μM	Human serum
Binding of a biotinylated aptamer to target in the sample and reaction with AuNPs-streptavidin conjugate, then subsequent capturing by the antibody at the test line	Osteopontin	AuNPs	Osteopontin antibody	Complementary ssDNA	0.1 ng ml^{-1}	10–500 ng ml^{-1}	Human serum
Sandwich LFA based on biotin—1° aptamer immobilized on streptavidin coated membrane as a capturing probe and 2° aptamer conjugated with AuNPs as a signaling probe	Vaspin	AuNPs	Streptavidin-biotinylated aptamer	Streptavidin-biotinylated complementary aptamer	0.105 nM	0.10–25 nM	Human serum
Combining aptamer-exonuclease III-assisted amplification with LFA	*E. coli* O157:H7	AuNPs	Biotinylated poly T probe	Biotinylated complementary sequence to the AuNPs probes	7.6×10^1; 8.35×10^2 cfu ml^{-1}	10^2–10^6 cfu ml^{-1}	Culture media; Milk
Aptamer-gated release of TMB as signal molecule and HRP activity to generate signal	*L. monocytogenes*	Silica nanoparticle	Immobilized HRP	No control line	53 cells ml^{-1}	nr	Chicken

Sandwich LFA for the detection of whole virus particles	Avian influenza H5N2	AuNPs	Biotin modified primary aptamer	Biotin modified poly A sequence	1.2×10^6 EID_{50} ml^{-1}	1.2×10^6–10^7 EID_{50} ml^{-1}	Duck's feces
A dual recognition element LFA using both aptamer and antibody	Influenza virus (A/H3N2/Panama/2007/99)	AuNPs	Streptavidin	Antibody	2×10^6 virus particle	—	—
Pre-enrichment with magnetic nanoparticles conjugated with aptamer–ssDNA1and detection of released ssDNA1using LFA strip and AuNPs capture probe	*Salmonella* Typhimurium	AuNPs	Streptavidin-biotin modified ssDNA complementary with ssDNA1	Streptavidin-biotin modified poly A ssDNA complementary with poly T ssDNA on AuNPs surface	4.1×10^2 cfu ml^{-1}	8.6×10^2–8.6×10^7 cfu ml^{-1}	Milk
Complex formation between AuNPs-aptamer1 conjugate, analyte and apatmer 2 immobilized on the test line	*Salmonella* Typhimurium; *E. coli O157:H7; Staphylococcus aureus*	AuNPs	Streptavidin-biotin modified aptamer2	Streptavidin-biotin modified complementary DNA with AuNPs-aptamer conjugate	5×10^3; 3×10^4; 2×10^4 cfu ml^{-1}	nr	Food samples
Desorption of specific aptamer from AuNPs surface in the presence of target molecule	Cortisol	AuNPs	Cysteamine	—	1 ng ml^{-1}	nr	Sweat
Dissociation of specific aptamer from duplex probe conjugated with AuNPs in the presence of target	Cortisol	AuNPs	BiotinylatedDNA probe	Biotin-modified poly A probe	0.37 ng ml^{-1}	0.5–15 ng ml^{-1}	Saliva
Dissociation of specific aptamer from duplex probe conjugated with AuNPs in the presence of target	Progesterone	AuNPs	Streptavidin	—	5 nM	nr	Water

(*Continued*)

Table 1.4. (*Continued*)

Strategy	Analyte	Label	Test line	Control line	LOD	Detection range	Matrix
Magnetic sepration of analyte by aptamer-cDNA duplex conjugated with magnetic microspheres; then detection of cDNA by LFA strip	Kanamycin	AuNPs	Streptavidin-biotin-capture DNA1	Streptavidin-biotin-capture DNA2	4.96 nm	5–500 nM	Milk, honey
Competitive reaction between analyte in sample and analyte-career protein conjugate on the test line for binding to AuNPs-aptamer	Oxytetracycline	AuNPs	Oxytetracycline-carrier protein	Biotin-modified complementary probe	5 ng ml^{-1}	nr	Milk
Competitive reaction between analyte in sample and C-reactive protein conjugated with biotin for binding to AuNPs-aptamer-mFc	Ampicillin	AuNPs	Streptavidin	α-mouse antibody	185 mg l^{-1}	nr	Milk
Complex formation between analyte in sample, labeled DNA on conjugate pad and capture DNA on the test line	Ampicillin; Kanamycin	Hexachloro-6-carboxyflu orescein	Biotinylated ampicillin/ kanamycin capture DNA	—	0.06; 0.015 ng l^{-1}	0.5–500; 0.5–1000 ng l^{-1}	Water

aptamer-based dot-blot for detection of human cardiac troponin I using a biotinylated aptamer that was conjugated with streptavidin-capped AuNPs. Based on development of a red dot (depicting the aptamer-target binding), authors reported detection as low as 5 ng ml^{-1} of human cardiac troponin I in plasma [37].

1.3.3 Aptamer based electrochemical system for POCT

Aptamer-based electrochemical biosensors based on micro-fabricated devices offer small size, easy portability, low cost, and high sensitivity often requisite in POCT applications. A typical electrochemical aptasensor consists of (i) a bioreceptor that selectively recognizes and binds the target (e.g. aptamer), (ii) a transducer to convert biological recognition events into electrical signals through reduction or oxidation reactions (e.g. paper-based electrodes, screen-printed electrodes), and (iii) electronics and a display to process the provide visual/value-based assay outcome. Conductometric, amperometric, and electrochemical impedance spectroscopy (EIS) are some of the commonly used electrochemical techniques in aptamer-based electrochemical sensors. The commercial glucometer is the best example of a POCT. In the present time, glucometers are the most valued POC diagnostic equipment as a tremendously large number of people all over the world relies on these small, inexpensive, user-friendly, and highly accurate devices to manage their blood sugar levels. Interestingly, the commercial glucometers can also be repurposed to measure/analyze/detect a variety of other non-glucose-based targets [38–40]. The ability to repurpose glucometers for other targets, with aptamers as biorecognition elements, and connect to smartphones through Bluetooth, has proved to quite successful for detection of SARS-CoV-2 in the COVID-19 pandemic period [41]. A recent study by Singh *et al* [41] demonstrated development of an aptamer-based SARS-CoV-2 POCT that costs significantly little ($3.20/test), while retaining rapid (results available within 1 h) and accurate (100% sensitivity; positive percent agreement) diagnostic abilities (figure 1.5).

In another similar study, Joe *et al* reported fabrication of a portable mini-potentiostat for detection of variety of targets including vaspin (type 2 diabetes biomarker) and thrombin (biomarker for pulmonary metastasis and cardiovascular diseases) for POCT from real samples [42]. One more example of the application of aptamer-based electrochemical POCTs is the demonstration of an aptamer-based inexpensive electrochemical sensor for real-time monitoring of the mycotoxin ochratoxin A in a flowing stream of foodstuffs [43]. Overall, the past decade has witnessed development of multiple aptamer-based electrochemical sensors for POCT applications.

1.4 Conclusions

Undoubtedly, aptamers have proved to be on par with conventional antibodies for detection of multiple analytes. This is evident from a large array of colorimetric, fluorescence- and chemiluminescence-based, and electrochemical methods developed using aptamers as recognition molecules. Aptamer-based POCTs are continually evolving, starting from the earliest simple ALISA/ELASA/ELONA, to LFAs, and then electrochemical-based systems with digital readout facility. Despite this,

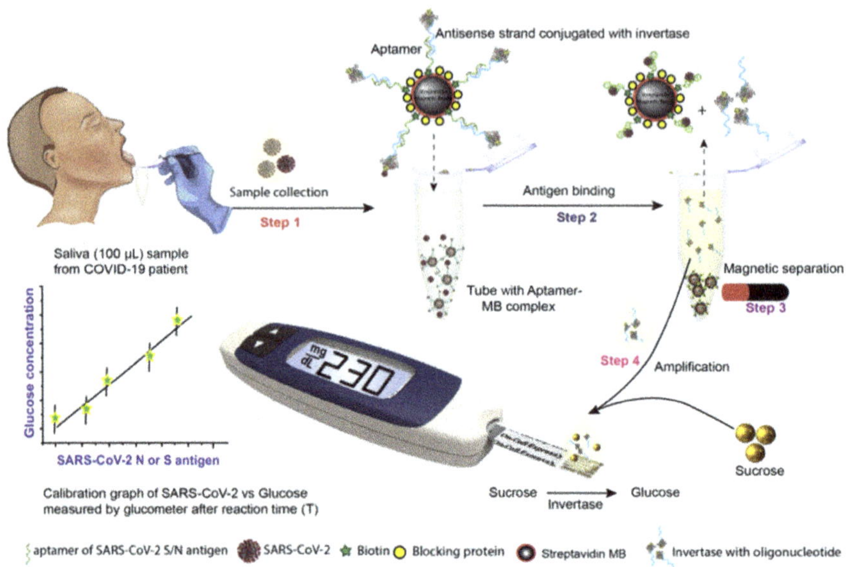

Figure 1.5. Overview of an aptamer-based POCT for SARS-CoV-2. Biotinylated aptamer to N or S proteins is conjugated to streptavidin-coated magnetic beads (MB) and pre-hybridized with a complementary antisense oligonucleotide strand that is covalently attached to an invertase enzyme. Addition of viral antigen sample (saliva; step-1) resulted in aptamer binding with SARS-CoV-2 virion, releasing invertase-antisense oligonucleotide (Step 2). MB conjugated aptamer-antigen complex were then collected through a magnet (Step 3). The remained antisense-invertase are collected and incubated with sucrose which convert it to glucose for direct readout using a glucometer (Step 4). The glucose concentration is correlated with the SARS-CoV-2 N or S protein concentration. Reproduced with permission from [41]. Copyright (2021) Elsevier.

aptamer-based POCTs for rapid diagnostic purposes are still scarce and lackluster, and at an early stage of development, particularly for clinical diagnostic utility. Developing aptamer-based POCTs, for example those based on lateral flow assays and dot-blot assays, may require identification of bottlenecks that possibly impede the transition of aptamer-based assays into POCTs. It should be ensured that the fabrication of POCT devices should be facile and easily executable for a high-throughput purpose, the POCT device should be equipped with a convenient readout system, nuclease resistant aptamers (created through base modification) should be used, and sensitivity and high specificity of POCTs should be maintained. Given enough boost, effort and time investment, aptamer-based POCTs can pave their trajectory to being one of the most sought-after POCTs. However, the future goal of developing aptamer-based POCTs should strictly comply with the ASSURED criterion to enable simple, rapid and cost-effective diagnostics.

Acknowledgments

Research in the laboratory of the corresponding author is supported by funds from the Science and Engineering Research Board grant (No. ECR/2017/003 179). Authors declare no conflict of interest.

References

[1] Schurer H, Stembera K, Knoll D, Mayer G, Blind M, Förster H H, Famulok M, Welzel P and Hahn U 2001 Aptamers that bind to the antibiotic moenomycin A *Bioorg. Med. Chem.* **9** 2557–63

[2] Geiger A, Burgstaller P, von der Eltz H, Roeder A and Famulok M 1996 RNA aptamers that bind L-arginine with sub-micromolar dissociation constants and high enantioselectivity *Nucleic Acids Res.* **24** 1029–36

[3] Bock L C, Griffin L C, Latham J A, Vermaas E H and Toole J J 1992 Selection of single-stranded DNA molecules that bind and inhibit human thrombin *Nature* **355** 564–6

[4] Dobbelstein M and Shenk T 1995 In vitro selection of RNA ligands for the ribosomal L22 protein associated with Epstein-Barr virus-expressed RNA by using randomized and cDNA-derived RNA libraries *J. Virol.* **69** 8027–34

[5] Sefah K, Shangguan D, Xiong X, O'Donoghue M B and Tan W 2010 Development of DNA aptamers using Cell-SELEX *Nat. Protoc.* **5** 1169–85

[6] Tuerk C and Gold L 1990 Systematic evolution of ligands by exponential enrichment: RNA ligands to bacteriophage T4 DNA polymerase *Science* **249** 505–10

[7] Ellington A D and Szostak J W 1990 In vitro selection of RNA molecules that bind specific ligands *Nature* **346** 818–22

[8] Robertson D L and Joyce G F 1990 Selection *in vitro* of an RNA enzyme that specifically cleaves single-stranded DNA *Nature* **344** 467–8

[9] Ahirwar R, Vellarikkal S K, Sett A, Sivasubbu S, Scaria V, Bora U, Borthakur B B, Kataki A C, Sharma J D and Nahar P 2016 Aptamer-assisted detection of the altered expression of estrogen receptor alpha in human breast cancer *PLoS One* **11** e0153001

[10] Stoltenburg R, Reinemann C and Strehlitz B 2007 SELEX–a (r)evolutionary method to generate high-affinity nucleic acid ligands *Biomol. Eng.* **24** 381–403

[11] Kupakuwana G V, Crill J E, McPike M P and Borer P N 2011 Acyclic identification of aptamers for human alpha-thrombin using over-represented libraries and deep sequencing *PLoS One* **6** e19395

[12] Kumar Kulabhusan P, Hussain B and Yüce M 2020 Current perspectives on aptamers as diagnostic tools and therapeutic agents *Pharmaceutics* **12** 646

[13] Thiviyanathan V and Gorenstein D G 2012 Aptamers and the next generation of diagnostic reagents *Proteomics. Clin. Appl.* **6** 563–73

[14] Healy M J, Lewis D S, Kurz M, Boomer M R, Thompson M K, Wilson C and McCauley T G 2004 Pharmacokinetics and biodistribution of novel aptamer compositions *Pharm. Res.* **21** 2234–46

[15] Silverman S K 2004 Deoxyribozymes: DNA catalysts for bioorganic chemistry *Org. Biomol. Chem.* **2** 2701–6

[16] Ng E W M, Shima D T, Calias P, Cunningham E T, Guyer D R and Adamis A P 2006 Pegaptanib, a targeted anti-VEGF aptamer for ocular vascular disease *Nat. Rev. Drug Discov.* **5** 123–32

[17] Louis S, Green D J, Bell C, Beebe L A, Feistner B D, Gill S C, Jucker F M and Janjic N 1995 Nuclease-resistant nucleic acid ligands to vascular permeability factor/vascular endothelial growth factor *Chem. Biol.* **2** 13

[18] Klussmann S, Nolte A, Bald R, Erdmann V A and Furste J P 1996 Mirror-image RNA that binds D-adenosine *Nat. Biotechnol.* **14** 1112–5

[19] Keefe A D and Cload S T 2008 SELEX with modified nucleotides *Curr. Opin. Chem. Biol.* **12** 448–56

[20] Richardson F C, Tennant B C, Meyer D J, Richardson K A, Mann P C, Mcginty G R, Wolf J L, Zack P M and Bendele R A 1999 An evaluation of the toxicities of 2′-fluorouridine and 2′-fluorocytidine-HCI in F344 rats and woodchucks (*Marmota monax*) *Toxicol. Pathol.* **27** 607–17

[21] Ahirwar R 2021 Recent advances in nanomaterials-based electrochemical immunosensors and aptasensors for HER2 assessment in breast cancer *Microchim. Acta* **188** 317

[22] Ahirwar R, Khan N and Kumar S 2021 Aptamer-based sensing of breast cancer biomarkers: a comprehensive review of analytical figures of merit *Expert Rev. Mol. Diagn.* **21** 703–21

[23] Chen A and Yang S 2015 Replacing antibodies with aptamers in lateral flow immunoassay *Biosens. Bioelectron.* **71** 230–42

[24] Chua A, Yean C Y, Ravichandran M, Lim B and Lalitha P 2011 A rapid DNA biosensor for the molecular diagnosis of infectious disease *Biosens. Bioelectron.* **26** 3825–31

[25] Dhiman A, Kalra P, Bansal V, Bruno J G and Sharma T K 2017 Aptamer-based point-of-care diagnostic platforms *Sensors Actuators* B **246** 535–53

[26] Gopinath S C B, Lakshmipriya T, Chen Y, Phang W-M and Hashim U 2016 Aptamer-based 'point-of-care testing' *Biotechnol. Adv.* **34** 198–208

[27] Sharma T K, Bruno J G and Dhiman A 2017 ABCs of DNA aptamer and related assay development *Biotechnol. Adv.* **35** 275–301

[28] Koczula K M and Gallotta A 2016 Lateral flow assays *Essays Biochem.* **60** 111–20

[29] Bahadır E B and Sezgintürk M K 2016 Lateral flow assays: principles, designs and labels *TrAC, Trends Anal. Chem.* **82** 286–306

[30] Xu H, Mao X, Zeng Q, Wang S, Kawde A-N and Liu G 2009 Aptamer-functionalized gold nanoparticles as probes in a dry-reagent strip biosensor for protein analysis *Anal. Chem.* **81** 669–75

[31] Majdinasab M, Badea M and Marty J L 2022 Aptamer-based lateral flow assays: current trends in clinical diagnostic rapid tests *Pharmaceuticals (Basel)* **15** 90

[32] Wang L, Ma W, Chen W, Liu L, Ma W, Zhu Y, Xu L, Kuang H and Xu C 2011 An aptamer-based chromatographic strip assay for sensitive toxin semi-quantitative detection *Biosens. Bioelectron.* **26** 3059–62

[33] Ranganathan V, Srinivasan S, Singh A and DeRosa M C 2020 An aptamer-based colorimetric lateral flow assay for the detection of human epidermal growth factor receptor 2 (HER2) *Anal. Biochem.* **588** 113471

[34] Schüling T, Eilers A, Scheper T and Walter J 2018 Aptamer-based lateral flow assays *AIMS Bioeng.* **5** 78–102

[35] Citartan M 2021 Aptamers as the powerhouse of dot blot assays *Talanta* **232** 122436

[36] Wang Y, Ye Z and Ying Y 2013 Detection of immunoglobulin E using an aptamer based dot-blot assay *Chin. Sci. Bull.* **58** 2938–43

[37] Dorraj G S, Rassaee M J, Latifi A M, Pishgoo B and Tavallaei M 2015 Selection of DNA aptamers against Human Cardiac Troponin I for colorimetric sensor based dot blot application *J. Biotechnol.* **208** 80–6

[38] Du Y, Hughes R A, Bhadra S, Jiang Y S, Ellington A D and Li B 2015 A sweet spot for molecular diagnostics: coupling isothermal amplification and strand exchange circuits to glucometers *Sci Rep.* **5** 11039

[39] Taebi S, Keyhanfar M and Noorbakhsh A 2018 A novel method for sensitive, low-cost and portable detection of hepatitis B surface antigen using a personal glucose meter *J. Immunol. Methods.* **458** 26–32

[40] Zhang J, Lan T and Lu Y 2020 Translating *in vitro* diagnostics from centralized laboratories to point-of-care locations using commercially-available handheld meters *Trends Anal. Chem. TRAC.* **124**

[41] Singh N K, Ray P, Carlin A F, Magallanes C, Morgan S C, Laurent L C, Aronoff-Spencer E S and Hall D A 2021 Hitting the diagnostic sweet spot: point-of-care SARS-CoV-2 salivary antigen testing with an off-the-shelf glucometer *Biosens. Bioelectron.* **180** 113111

[42] Joe C, Lee B H, Kim S H, Ko Y and Gu M B 2022 Aptamer duo-based portable electrochemical biosensors for early diagnosis of periodontal disease *Biosens. Bioelectron.* **199** 113884

[43] Somerson J and Plaxco K W 2018 Electrochemical aptamer-based sensors for rapid point-of-use monitoring of the mycotoxin ochratoxin a directly in a food stream *Molecules* **23** 912

Chapter 2

Point-of-care systems: brief history to recent advances in the field of cancer

Sayali Mukherjee and Tanushree Sharma

Globally, cancer is the second most common cause of death and is responsible for around 1 in 6 deaths. With the global incidence of cancer on the rise, it is vital to discover and invest in novel technologies for its effective management and treatment. There is a widely accepted understanding that early detection and screening are crucial in improving the chances of successful treatment and management of cancer but the current technologies for cancer cures are time-consuming, invasive and costly in nature, which deters most of the patients from availing timely diagnosis. Point-of-care systems have played a vital role in revolutionizing the delivery of cancer care by providing cost-effective and rapid prognostic and diagnostic tools at or nearby patient's primary care. They aid in acquiring a patient's clinical information in a resource-limited setting with fast, sensitive and economical diagnostic tools, which aids in timely diagnosis and enhancement of well-being of the patients and reduced cancer death rate. The ongoing development and investment in novel point-of-care technologies are crucial in the fight against cancer, enabling faster and more accurate diagnosis, personalized treatment, and ultimately, improving patient outcomes.

2.1 Introduction

Point-of-care (POC) systems encompass the technological advancements that aim at providing fast and accurate test results at the patient's primary care so that the right cure can be provided at the earliest possible time [1]. It is a patient-centered approach that prioritizes the patient over the healthcare provider [2]. The idea behind POC is that the healthcare system should be centered around the patient, with diagnostic and treatment options that are convenient, easily accessible, and affordable. In recent years, there has been a growing interest in this approach as it encourages the utilization of precise and fast diagnostic tools that can be applied on

doi:10.1088/978-0-7503-5012-9ch2

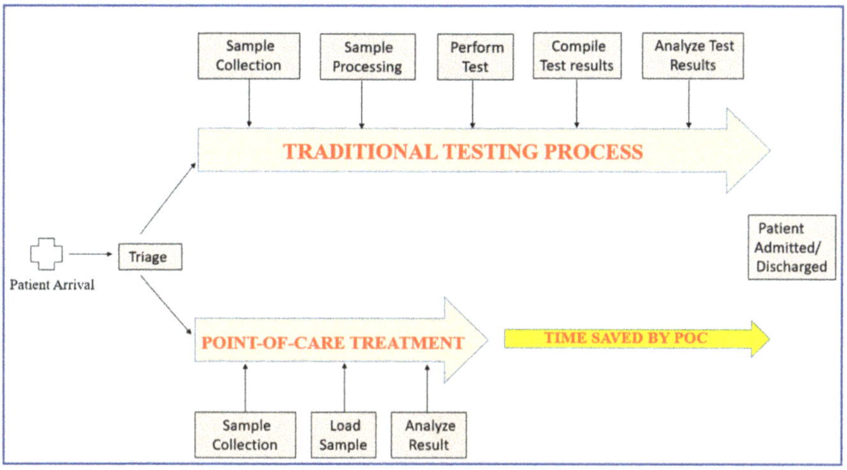

Figure 2.1. Rapid turn-around-time in case of point-of-care treatment over traditional testing approach.

or close to the location of patient care, instead of depending on centralized laboratories or diagnostic centers.

POC analysis refers to acquiring clinical data at the site of the patient's primary examination, which reduces turn-around time (TAT), the time elapsed between sample collection and test result procurement (figure 2.1). This user-friendly approach enables appropriate and timely diagnosis. POC testing is also known as near-patient testing, alternate-site testing or extra-laboratory testing as it involves the conduction of diagnostic tests outside the traditional laboratory environment. It is distinguished by its close proximity to the patient, its ability to provide quantitative or semi-quantitative measurements, rapid turn-around time, and the absence of sample preparation or pipetting. The approach employs dedicated analytical instruments that are user-friendly and preloaded with reagents, which allows for immediate therapeutic action to be taken based on the results obtained.

Although advances made in POC systems are underexploited, early successes have shown that it holds significant promise for detection, diagnosis, and treatment of cancer. Previously the diagnostic system was hospital- and laboratory-centric, involving the use of expensive equipment and trained personnel to operate them, which was highly capital intensive. But the transition towards POC systems has led to the incorporation of durable, miniaturized and simplified tests, which not only cut down upon the overall cost of materials, equipment's and trained personals but also provide accurate real-time diagnostic results. Thus, POC systems enable the rapid movement through a 'test and treat cycle', which aids in accurate and timely diagnosis [3].

POC systems have played a pivotal role in strengthening the healthcare industry throughout the world. They have played a major role in uplifting the healthcare system of developing countries. The developing countries, due to large population size, low availability of healthcare personnel and strained financial status, are unable to deliver quality care. POC systems have greatly helped in uplifting the healthcare

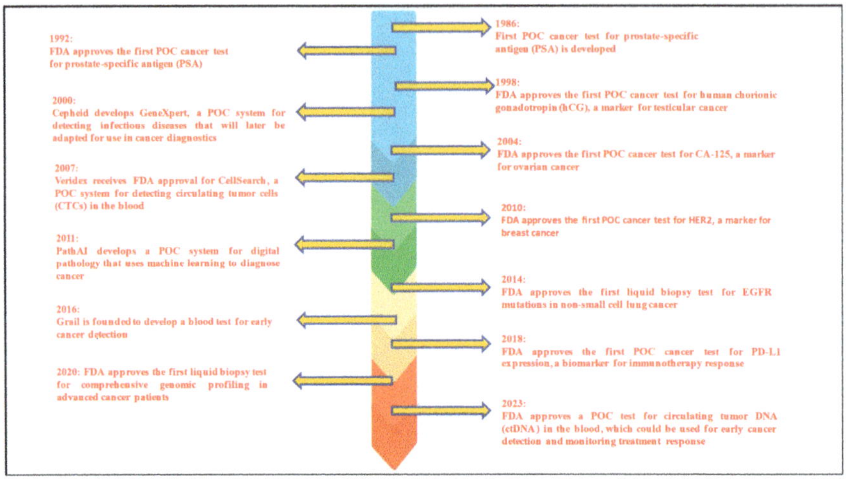

Figure 2.2. Timeline of key milestones in the development of point-of-care (POC) cancer diagnostics.

status of such developing countries. The first POC testing was done in 1962 for the fast analysis of blood glucose levels [4], and later on in 1977 for the fast pregnancy tests [5]. Following this was the development of POC devices for monitoring cardiac markers and coagulation tests in the 1980s [6]. Since then, there has been a steady growth in the number and variety of POC devices available for a range of tests, including infectious diseases, cancer, and genetic testing. The evolution of technology has enabled the development of more sophisticated and accurate POC devices, with the potential to improve patient care and outcomes. Thus, POC systems have become an integral part of healthcare systems and have also paved the way for personalized diagnostics as shown in figures 2.2 and 2.3.

2.2 Cancer incidence and need for early diagnosis

Cancer poses a significant hindrance to the increasing life expectancy globally and is the second most prevalent cause of death [7]. It is a significant contributor to both mortality and morbidity throughout the globe irrespective of the magnitude of human development [8]. In 2019, the World Health Organization (WHO) published a report that presented the findings that cancer was responsible for majority of deaths, before 70 years of age, in 112 out of 183 countries worldwide. Several factors including ageing, population surge, exposure to carcinogenic environment, unhealthy habits and socio-economic development reflect upon the growing burden of cancer incidence and death [9].

The global cancer incidence is surging each year. In 2020, the International Agency for Research on Cancer furnished a report based on the GLOBOCAN Cancer Statistics 2020 (table 2.1), on the increasing burden of cancer. In 2020, there was a reported estimation of 19.3 million novel cancer incidences and 10.0 million fatalities caused by cancer (excluding the non-melanoma skin cancer). The GLOBOCAN 2020 statistics, based on distribution by world region, showed that

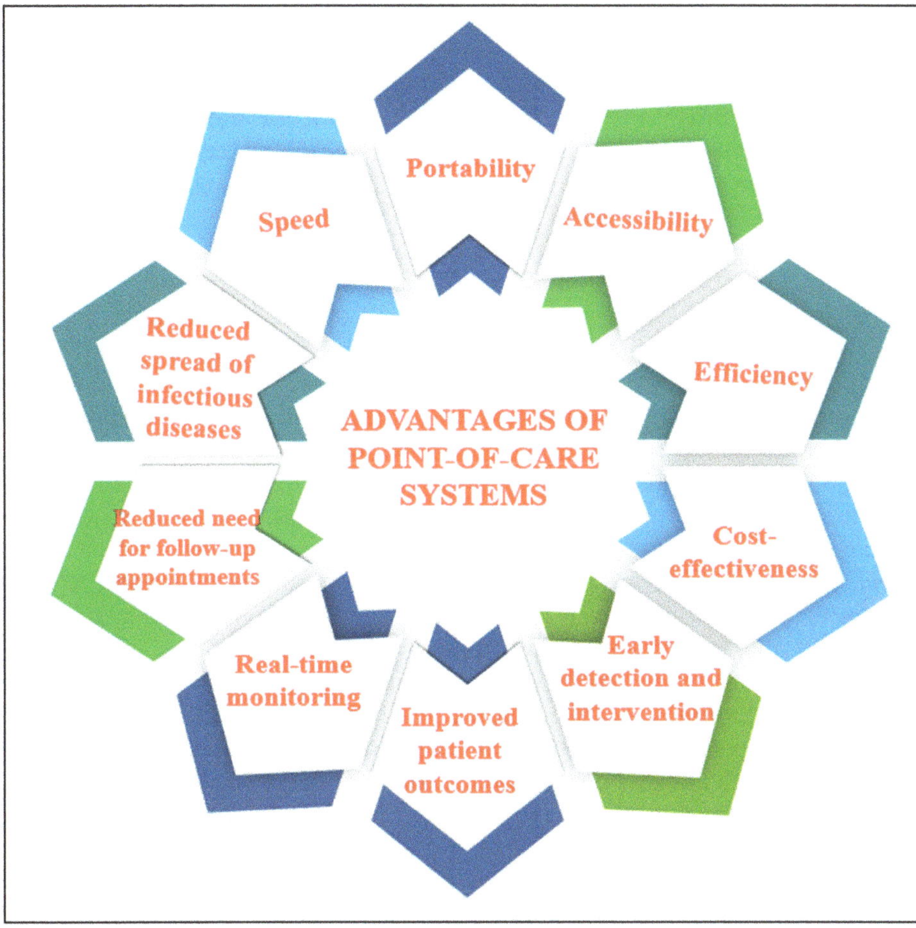
Portability
Speed
Accessibility
Reduced spread of infectious diseases
Efficiency
ADVANTAGES OF POINT-OF-CARE SYSTEMS
Reduced need for follow-up appointments
Cost-effectiveness
Early detection and intervention
Real-time monitoring
Improved patient outcomes

Figure 2.3. Advantages of point-of-care (POC) systems in cancer diagnostics.

Table 2.1. Estimated incidence rates from the Global Cancer Observatory for the year 2020, of the most common cancer types worldwide.

Rank	Cancer type	Estimated new cases in 2020	Incidence rate (per 100,000)
1	Lung and Bronchus	2 206 771	29.8
2	Breast	2 261 419	24.4
3	Prostate	1 414 259	15.2
4	Colorectal	1 931 590	20.7
5	Stomach	1 089 103	11.7
6	Liver	905 677	9.7
7	Oesophageal	604 139	6.5
8	Cervical	604 127	6.5
9	Bladder	573 278	6.2
10	Non-Hodgkin Lymphoma	573 276	6.2

for both the sexes combined, around 50% of the new cancer incidences and 58.3% of cancer mortalities occurred in Asia, where almost 59.5% of global population resides. The region of Europe had the second-highest number of cancer cases overall, 22.8%, and cancer deaths, 19.6%, representing almost 9.7% of world population. America came next in line, with the third highest number of cancer cases, accounting for 20.9% of cancer incidences and 14.2% cancer mortalities. Asia (583%) and Africa (7.2%) accounted for the highest share of cancer deaths because of distribution of different types of cancer and higher fatality rates [10].

Considering the prevalence of various types of cancer, female breast cancer accounted for the major share of newly diagnosed cancer cases, estimating around 11.7% of the total cases. This was closely trailed by lung (11.4%), colorectal (10.0%), prostate (7.3%) and stomach (5.6%) cancer. Lung cancer accounted for the major share of mortality (18.0%) followed by colorectal (9.4%), liver (8.3%), stomach (7.7%) and breast (6.9%) cancer. Lung cancer was also found to be the most frequent occurring and principal cause of mortality in men. In men, lung cancer was identified as the most frequent occurring and principal cause of fatality. On the other hand, breast cancer was identified as the most frequently diagnosed cancer and the principal cause of mortality among women. Additionally, colorectal and lung cancers were the leading cancer types in terms of frequency, while in terms of mortality, the situation was reversed for women [10].

Studies on cancer prediction have shown that the future burden of cancer will continue to rise. Assuming that the cancer rates measured in 2020 stay constant, it is projected that there will be approximately 28.4 million novel cancer cases around the globe by 2040, which is a significant increase from the initial 19.3 million cases stated in 2020 [10]. Therefore, incidences of global cancer point towards the construction of a suitable and sustainable structure for the discharge of affirmed preventive cancer care diagnostic approaches worldwide for effective cancer treatment. The astounding heterogeneity of cancer continually hints towards the underlying causes and fortifies the demand for a global upsurge for disease control endeavors. POC systems and their attuned integration in national health planning ventures can aid in the global reduction of future cancer burden and also serve to narrow down the existing cancer inequities between developing and developed countries as observed today.

Studies have made it evident that the ease of diagnosis and survival rates differ among different types of cancer and that the survival rates decline by 40% once the cancer reaches the metastatic stage [11]. Additionally, low survival rate cancers such as pancreas, colon, liver, and lung cancer demand early diagnosis, but diagnosis is delayed due to unavailability of suitable screening tools. Highly sensitive and accurate POC diagnostic tools are thus required for early screening and detection of cancer biomarkers at the patient's primary care site. Recently, micro- and nanofabrication technologies, coupled with various sensing platforms, have shown promise in developing rapid, economical, and reliable POC-based cancer diagnostic tools (table 2.2). For example, paper-based microfluidic devices have been used for the detection of several cancer biomarkers, such as prostate-specific antigens (PSAs), carcinoembryonic antigens (CEAs), and α-fetoproteins (AFPs) [12]. These devices are low-cost, disposable, and require minimal sample volume. Additionally,

Table 2.2. Point-of-care systems developed for some common cancers.

Cancer types	POC devices used for detection
1. Breast	Oncotype DX, Breast Cancer Index (BCI), MammaPrint, Terahertz Spectroscopy (THz), Digital Breast Tomosynthesis (DBT), iBreastExam
2. Lung and Bronchus	Bronchoalveolar lavage (BAL), Brevium, LungScope™, Lung cancer breathalyzer (LCB)
3. Colorectal	Colorectal cancer rapid test kit, Computed tomography (CT) colonography, Stool DNA test (Cologuard), Fecal immunochemical test (FIT)
4. Prostate	Prostate Health Index (phi) test, 4Kscore test, ExoDx Prostate (IntelliScore) test, Prostate cancer gene 3 (PCA3) test
5. Stomach	MagiSense COVID-19 IgG/IgM Rapid Test Cassette, BreathID Hp Lab System
6. Liver	Alpha-fetoprotein (AFP) rapid test kits, NanoVelcro Chip, Handheld Raman spectroscopy, OncoE6™ Cervical Test
7. Esophageal	Spectroscopy-based devices (VLE device and Niris Imaging System), Confocal laser endomicroscopy (CLE) devices (Cellvizio system and GastroFlex system)
8. Bladder	NMP22 BladderChek, UroVysion, BTA TRAK, Xpert Bladder Cancer Monitor
9. Non-Hodgkin Lymphoma	Alere Determine™ HIV-1/2 Ag/Ab Combo, GeneXpert® System, Accu-Chek® Inform II System
10. Pancreatic	MiCheck, CancerSEEK, Cytosponge

microelectromechanical systems (MEMS)-based biosensors have also been developed for the detection of several cancer biomarkers, such as human epidermal growth factor receptor 2 (HER2), CEA and PSA [13]. They offer high sensitivity, specificity, and selectivity, making them promising candidates for POC cancer diagnosis. Apart from this, nanoparticle-based biosensors, utilizing the unique optical, magnetic, and electrical properties of nanoparticles to detect cancer biomarkers such as miRNAs, proteins, and DNA, are also being integrated into portable diagnostic devices [14]. These technologies are portable, usea small quantity of samples and reagents, have reduced screening time and render multiplexed ultrasensitive analysis to better diagnostic and prognostic methods (table 2.2).

Thus, early diagnosis of cancer is considered to be a public primacy, with patient's primary site a preferred setting to carry out initial diagnostic tests [15]. This has indeed led to a predisposition to develop enhanced diagnostic tools and screening tests that can be useable at the patient's primary care site. Over the years, sustained and substantial investments in technological and therapeutic advancements of novel biomarkers has greatly benefited in improving the accuracy and timeliness of cancer diagnostic tools that could be put to use at patient's primary care site for early screening and cancer detection [16].

While ongoing technological advancements are rapidly coming up with a new array of diagnostic tools such as biomarkers, lab-on-a chip devices, microfluidic devices, wearable sensors, imaging devices, biosensors, artificial intelligence algorithms [17], the vast majority of them are apparently failing in initial cancer screening methodology because of their lack of adequacy to work in low prevalence populations, which is their ultimate target [13], the supposed 'spectrum effect'. Thus, a screening test which is being developed in a population at high risk of a disease will typically exhibit low sensitivity and high specificity when put to use within a population at low risk of a disease [18]. This results in high rates of false-positive tests. Alternatively, it has also been seen that the diagnostic tests have been marketed and inappropriately applied too soon which has resulted in catastrophic effects. One well-known example is the application of prostate specific antigen (PSA) screening test within the population prior to the screening trials [19]. Thus, rigorous evaluation of novel POC diagnostic tools and tests is required across a diverse range of medical disciplines before their vast implementation at the population level.

2.3 Biomarkers in cancer detection

Biomarkers are indicators of biological, pathogenic, and pharmacological effects to a therapeutic intervention [20]. They are usually defined as biochemical substances elicited by cancerous cells whose precise qualitative and quantitative measurement would lead to cancer detection and know-how about the extent of malignancy [21]. They can be identified in sample matrices like plasma, urine, tissue, serum, whole blood, etc [22]. The biomarkers could be endogenous products of cancerous cells or products of genes switched on due to cancerous cells. They could also encompass intracellular molecules like proteins, which may be found in tissues or released into blood circulation and hence appear in serum or plasma. They function as significant indicators of cancer, and development of POC systems based on the principle of precise detection of biomarkers would aid in early diagnosis and timely cancer cures (figure 2.4) [23].

Biomarkers play a crucial role in comprehending the spectrum of carcinomas. They have gained widespread applications in epidemiology, screening, prognosis, diagnosis and randomized clinical trials. They have been used to detect the underlying cause of disease pathogenesis as they are based on the altered constitution of bodily fluids and tissues. They provide a standardized classification of diseases and their related risk factors. The goal in cancer research currently revolves around the discovery of biomarkers associated with different cancers. Their discovery would eventually lead to development of novel therapeutic strategies which could be used in the identification and cure of disease pathogenesis. With the development of omic technologies like metabolomics, proteomics, etc, the discovery of biomarkers has become a fairly achievable task. These technologies have facilitated easy identification of biomarkers and associated signaling molecules involved in several metabolic processes. They have also enabled the observation of

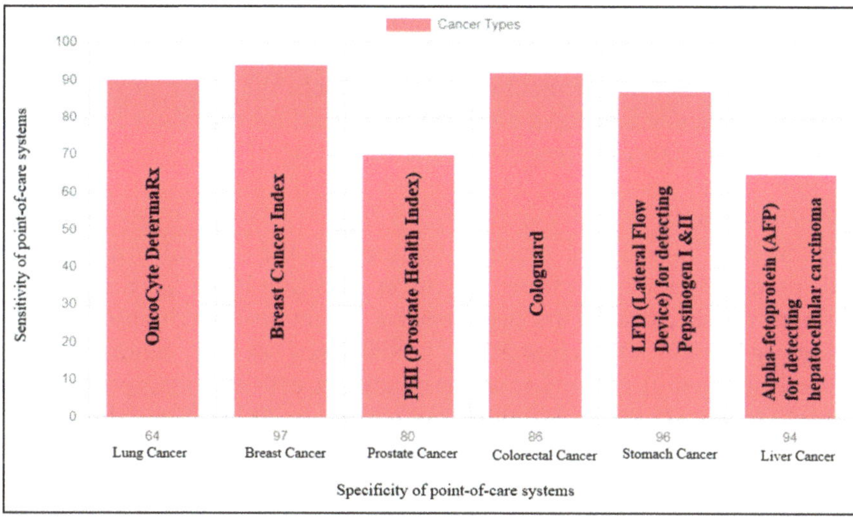

Figure 2.4. Bar graph highlighting the sensitivity and specificity of different POC systems for detecting several cancer types.

functional disturbances, cellular and molecular mechanisms, whose precise study would aid in cancer-targeted therapeutic strategies.

Biomarkers are the fundamental unit of ultrasensitive POC devices which are 'fit-for-purpose', in clinical settings, appropriately implemented for cancer detection at the patient's bedside. Currently, detection of the biomarker complements histopathology by providing additional information that aids in the selection of the best diagnostic approach [24, 25]. However, biomarkers are not yet considered as a stand-alone entity for providing a definitive diagnosis as they lack specificity, a critical requirement in clinical diagnosis [26]. This can be attributed to the existence of tumoral heterogeneity exhibited by patients [26]. In addition, another feature that restricts the use of biomarker as a stand-alone entity for definitive diagnosis is the false-positive results exhibited by them. For example, patients possessing a benign disease sometimes exhibit low biomarker levels which fall below the detection limit and obstruct early-stage cancer detection [27]. In such cases, enhancing technical diagnostic approaches, which would aim at ultrasensitive detection and delineation of biomarkers via in-depth analysis of post-translational modifications and widening the scale of biomarkers to encompass metabolites such as DNA, RNA, proteins, lipids, exosomes, circulating tumor cells, etc, may facilitate the development of finer technologies based on biomarkers and lay foundations for it to become the novel gold-standard in cancer diagnosis [28, 29].

2.3.1 Nucleic acid biomarkers

A number of nucleic acid components like DNA, RNA or miRNAs have been proposed as promising candidates for cancer biomarkers but they often require a detailed standardization and confirmation based on multicentred studies before being put to use in a clinical utility. Currently no nucleic acid biomarker has been robust enough to serve as a stand-alone diagnostic tool, but when used in combination with other nucleic acid biomarker panels, they have proved to improve the diagnostic efficiency and have also facilitated patient stratification and aided in the improvement of cancer-targeted treatments.

2.3.1.1 Cell-free DNA

Currently, there is insufficient evidence to support the clinical utility of cell-free DNA as a potential biomarker for early cancer detection but it has attracted a lot of scientific curiosity because of its non-invasive detection and disease pathogenesis monitoring potential. The circulating DNA-based cancer biomarkers exhibit enhanced specificity and stability towards cancerous cells enabling precise detection of cancerous stage and extent of malignancy which would aid in deciding the correct diagnostic approach.

The first report on cell-free DNA as a potential biomarker was published in the year 1948 by Mandel and Metais. They delineated the occurrence of circulating nucleic acids in the blood of healthy individuals, and suggested that they may be derived from normal tissue turnover [30]. In the following years, many studies confirmed the presence of cell-free DNA in the blood of cancer patients, and demonstrated that it could be used as a biomarker for cancer detection, monitoring, and treatment response [31]. Cell-free DNA refers to the small fragments of DNA that are released in the bloodstream by normal and cancerous cells. These fragments can be detected and analysed through a variety of techniques, including next-generation sequencing and digital PCR. The quantity and qualities of cell-free DNA may differ based on various factors, including the kind and progression of cancer, as well as lifestyle and age.

Although the clinical utility of cell-free DNA as a potential biomarker for early cancer detection is still debatable, it has shown promise in several studies. For example, a 2014 study, which analysed the levels of cell-free DNA in the blood of patients with several classes of cancer, demonstrated that the levels were higher in individuals with advanced stages of cancer compared to those with early-stage cancer [32]. Another study aimed at determining the sensitivity and specificity of cell-free DNA as a biomarker for early diagnosis of non-small cell lung cancer, found that it was a promising biomarker for early detection [33]. Furthermore, a study aimed at investigating the utility of cell-free DNA as a biomarker for colorectal cancer detection in a prospective group of patients, found that the levels of cell-free DNA were significantly elevated in patients with colorectal cancer compared to healthy controls, and that it could be a useful biomarker for early cancer detection [34]. Yet another study, aimed at investigating the feasibility of using cell-free DNA, in the saliva and plasma of patients with head and neck squamous cell cancer, as a biomarker for early detection, found that cell-free DNA was detectable in both saliva and plasma samples, and that it could be a promising biomarker for early detection of this type of cancer [35]. Recent studies have also established them as suitable biomarkers for prostate cancer detection as their expression increases threefold in it [36]. Importantly, cell-free DNA has served as a suitable and specific biomarker for correlating various pathological stages of cancer [37].

However, cell-free DNA cannot be considered as a stand-alone cancer-specific marker due to unavailability of reference DNA concentrations in controls. Thus, quantification of cell-free DNA alone cannot be considered as a tumor-specific biomarker [38]. Recent studies have detected circulating mutant tumor DNA (ct-DNA), representing the entire genetic make-up of a tumor, in the blood sample of cancer patients. POC systems targeting the precise quantification of ct-DNA coupled with cell-free DNA pose tremendous therapeutic potential in cancer management, treatment and control [39]. Such POC systems, further coupled with sequencing technologies, would aid not only in precise cancer detection and diagnosis but would also pave the way for personalized treatment approaches.

2.3.1.2 Hypermethylation events

Research studies have indicated that the process of tumorigenesis frequently causes extensive DNA methylation events in the cell, which involve global hypomethylation of the genome and localized hypermethylation of several CpG (5′-cytosine-phosphate-guanine-3′) islands present on gene promoters and first exons. These epigenetic alterations occur in the early stages of cancer and can be used as promising biomarkers for timely diagnosis of cancer [40].

Several researches have highlighted the potential of hypermethylation events as biomarkers for various types of cancers, including colorectal cancer (CRC), gastric cancer, lung cancer, and prostate cancer. One such hypermethylation event is known to occur in prostate cancer and serves as an important biomarker for its early detection and timely cure. In prostate cancer, hypermethylated CpG islands are found in the promoter region of GSTP1 (Glutathione S-transferase P) encoding gene, which is a tumor-suppressor gene carrying out several detoxification functions within the cell. The hypermethylated CpG islands lead to loss of gene function, thus serving as an essential biomarker in prostate carcinogenesis. This epigenetic modification has been extensively investigated and put to use as a nucleic acid biomarker for diagnosis of prostate cancer [41]. Another study showed that a panel of four hypermethylated genes (HLTF, SFRP2, TWIST1, and SLC5A8) in plasma samples could accurately distinguish CRC patients from healthy controls with high sensitivity and specificity [42]. In yet another study it was effectively demonstrated that a panel of four hypermethylated genes (SEPT9, ALX4, TAC1, and NPY) could effectively detect early-stage CRC with a sensitivity of 70.6% and a specificity of 86.7% [43].

Apart from CRC, hypermethylation events have also been investigated as potential biomarkers for other types of cancers. For example, research carried out by Chen *et al* has demonstrated that a panel of three hypermethylated genes (RASSF1A, CDH13, and APC) in plasma samples could accurately detect gastric cancer with a sensitivity of 90.5% and specificity of 89.7% [44]. Yet another research paper by Xu *et al* showed that a panel of three hypermethylated genes (SHOX2, SOX17, and TAC1) in plasma samples could accurately detect lung cancer with sensitivity and specificity of 83.3% and 82.4%, respectively [45].

Thus, hypermethylation events act as essential biomarkers for early cancer detection. The therapeutic tests based on the principle of detection of hypermethylated biomarkers are highly specific and accurate as they target specific gene loci which reduces the chances of false-positive results. This feature enables the rapid development of POC systems based on detecting DNA methylation changes. POC systems revolving around the rapid detection of hypermethylation events would lead to development of non-invasive, easy, economical and rapid diagnostic tests at the patient's primary care site. This would eventually lead to early cancer diagnosis and cures.

2.3.1.3 Circulating microRNAs (miRNAs)

Recent studies have highlighted the robust role played by miRNAs, another class of nucleic acid biomarkers that have been studied for their potential in cancer detection. miRNAs are small non-coding RNAs that serve an essential function in gene expression regulation by binding to target messenger RNAs and inhibiting their translation or promoting their degradation. They were first established as cancer biomarkers in 2008 when they were used to detect the presence of diffused large B cell lymphoma in serum of cancer patients [46]. They are highly accessible nucleic acid biomarkers as they are present in various bodily fluids, including blood, urine, and saliva, in stable forms protected from degradation by being encapsulated in exosomes or bound to RNA-binding proteins. They are highly tissue specific and can be used to grade disease progression and cancer stage.

Several researches have shown that the expression profiles of circulating miRNAs are deregulated in cancer patients in comparison to healthy individuals, suggesting that they could be used as potential biomarkers for cancer detection. For example, a study on colorectal cancer (CRC) identified a panel of four miRNAs (miR-21, miR-92a, miR-29a, and miR-143) that were significantly upregulated in the serum of individuals with CRC in comparison to healthy groups, thus indicating that the identified miRNA panel had the potential to serve as a non-invasive diagnostic tool for early detection of CRC [47]. Another study identified a panel of three miRNAs (miR-21, miR-205, and miR-214) that were significantly upregulated in the serum of patients with ovarian cancer in comparison to the healthy groups, thus showing that the identified miRNA panel had the potential to serve as a non-invasive diagnostic tool for ovarian cancer [48].

Thus, multi-marker panels of miRNAs provide a non-invasive approach to serve as an important biomarker for various cancers including CRC [47], ovarian cancer [48], breast carcinoma [49], renal fibrosis [50], etc. They serve as an important class of biomarkers, as cancer being a heterogenous disease can be easily detected using the multi-point approach put forth by miRNAs.

2.3.2 Protein biomarkers

Early detection and diagnosis of cancer have promising potential through cancer diagnostics based on the accurate detection of protein biomarkers. However, currently the protein biomarkers are insufficient for diagnostic specificity as compared to nucleic acid biomarkers. Liquid biopsy is the most plausible approach for easy quantification of protein biomarkers. It provides the most plausible way to assess the health of tissues by detecting the presence of protein biomarkers associated with tumor in bodily fluids like serum, blood, saliva, etc. It is an easy approach for large-scale screening and precise detection of the diseased state.

For example, in the case of tumors, the blood sample can be screened for tumor disseminated cells. These cells can then be used to study the precise proteomics of carcinogenic cells. This approach would provide tumor-specific biomarkers, which could further be used to carry out early cancer detection studies. Despite the technological advancements the field encompassing protein biomarkers has progressed slowly. But studies have shown that protein biomarkers possess the highest specificity to detect cancer and grade its malignancy. Carcinogenic cells undergo maximum necrotic events due to their poor vascularization and uncontrolled growth [36]. These necrotic events lead to the release of cell's protein content in the bloodstream. Thus, diagnostic tools aimed at accurately assessing tumor-specific proteins would aid in early cancer detection.

Recent research has gained success in specifically detecting proteins associated with certain tumors. For example, Troponin is used as a protein biomarker for diagnosing acute myocardial infarction. A POC device called the Triage Cardiac Panel, which measures troponin levels, has been shown to have high diagnostic accuracy in several studies [51]. Another protein biomarker called C-reactive protein (CRP) is used to indicate the presence of inflammation in the body. A POC device called the Afinion™ CRP has been developed to measure CRP levels in just a few minutes using a fingerstick blood sample [52]. Another such protein biomarker is prostate-specific antigen (PSA), which is used for prostate cancer screening. SIA PSA Rapid Test, a POC device, is used to measure PSA levels [53]. Apart from this, another protein biomarker called brain natriuretic peptide (BNP) is used for diagnosing heart failure. The Alere™ Natriuretic Peptide Test is a POC device that measures BNP levels and has been shown to have high diagnostic accuracy [54]. Another such protein biomarker is alpha-fetoprotein (AFP), which is used for diagnosing liver cancer. The AFP-L3% test is a POC device that measures the percentage of AFP that is the specific form associated with liver cancer. It has been shown to have high diagnostic accuracy in several studies [55].

Thus, POC systems should aim at precisely detecting these protein biomarkers. Detection of these tumor-specific protein biomarkers at the patient's primary care site using novel POC diagnostic tools would lead to early detection of cancer, which would further aid in timely and accurate diagnosis. Currently, translational research is focussing to bridge the gap between laboratory-derived and clinical utility protein biomarkers. It has aided in the development of protein biomarkers possessing theranostic capabilities, biomarkers possessing predictive, prognostic as well as diagnostic potential.

2.3.3 Circulating tumor cells (CTCs)

Circulating tumor cells (CTCs) are a small subset of cancerous cells that have separated from the primary tumor and entered the bloodstream or lymphatic system, potentially leading to metastasis in distant organs [56]. As a biomarker, they show promise for early cancer detection. They employ a non-invasive approach for cancer screening as compared to tissue biopsy but their detection poses a significant challenge. As mentioned, they are a rare group of cancer cells, usually found in low numbers, i.e. around 10 ml^{-1} of blood or 0.01%. Their separation and identification from millions of white and red blood cells poses a significant challenge. Their identification becomes even more challenging because of their heterogenous nature. They possess variable physical and chemical characteristics. They differ in shape, size, expression of surface proteins, etc. The heterogeneity of these cells depends on its primary cancer type and stage, which makes their detection a laborious task requiring highly specific and ultrasensitive diagnostic tools.

Despite existing in very low numbers CTCs are considered to be a beneficial group of biomarkers. They are present in the circulatory system and POC systems employing precise diagnostic techniques such as immunomagnetic separation would lead to their specific isolation, which would aid in early cancer detection and diagnosis. POC systems employing CTC detection serve as a highly specific and sensitive recognition method in cancer diagnosis. In general, detection of CTCs includes four steps; capture, enrichment, detection, and final release. First, blood samples are collected from individuals suspected to have cancer. Then, the blood sample is processed to isolate the CTCs from the background of normal blood cells. This is achieved using various techniques such as immunomagnetic separation, filtration, and microfluidic devices. Once the CTCs are isolated, they are characterized using various techniques such as fluorescence microscopy, flow cytometry, and molecular assays to confirm their identity as cancer cells. Finally, the number and characteristics of CTCs are analysed to determine their potential use as biomarkers for cancer diagnosis and treatment monitoring.

Detection and isolation of CTCs require highly specialized tests. One of the first CTC detection tests is CELLSEARCH, which has been successfully implemented in cancer diagnosis [57]. The test aims at the detection of CTCs, possessing epithelial cell adhesion molecules, extracted from blood samples with the help of magnetic beads carrying functionalized anti-epithelial cell adhesion molecule antibodies (anti-EpCAM) [58]. The test has been successfully carried out for metastatic colorectal, prostate and breast cancer identification [57]. Isolation of CTCs from blood samples not only directs towards the presence of cancer, but also sheds light on the grade of malignancy and whether any therapeutic intervention would be beneficial or not [59]. In addition, the extent of CTCs also points towards the mortality index as it is directly related to the number of CTCs present in a blood sample. Although CTC detection tests are highly sensitive, their specificity can be further increased by the use of antibodies against multiple CTC-derived biomarkers.

Apart from the detection of CTCs using anti-EpCAM antibodies, nanoparticles have also been incorporated in CTC research. Nanoparticles have a high surface area to volume ratio, which facilitates selective and precise capture of CTCs. For example, coupling of graphene oxide quantum dots with magnetic nanoplatforms forms a functionalized nanostructured substrate with anti-Glypican 3 antibody, which is used for the specific detection of CTCs of liver cancer [60]. Apart from this, an electrochemical sensing strategy has also been developed for capturing CTCs in blood. It is based on aptamer-functionalized and magnetic graphene nanosheets of gold nanoparticle array. Centrifugo-magnetophoretic systems have also been employed for POC detection of CTCs. Such systems use centrifugal force to isolate CTCs bound to magnetic microbeads. Another CTC based approach has been employed in the identification of prostate cancer. It is a liquid biopsy method based on the approach of single-cell mRNA cytometry. In this approach, magnetic iron oxide nanoparticles tagged with probes carry out magnetic clustering by targeting cellular mRNA. This magnetic clustering enables the rapid capture of cells on microfluidic devices. Thus, mRNAs in CTCs can be directly detected using this approach [61].

Capturing CTCs by rapid enforcement of these techniques would enable precise cancer detection along with its severity and grade of malignancy. This would further aid in deciding the appropriate therapeutic approach.

2.3.4 Exosomes

Exosomes are small extracellular vesicles which are secreted by cells and contain various biomolecules, including nucleic acids. They have emerged as a promising class of biomarkers for cancer detection due to their stability and specificity. Exosomes can be isolated from various biofluids and their molecular content can be analyzed to identify cancer-specific nucleic acid biomarkers. Current advancements in nanotechnology have led to the development of point-of-care devices that use exosomes as biomarkers for early cancer detection. These devices offer rapid and sensitive detection, and can potentially be used for real-time monitoring of cancer progression and treatment response.

Several researches have highlighted the critical role played by exosomes in cancer progression [62]. Recent research has shown that the double-stranded DNA of exosomes can be used to detect any mutational event of carcinogenic cells [63]. Studies on exosomes have shown that during oncogenic development there is a 20-fold increase in exosomal DNA as compared to normal cells, thus serving as a potential biomarker for early cancer detection. For example, researchers recently developed a point-of-care system for precise detection of exosomes from urine samples of bladder cancer patients. The system used a microfluidic chip that was coated with an antibody against CD63, a protein that is present on the surface of exosomes. The chip was functionalized with a DNAzyme that could specifically recognize and cleave the target RNA sequence in the exosomes. The DNAzyme was conjugated with gold nanoparticles that could amplify the signal and provide a visual readout. The researchers tested the system using urine samples from 25 bladder cancer patients and 20 healthy controls. The system showed sensitivity and specificity of 96% and 90%, respectively, for detection of bladder cancer exosomes [62]. The system also showed a linear correlation between the concentration of exosomes and the severity of bladder cancer. Thus, the study clearly highlighted the potential of exosome-based biomarkers for non-invasive and early detection of cancer.

2.4 Point-of-care systems in cancer diagnosis

2.4.1 Paper-based

Clinical diagnostics are a cardinal component of the healthcare industry across the globe. Around 5.8 billion of the world's population lives in average-income or low-income and poor-resource settings. This obstructs their access to expensive and high-end medical instruments required for proper and timely disease diagnosis. Hence, an uplift in technological advancements aiming towards the development of economical, portable, easily accessible and simple POC diagnostic devices is needed, which would aid in better healthcare delivery with rapid prognostic and diagnostic approaches. The POC diagnostic tools go beyond the conventional testing methodologies. They make a drastic shift from the traditional laboratory environment to the patient's primary care site, which aids in accurate detection and timely diagnosis of cancer. It is believed that there would be a rapid rise in the market of POC diagnostics, around an annual growth rate of 9.3% due to their pivotal role in clinical settings.

Currently, paper-based POC diagnostic tools are acquiring the center stage because of their easy fabrication, affordability, sensitivity, reproducibility, low sample requirement and accurate detection [64]. The first paper-based POC diagnostic tool was developed by Whitesides *et al* in 2007. This tool was designed to detect liver function by measuring levels of alanine aminotransferase (ALT), an enzyme that is often elevated in liver disease. The diagnostic tool consisted of a paper strip containing a series of zones that were preloaded with different reagents. The test was performed by adding a small sample of blood to the paper strip, which would then wick through the different zones. Each zone contained a different reagent that would react with ALT, producing a color change that could be visually detected [65]. This paper-based POC diagnostic tool was significant because it was simple to use, inexpensive, and did not require any specialized equipment or training to operate. It also had the potential to be adapted for other diagnostic tests by simply swapping out the reagents in the different zones of the paper strip.

One essential advantage of paper-based POC systems is their simplicity, as they require minimal training and technical expertise to operate. These systems are based on lateral flow assay (LFA) technology, which uses paper as the substrate for the immobilization of biomolecules such as antibodies or DNA probes. Paper-based POC systems for cancer detection have been developed using a range of biomarkers, including proteins, nucleic acids, and cells.

Since the development of this first paper-based POC diagnostic tool, many other researchers have developed similar paper-based diagnostic tools for a variety of applications, including infectious disease testing, cancer biomarker detection, and environmental monitoring. These paper-based diagnostic tools have the potential to revolutionize healthcare in low-resource settings, where access to traditional diagnostic tests is limited.

For instance, a paper-based POC system was developed for the precise detection of the prostate-specific antigen (PSA), a protein biomarker for prostate cancer. The system employed a lateral flow immunoassay (LFIA) format, where antibodies against PSA were immobilized on the paper substrate. The system was able to detect PSA in spiked human serum samples with a limit of detection (LOD) of 0.1 ng ml^{-1}, which is comparable to standard laboratory-based immunoassays [66]. In another study, a paper-based POC system was developed for the detection of circulating tumor cells (CTCs), which are a potential biomarker for the diagnosis and monitoring of cancer. The system used a combination of immunoaffinity and size-based filtration to capture and detect CTCs from blood samples. The captured cells were then visualized using fluorescent microscopy. The system was able to detect as few as 10 CTCs ml^{-1} of blood in spiked samples [67]. Recently, a paper-based POC system was developed for the detection of microRNAs (miRNAs), which are small non-coding RNA molecules, critical in cancer development and progression. The system employed a hybridization-based approach, where capture probes for miRNAs were immobilized on the paper substrate. The system was able to detect miRNA-21, a biomarker for lung cancer, with a LOD of 0.1 fM in spiked buffer samples and 100 pM in human serum samples [68].

Furthermore, paper-based POCs can also be used to detect nucleic acid biomarkers, such as cell-free DNA and exosomes, using isothermal amplification techniques like loop-mediated amplification (LAMP) or recombinase polymerase amplification (RPA). For instance, a paper-based device was developed for the detection of circulating cell-free DNA from non-small cell lung cancer (NSCLC) patients using LAMP amplification [69]. Another study reported the development of a paper-based device for the detection of exosomes in the urine of bladder cancer patients using RPA amplification [70].

Overall, paper-based POC systems show great promise for cancer detection due to their simplicity, portability, and affordability. These systems can be easily put to use for the detection of various biomarkers using diverse amplification techniques, making them a versatile tool for early cancer diagnosis. However, further studies are needed to validate their accuracy and sensitivity in detecting cancer biomarkers in real-world settings.

2.4.2 Printed electrode-based

Electrode-based POC systems are diagnostic tools that employ electrochemical sensing techniques for detecting specific biomolecules in biological samples. These systems use printed electrodes, which are fabricated by printing conductive ink on a substrate, such as paper or plastic, and functionalizing them with biomolecules specific to the target analyte. When a sample is added, the target analyte binds to the biomolecule on the electrode surface, causing a change in the electrical signal that can be detected and quantified.

In cancer diagnosis, electrode-based POC devices have been developed to accurately detect a variety of cancer biomarkers, including proteins, nucleic acids, and exosomes. For example, an electrochemical immunosensor was developed for the detection of prostate-specific antigen (PSA), a biomarker for prostate cancer. The sensor was based on a gold nanoparticle-modified screen-printed carbon electrode and anti-PSA antibody immobilized on the surface of the electrode.

The sensor showed high sensitivity and specificity in detecting PSA in human serum samples [71]. Another study reported the development of a nanostructured electrode-based platform for the detection of circulating tumor cells (CTCs). The platform was based on the use of gold nanorods immobilized on a gold electrode. The CTCs were captured on the surface of the electrode via antibody-antigen interactions. The platform showed high sensitivity and specificity in detecting CTCs in blood samples from cancer patients [72]. Another electrode-based POC system encompassed the development of a DNA sensor for the detection of a cancer-related mutation in the KRAS gene. The sensor was based on a graphene oxide-modified glassy carbon electrode and a peptide nucleic acid probe specific to the KRAS mutation. The sensor showed high sensitivity and specificity in detecting the KRAS mutation in cancer cell lines and patient samples [73]. Apart from this, an impedimetric biosensor was also developed for the detection of carcinoembryonic antigen (CEA), a biomarker for colorectal cancer. The biosensor was based on a gold electrode modified with a self-assembled monolayer of thiolated polyethylene glycol and anti-CEA antibody. The biosensor showed enhanced sensitivity and specificity in detecting CEA in human serum samples [74].

Overall, electrode-based POC systems offer several advantages over traditional laboratory-based methods, including low cost, rapid turn-around time, and portability. These systems have the potential to revolutionize cancer diagnosis and improve patient outcomes by enabling early cancer detection and personalized treatment approaches.

2.4.3 Smartphone based

Smartphone-based POC systems are becoming increasingly popular due to their portability, affordability, and user-friendliness. They enable the integration of diagnostic devices with smartphones, allowing for real-time monitoring of health parameters, remote data sharing, and analysis.

For examples, HemeChip, a smartphone-based POC system has been developed for the diagnosis of blood cancers, including leukaemia and lymphoma. The system consists of a microfluidic chip that separates cancer cells from blood samples, and a smartphone-based imaging system that analyses the cells using image processing algorithms. The system has shown high sensitivity and specificity in detecting cancer cells, and can be used for early diagnosis and monitoring of disease [75]. Similarly, POCkit, another smartphone-based POC system has been employed for the detection of cancer biomarkers, such as prostate-specific antigen (PSA) and alpha-fetoprotein (AFP), in blood samples. The system consists of a disposable microfluidic cartridge and a smartphone-based reader that measures the color change in the cartridge after the reaction between the biomarkers and the reagents. The system has shown high accuracy and can be used for early diagnosis of cancer [76]. Another smartphone-based POC system called mChip is used for the diagnosis of cervical cancer. The system consists of a microfluidic chip that separates cervical cells from a Pap smear sample, and a smartphone-based reader that analyses the cells using fluorescence imaging. The system has shown high sensitivity and specificity in detecting cervical cancer cells, and can be used for early diagnosis and screening of the disease [77]. Oscan, is yet another smartphone-based POC system, used for the diagnosis of oral cancer. The system consists of a handheld device that captures images of the oral cavity and a smartphone-based software that analyses the images using machine learning algorithms. The system can detect early-stage oral cancer lesions with high accuracy, and can be used for early diagnosis and screening of the disease [78].

Overall, smartphone-based POC systems have shown great potential in cancer diagnosis due to their portability, affordability, and user-friendliness. With further development and optimization, these systems have great potential to revolutionize cancer treatment approaches and facilitate positive patient outcomes.

2.5 Recent advances in the application of POC in cancer

In 2020, it was estimated that approximately 19.3 million new cases of cancer and 10 million cancer-related deaths occurred globally, making cancer a primary contributor to mortality rates. Early detection and diagnosis are critical in reducing cancer-related mortality rates. POC testing has emerged as a promising approach for early cancer diagnosis, as it facilitates rapid and accurate diagnosis in a cost-effective manner with minimal infrastructure requirements.

Recent advances in the application of POC systems in cancer have greatly improved cancer diagnosis and management. These advancements have been driven by innovations in technology, materials science, and engineering, leading to more efficient and accurate POC systems (figure 2.5). POC systems have been developed for various cancer types, including breast, lung, prostate, and colorectal cancer. These systems have been designed to be portable, user-friendly, and cost-effective, making them ideal for use in resource-limited settings. They have also been utilized in monitoring cancer treatment response and detecting cancer recurrence. Furthermore, POC systems have been integrated with artificial intelligence and machine learning algorithms to improve diagnostic accuracy and provide personalized treatment recommendations. These

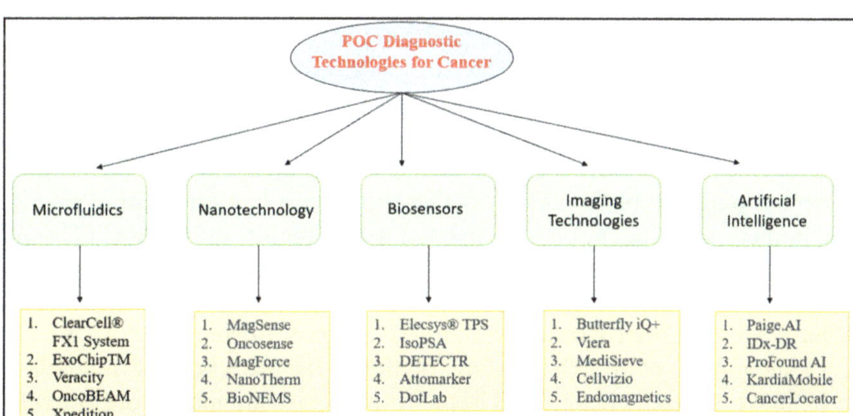

Figure 2.5. Multiple innovative technologies for POC diagnostic applications in cancer.

recent advances in POC devices have the potential to greatly improve cancer patient outcomes and lower healthcare costs.

There have been numerous recent advancements in the application of POC systems in cancer diagnosis and treatment. Some of them include:

1. Development of a paper-based microfluidic chip for rapid screening of circulating tumor cells (CTCs) in whole blood. The chip uses inkjet printing technology to print capture antibodies on the paper surface, which selectively bind to CTCs in the blood sample. The captured CTCs can then be visualized and counted using fluorescence microscopy. This approach has the potential to be used for early cancer detection and monitoring of cancer progression [79].
2. Use of an electrochemical sensor based on graphene quantum dots and gold nanoparticles for detection of prostate-specific antigen (PSA), a biomarker for prostate cancer. The sensor showed high sensitivity and specificity towards PSA detection in human serum samples, and the results were obtained within 10 min. This approach can be potentially used for early diagnosis of prostate cancer in resource-limited settings [80].
3. Development of a smartphone-based diagnostic platform for detecting cancer-associated exosomes in urine samples. The platform uses a lateral flow immunoassay strip and a smartphone camera for quantitative detection of exosomes in the urine sample. The results can be obtained within 30 min and the platform has shown high sensitivity and specificity towards exosome detection in urine samples from bladder cancer patients [81].
4. Use of a microfluidic chip for isolation and analysis of extracellular vesicles (EVs) from cancer patients' blood samples. The chip uses a combination of size-based and immunoaffinity-based isolation methods for highly efficient EV isolation, followed by on-chip analysis of EVs using a combination of optical and electrical detection methods. This approach has the potential to be used for liquid biopsy-based cancer diagnosis and monitoring [82].
5. Development of a biosensor based on a nanocomposite of gold nanoparticles and graphene oxide for detection of carcinoembryonic antigen (CEA), a biomarker for colon and lung cancer. The biosensor showed high sensitivity towards CEA detection in human serum samples, with a detection limit of 0.03 ng ml^{-1}. This approach can be potentially used for early diagnosis and monitoring of colon and lung cancer [83].
6. Use of a microfluidic chip for isolation and analysis of CTCs from breast cancer patients' blood samples. The chip uses a combination of microfluidic channels and magnetic nanoparticles for highly efficient CTC isolation, followed by on-chip analysis of CTCs using immunofluorescence staining and microscopy. This approach has the potential to be used for liquid biopsy-based breast cancer diagnosis and monitoring [84].
7. Development of a POC testing platform for detection of multiple cancer biomarkers in saliva samples. The platform uses a combination of electrochemical sensors and microfluidic channels for simultaneous detection of multiple biomarkers, including interleukin-6, alpha-fetoprotein, and carcinoembryonic

antigen. The platform has shown high sensitivity and specificity towards biomarker detection in saliva samples from cancer patients [85].

8. Development of CRISPR-Cas based diagnostic tools. The CRISPR-Cas system has been repurposed for diagnostic applications by utilizing the Cas enzyme's ability to cleave specific nucleic acid sequences. This technology has been used to develop rapid and sensitive diagnostic tools for cancer. For example, a CRISPR-Cas12a based assay was developed for the detection of mutations in the TP53 gene, which is commonly mutated in many types of cancer. The assay was able to detect mutations with high specificity and sensitivity in as little as 20 min using a simple paper-based device [86].
9. Artificial intelligence (AI) has also shown great potential in revolutionizing cancer diagnosis and treatment. The integration of AI into POC devices has enabled the development of faster, more accurate, and cost-effective diagnostic tools. AI algorithms can analyse large amounts of patient data, including medical records, imaging data, and genetic information, to generate personalized cancer diagnosis and treatment plans. For instance, a recent study reported the development of a smartphone-based AI diagnostic tool for the detection of skin cancer, with an accuracy of 90.2% [87].
10. Wearable sensors have emerged as a promising tool for POC cancer detection, monitoring, and treatment. These sensors can continuously monitor biomarkers in real-time, providing valuable insights into a patient's health status. For instance, a recent study demonstrated the use of a wearable sweat sensor for non-invasive monitoring of glucose, lactate, and cortisol levels in cancer patients [88]. Another study reported the use of a wearable graphene-based sensor for the detection of prostate-specific antigen (PSA), a biomarker for prostate cancer [89]. These wearable sensors have the potential to improve cancer management by providing real-time, personalized data to healthcare providers and patients.

Thus, recent advances in the application of POC in cancer have shown tremendous potential in improving cancer detection, monitoring, and treatment outcomes. These advancements offer several advantages over traditional diagnostic methods, such as portability, low cost, and ease of use, i.e. suitable for a resource-limited setting. Further research and development in this field will continue to drive innovation and improve cancer care worldwide.

2.6 Limitations and challenges in using POC in cancer diagnostics

POC devices have emerged as a promising tool in cancer diagnostics, offering faster and more accurate diagnosis, monitoring, and treatment. However, despite the potential benefits, the use of POC devices in cancer diagnostics still faces several limitations and challenges. These limitations and challenges can arise from different stages of the POC process, including sample collection, processing, analysis, and interpretation. It is essential to identify these limitations and challenges to improve the development and implementation of POC devices in cancer diagnostics.

Some of the limitations and challenges in using POC in cancer diagnostics include:

1. Limited sensitivity and specificity: Despite the considerable progress made in the sensitivity and specificity of POC tests, there is still scope for enhancement. The occurrence of false positives and false negatives can result in inaccurate diagnoses and delayed treatment, potentially leading to severe repercussions for patients.
2. Technical limitations: Some point-of-care devices require extensive user training, which can limit their use in resource-limited settings where healthcare workers may not have the necessary expertise. Additionally, some tests may be affected by factors such as temperature, humidity, or the presence of other substances in the sample.
3. Regulatory challenges: POC devices must meet regulatory requirements in order to be approved for use in clinical settings. This can be a lengthy and expensive process, and some devices may not be able to meet the necessary standards.
4. Cost: While POC tests can be less expensive than traditional laboratory-based tests, they still require a certain level of investment in terms of equipment and supplies. This can be a barrier to their adoption in resource-limited settings.
5. Data management: POC tests generate large amounts of data that need to be managed and stored. This can be a challenge in settings where electronic health records are not widely used or where there are limited resources for data management.
6. Limited scope: Some POC tests are designed to detect only a specific type of cancer or a specific biomarker. This can limit their utility in clinical settings where a broader range of tests may be needed.
7. Access to care: POC tests may not always be readily available in all healthcare settings, which can limit their usefulness in some populations. Additionally, some patients may not have access to healthcare facilities where POC tests are available.

While POC diagnostics offer several advantages in cancer diagnosis, there are also certain limitations and challenges that must be addressed. Further research is needed to improve the sensitivity and specificity of POC tests, establish standardization and regulatory oversight, develop and validate appropriate biomarkers, and increase accessibility and affordability of POC tests.

2.7 Conclusion

In conclusion, the field of POC systems for cancer diagnosis and management has evolved significantly over the past few decades. From the earliest development of lateral flow assays to the recent emergence of highly sensitive biosensors and microfluidic devices, the advances in POC technology have greatly improved cancer care and management. These POC systems have the potential to revolutionize cancer diagnosis and treatment by offering rapid and reliable results, reducing healthcare costs, and improving patient outcomes.

The brief history of POC systems has shown that the technology has come a long way, but there are still challenges to be addressed. The development of more sensitive and specific diagnostic assays, the integration of multiple biomarkers for improved accuracy, and the need for more user-friendly and cost-effective devices are among the major challenges that need to be addressed. Despite these challenges, the recent advances in POC systems for cancer diagnosis and management hold great promise. The incorporation of nanotechnology, microfluidics, and smartphone technology has laid the groundwork for the advancement of highly sensitive, rapid, and low-cost POC devices that are useful in a resource-limited setting. These devices can potentially transform cancer care by enabling early detection, monitoring treatment response, and improving patient outcomes.

In summary, the field of POC systems for cancer diagnosis and management is rapidly evolving, and the recent advances in technology hold great promise for improving cancer care and management. With continued research and development, POC systems are poised to become an essential tool in the fight against cancer, particularly in resource-limited settings where access to traditional diagnostic methods is limited.

References

[1] Konwar A N and Borse V 2020 Current status of point-of-care diagnostic devices in the Indian healthcare system with an update on COVID-19 pandemic *Sens. Int.* **1** 100015

[2] Price C P and John A S 2012 *Point-of-Care Testing: Making Innovation Work for Patient-Centered Care* (American Association for Clinical Chemistry)

[3] Pai M, Ghiasi M and Pai N P 2015 Point-of-care diagnostic testing in global health: what is the point *Microbe* **10** 103–7

[4] Olansky L and Kennedy L 2010 Finger-stick glucose monitoring: issues of accuracy and specificity *Diabetes Care* **33** 948–9

[5] National Institutes of Health 2014 The History of the Pregnancy Test Kit, A Timeline of Pregnancy Testing (http://history.nih.gov/exhibits/thinblueline/timeline.html) (Accessed: April 10 2020)

[6] Luppa P B, Müller C, Schlichtiger A and Schlebusch H 2011 Point-of-care testing (POCT): Current techniques and future perspectives *TrAC Trends Anal. Chem.* **30** 887–98

[7] Bray F, Laversanne M, Weiderpass E and Soerjomataram I 2021 The ever-increasing importance of cancer as a leading cause of premature death worldwide *Cancer* **127** 3029–30

[8] World Health Organization (WHO) 2020 Global Health Estimates 2020: Deaths by Cause, Age, Sex, by Country and by Region 2000-2019 (https://who.int/data/gho/data/themes/mortality-and-global-health-estimates/ghe-leading-causes-of-death) (Accessed: 11th December 2020)

[9] Omran A 1971 The epidemiologic transition: a theory of the epidemiology of population change *MILBANK* Q **49** 4

[10] Sung H, Ferlay J, Siegel R L, Laversanne M, Soerjomataram I, Jemal A and Bray F 2021 Global cancer statistics 2020: GLOBOCAN estimates of incidence and mortality worldwide for 36 cancers in 185 countries *CA Cancer J Clin.* **71** 209–49

[11] Jamil A and Kasi A 2021 Pneumatocele *Stat Pearls* (Stat Pearls Publishing)

[12] Nishat S, Jafry A T, Martinez A W and Awan F R 2021 Paper-based microfluidics: Simplified fabrication and assay methods *Sensors Actuators* B **336** 129681
[13] Nazir S and Kwon O S 2022 Micro-electromechanical systems-based sensors and their applications *Appl. Sci. Converg. Technol.* **31** 40–5
[14] Ibrahim N, Jamaluddin N D, Tan L L and Mohd Yusof N Y 2021 A review on the development of gold and silver nanoparticles-based biosensor as a detection strategy of emerging and pathogenic RNA virus *Sensors* **21** 5114
[15] Rubin G *et al* 2015 The expanding role of primary care in cancer control *Lancet Oncol* **16** 1231–72
[16] Lyratzopoulos G, Vedsted P and Singh H 2015 Understanding missed opportunities for more timely diagnosis of cancer in symptomatic patients after presentation *Br. J. Cancer* **12** S84–91
[17] Phillips K A, Van Bebber S and Issa A M 2006 Diagnostics and biomarker development: priming the pipeline *Nat. Rev. Drug Discov.* **5** 463–9
[18] Usher-Smith J A, Sharp S J and Griffin S J 2016 The spectrum effect in tests for risk prediction, screening, and diagnosis *Brit. Med. J.* **353**
[19] Pinsky P F, Prorok P C and Kramer B S 2017 Prostate cancer screening-a perspective on the current state of the evidence *New Engl. J. Med.* **376** 1285–9
[20] Hwang V J and Weiss R H 2016 Metabolomic profiling for early cancer detection: current status and future prospects *Expert Opin. Drug Metab. Toxicol.* **12** 1263–5
[21] Malati T 2007 Tumour markers: an overview *Indian J. Clin. Biochem.* **22** 17–31
[22] Füzéry A K, Levin J, Chan M M and Chan D W 2013 Translation of proteomic biomarkers into FDA approved cancer diagnostics: issues and challenges *Clin. Proteom.* **10** 1–4
[23] Srinivas P R, Kramer B S and Srivastava S 2001 Trends in biomarker research for cancer detection *Lancet Oncol.* **2** 698–704
[24] Biomarkers Definitions Working Group 2001 Biomarkers and surrogate endpoints: preferred definitions and conceptual framework *Clin. Pharmacol. Ther.* **69** 89–95
[25] Cheah A L, Goldblum J R and Billings S D 2013 Molecular diagnostics complementing morphology in superficial mesenchymal tumors *Semin. Diagn. Pathol.* **301** 95–109
[26] Fan X J *et al* 2014 Phosphorylated p38, a negative prognostic biomarker, complements TNM staging prognostication in colorectal cancer *Tumor Biol.* **35** 10487–95
[27] Hanash S M, Pitteri S J and Faca V M 2008 Mining the plasma proteome for cancer biomarkers *Natur* **452** 571–9
[28] Filella X and Foj L 2015 Emerging biomarkers in the detection and prognosis of prostate cancer *Clin. Chem. Lab. Med. (CCLM)* **53** 963–73
[29] Lin J, Li J, Huang B, Liu J, Chen X, Chen X M, Xu Y M, Huang L F and Wang X Z 2015 Exosomes: novel biomarkers for clinical diagnosis *Sci. World J.* **2015**
[30] Mandel P 1948 Les acides nucleiques du plasma sanguin chez 1 homme *CR Seances Soc. Biol. Fil.* **142** 241–3
[31] Leon S A, Shapiro B, Sklaroff D M and Yaros M J 1977 Free DNA in the serum of cancer patients and the effect of therapy *Cancer Res.* **37** 646–50
[32] Bettegowda C *et al* 2014 Detection of circulating tumor DNA in early-and late-stage human malignancies *Sci. Transl. Med.* **6** 224ra24
[33] Chen K Z *et al* 2016 Circulating tumor DNA detection in early-stage non-small cell lung cancer patients by targeted sequencing *Sci. Rep.* **6** 31985

[34] Mitchell M I, Ma J, Carter C L and Loudig O 2022 Circulating exosome cargoes contain functionally diverse cancer biomarkers: from biogenesis and function to purification and potential translational utility *Cancers* **14** 3350
[35] Wang Y *et al* 2015 Detection of somatic mutations and HPV in the saliva and plasma of patients with head and neck squamous cell carcinomas *Sci. Transl. Med.* **7** 293ra104
[36] Ellinger J, Müller S C, Wernert N, Von Ruecker A and Bastian P J 2008 Mitochondrial DNA in serum of patients with prostate cancer: a predictor of biochemical recurrence after prostatectomy *BJU Int.* **102** 628–32
[37] Schwarzenbach H, Alix-Panabières C, Müller I, Letang N, Vendrell J P, Rebillard X and Pantel K 2009 Cell-free tumor DNA in blood plasma as a marker for circulating tumor cells in prostate cancer *Clin. Cancer Res.* **15** 1032–8
[38] Schwarzenbach H, Hoon D S and Pantel K 2011 Cell-free nucleic acids as biomarkers in cancer patients *Nat. Rev. Cancer* **11** 426–37
[39] De Mattos-Arruda L, Cortes J, Santarpia L, Vivancos A, Tabernero J, Reis-Filho J S and Seoane J 2013 Circulating tumour cells and cell-free DNA as tools for managing breast cancer *Nat. Rev. Clin. Oncol.* **10** 377–90
[40] Kulis M and Esteller M 2010 DNA methylation and cancer *Adv. Genet* **70** 27–56
[41] Goessl C, Krause H, Müller M, Heicappell R, Schrader M, Sachsinger J and Miller K 2000 Fluorescent methylation-specific polymerase chain reaction for DNA-based detection of prostate cancer in bodily fluids *Cancer Res.* **60** 5941–5
[42] Wen L *et al* 2015 Genome-scale detection of hypermethylated CpG islands in circulating cell-free DNA of hepatocellular carcinoma patients *Cell Res.* **25** 1250–64
[43] Zhou J, Liu J, Gao Y, Shen L, Li S and Chen S 2021 miRNA-based potential biomarkers and new molecular insights in ulcerative colitis *Front. Pharmacol.* **12** 707776
[44] Martinez V G, Munera-Maravilla E, Bernardini A, Rubio C, Suarez-Cabrera C, Segovia C, Lodewijk I, Dueñas M, Martínez-Fernández M and Paramio J M 2019 Epigenetics of bladder cancer: where biomarkers and therapeutic targets meet *Front. Genet.* **10** 1125
[45] Wang S C, Liao L M, Ansar M, Lin S Y, Hsu W W, Su C M, Chung Y M, Liu C C, Hung C S and Lin R K 2021 Automatic detection of the circulating cell-free methylated DNA pattern of GCM2, ITPRIPL1 and CCDC181 for detection of early breast cancer and surgical treatment response *Cancers* **13** 1375
[46] Lawrie C H *et al* 2008 Detection of elevated levels of tumour-associated microRNAs in serum of patients with diffuse large B-cell lymphoma *Br. J. Haematol.* **141** 672–5
[47] Shaukat A and Levin T R 2022 Current and future colorectal cancer screening strategies *Nat Rev. Gastroenterol. Hepatol.* **19** 521–31
[48] Montagnana M, Benati M and Danese E 2017 Circulating biomarkers in epithelial ovarian cancer diagnosis: from present to future perspective *Ann. Transl. Med.* **5**
[49] Xiong D D, Lv J, Wei K L, Feng Z B, Chen J T, Liu K C, Chen G and Luo D Z 2017 A nine-miRNA signature as a potential diagnostic marker for breast carcinoma: an integrated study of 1,110 cases *Oncol. Rep.* **37** 3297–304
[50] Solé C, Moliné T, Vidal M, Ordi-Ros J and Cortés-Hernández J 2019 An exosomal urinary miRNA signature for early diagnosis of renal fibrosis in lupus nephritis *Cells* **8** 773
[51] Vasan R S 2006 Biomarkers of cardiovascular disease: molecular basis and practical considerations *Circulation* **113** 2335–62
[52] Duffy S P and Criner G J 2019 Chronic obstructive pulmonary disease: evaluation and management *Med. Clin.* **103** 453–61

[53] Lojanapiwat B, Anutrakulchai W, Chongruksut W and Udomphot C 2014 Correlation and diagnostic performance of the prostate-specific antigen level with the diagnosis, aggressiveness, and bone metastasis of prostate cancer in clinical practice *Prostate Int.* **2** 133–9

[54] Begic E, Hadzidedic S, Kulaglic A, Ramic-Brkic B, Begic Z and Causevic M 2019 SOMAscan-based proteomic measurements of plasma brain natriuretic peptide are decreased in mild cognitive impairment and in Alzheimer's dementia patients *PLoS One* **14** e0212261

[55] Pusta A, Tertis M, Graur F, Cristea C and Al Hajjar N 2022 Aptamers and new bioreceptors for the electrochemical detection of biomarkers expressed in hepatocellular carcinoma *Curr. Med. Chem.* **29** 4363–90

[56] Williams S C 2013 Circulating tumor cells *Proc. Natl Acad. Sci.* **110** 4861

[57] Cellsearch (https://cellsearchctc.com/) (Accessed: 21 March 2018)

[58] Riethdorf S *et al* 2007 Detection of circulating tumor cells in peripheral blood of patients with metastatic breast cancer: a validation study of the CellSearch system *Clin. Cancer Res* **13** 920–8

[59] Maheswaran S *et al* 2008 Detection of mutations in EGFR in circulating lung-cancer cells *New Engl. J. Med.* **359** 366–77

[60] Shi Y *et al* 2015 Multifunctional biocompatible graphene oxide quantum dots decorated magnetic nanoplatform for efficient capture and two-photon imaging of rare tumor cells *ACS Appl. Mater. Interfaces* **7** 10935–43

[61] Kirby D, Glynn M, Kijanka G and Ducrée J 2015 Rapid and cost-efficient enumeration of rare cancer cells from whole blood by low-loss centrifugo-magnetophoretic purification under stopped-flow conditions *Cytometry* A **87** 74–80

[62] Liang L G *et al* 2017 An integrated double-filtration microfluidic device for isolation, enrichment and quantification of urinary extracellular vesicles for detection of bladder cancer *Sci. Rep.* **7** 46224

[63] Thakur B K *et al* 2014 Double-stranded DNA in exosomes: a novel biomarker in cancer detection *Cell Res.* **24** 766–9

[64] Cheung S F, Cheng S K and Kamei D T 2015 Based systems for point-of-care biosensing *J. Lab. Autom.* **20** 316–33

[65] Martinez A W, Phillips S T, Carrilho E, Thomas S W, Sindi H and Whitesides G M 2008 Simple telemedicine for developing regions: camera phones and paper-based microfluidic devices for real-time, off-site diagnosis *Anal. Chem.* **80** 3699–707

[66] Nemiroski A, Christodouleas D C, Hennek J W, Kumar A A, Maxwell E J, Fernández-Abedul M T and Whitesides G M 2014 Universal mobile electrochemical detector designed for use in resource-limited applications *Proc. Natl Acad. Sci.* **111** 11984–9

[67] Li C, He W, Wang N, Xi Z, Deng R, Liu X, Kang R, Xie L and Liu X 2022 Application of microfluidics in detection of circulating tumor cells *Front. Bioeng. Biotechnol.* **10**

[68] Chu Y, Gao Y, Tang W, Qiang L, Han Y, Gao J, Zhang Y, Liu H and Han L 2021 Attomolar-level ultrasensitive and multiplex microRNA detection enabled by a nanomaterial locally assembled microfluidic biochip for cancer diagnosis *Anal. Chem.* **93** 5129–36

[69] Seok Y, Joung H A, Byun J Y, Jeon H S, Shin S J, Kim S, Shin Y B, Han H S and Kim M G 2017 A paper-based device for performing loop-mediated isothermal amplification with real-time simultaneous detection of multiple DNA targets *Theranostics* **7** 2220

[70] Franco R, Pedrosa P, Carlos F F, Veigas B and Baptista P V 2015 Gold nanoparticles for DNA/RNA-based diagnostics *Handbook of Nanoparticles* **7** 1339

[71] Alnaimi A, Al-Hamry A, Makableh Y, Adiraju A and Kanoun O 2022 Gold nanoparticles-MWCNT based aptasensor for early diagnosis of prostate cancer *Biosensors* **12** 1130

[72] Bhana S, Wang Y and Huang X 2015 Nanotechnology for enrichment and detection of circulating tumor cells *Nanomedicine* **10** 1973–90

[73] Liang Y, Xu Y, Tong Y, Chen Y, Chen X and Wu S 2022 Graphene-based electrochemical sensor for detection of hepatocellular carcinoma markers *Front. Chem.* **10** 883627

[74] Li J, Gao H, Chen Z, Wei X and Yang C F 2010 An electrochemical immunosensor for carcinoembryonic antigen enhanced by self-assembled nanogold coatings on magnetic particles *Anal. Chim. Acta.* **665** 98–104

[75] Beduk T, Beduk D, Hasan M R, Guler Celik E, Kosel J, Narang J, Salama K N and Timur S 2022 Smartphone-based multiplexed biosensing tools for health monitoring *Biosensors* **12** 583

[76] Zhang M, Cui X and Li N 2022 Smartphone-based mobile biosensors for the point-of-care testing of human metabolites *Mater. Today Bio.* **8** 100254

[77] Zhang S, Li Z and Wei Q 2020 Smartphone-based cytometric biosensors for point-of-care cellular diagnostics *Nanotechnol. Precis. Eng.* **3** 32–42

[78] Uthoff R D *et al* 2018 Point-of-care, smartphone-based, dual-modality, dual-view, oral cancer screening device with neural network classification for low-resource communities *PLoS One* **13** e0207493

[79] Zhang Y, Zhang X, Situ B, Wu Y, Luo S, Zheng L and Qiu Y 2021 Rapid electrochemical biosensor for sensitive profiling of exosomal microRNA based on multifunctional DNA tetrahedron assisted catalytic hairpin assembly *Biosens. Bioelectron.* **183** 113205

[80] Wang C, Xin D, Yue Q, Wan H, Li Q, Wang Y and Wu J 2023 A novel electrochemical IL-6 sensor based on Au nanoparticles-modified platinum carbon electrode *Front. Bioeng. Biotechnol.* **11** 1128934

[81] Zhu X, Su H, Liu H and Sun B 2023 A selectivity-enhanced fluorescence imprinted sensor based on yellow-emission peptide nanodots for sensitive and visual smart detection of λ-cyhalothrin *Anal. Chim. Acta.* **1255** 341124

[82] Abreu C M, Costa-Silva B, Reis R L, Kundu S C and Caballero D 2022 Microfluidic platforms for extracellular vesicle isolation, analysis and therapy in cancer *Lab Chip* **22** 1093–125

[83] Tai J, Fan S, Ding S and Ren L 2022 Gold nanoparticles based optical biosensors for cancer biomarker proteins: a review of the current practices *Front. Bioeng. Biotechnol.* **10** 877139

[84] Zhang X, Lu X, Gao W, Wang Y, Jia C and Cong H 2021 A label-free microfluidic chip for the highly selective isolation of single and cluster CTCs from breast cancer patients *Transl. Oncol.* **14** 100959

[85] Khan R S, Khurshid Z and Yahya Ibrahim Asiri F 2017 Advancing point-of-care (PoC) testing using human saliva as liquid biopsy *Diagnostics* **7** 39

[86] Kaminski M M, Abudayyeh O O, Gootenberg J S, Zhang F and Collins J J 2021 CRISPR-based diagnostics *Nat. Biomed. Eng.* **5** 643–56

[87] Farina E, Nabhen J J, Dacoregio M I, Batalini F and Moraes F Y 2022 An overview of artificial intelligence in oncology *Future Sci. OA* **8** FSO787

[88] Zafar H, Channa A, Jeoti V and Stojanović G M 2022 Comprehensive review on wearable sweat-glucose sensors for continuous glucose monitoring *Sensors* **22** 638

[89] Xu L, Wen Y, Pandit S, Mokkapati V R, Mijakovic I, Li Y, Ding M, Ren S, Li W and Liu G 2019 Graphene-based biosensors for the detection of prostate cancer protein biomarkers: a review *BMC Chem.* **13** 1–2

Chapter 3

Aptasensors for cancer diagnostics: an insight into immobilization strategies

Pushpesh Ranjan, Rudramani Tiwari, Lal Singh Banjara, Mohd Abubakar Sadique, Shalu Yadav, Raju Khan, S Krishnamoorthi, Ajay Kumar Meena and Subhash Chandra Verma

Aptamers are single-stranded oligonucleotides (RNA or DNA) that are artificially synthesized through the systematic evolution of ligands by the exponential enrichment (SELEX) method. Aptamer-based diagnostics holds great promise in biomedical applications such as the early detection of cancer biomarkers. In the fabrication of an aptasensor, several parameters including appropriate immobilization methods are crucial. However, the choice of the electrode surface is also important, as it directly influences the binding chemistry. The aptamers are immobilized through covalent attachments, physical adsorption, self-assembly of the monolayer, and affinity interactions to fabricate an aptasensor. These immobilization techniques are robust, reliable, simple and allow better binding of aptamers to retain their structural identity and functions, and offer a high-throughput detection platform. Nevertheless, the highly oriented aptamers on the electrode, which are achieved through direct immobilization, offer highly sensitive, selective, reproducible and cost-effective aptasensors. Nevertheless, the choice of materials and new advances in immobilization methods further improves the development of an aptasensor-based diagnostic platform for early detection of cancer biomarkers.

3.1 Introduction

The spotting and recognition of pathogenic agents are leading objectives in biomedical research and clinical diagnostics. Since pathogenic agents are present in low concentrations in human fluids (urine, serum, and blood), it is necessary to develop more sensitive and selective exposure methods for earlier diagnosis and more effective treatment of diseases. The World Health Organization (WHO) reports that the number of new cancer cases doubled from the year 2000 (10 million)

doi:10.1088/978-0-7503-5012-9ch3

to 2021 (20 million), with 10 million deaths [1]. The majority of cancer deaths are the result of failure in the pre-stage diagnosis of cancer cells due to their mortality rate [2]. These reports introduce us to an important challenge in molecular oncology for early diagnosis of disease [3]. Initial-stage detection and treatments improve the survival rate of patients. Development of improved detection approaches enables the advancement of new and early-stage diagnosis technologies. The best method of real diagnosis and pre-stage cures for cancer is possible by the detection of cancer biomarkers at the ultra-low level and the development of molecular probes that bind these biomarkers successfully [4]. So far, several platforms are reported for biomarker detection such as microarray [5], microbeads [6], nanoparticle-based platforms [7], electrochemical biosensing [8], electrochemiluminescence [9], optical biosensing [10] and enzymatic platforms [11]. Most of these methods are dependent upon the antibody-antigen interaction to show the disease progression by the generation of specific signals [12]. The major class of antibody-based biomarker probes is suitable only for tumor cells but immunogenicity and peptidase susceptibility are limited for their theranostic value [13, 14].

However, another detection platform known as aptasensors has been widely utilized for the sensitive detection of cancer biomarkers. The development of the systematic evolution of ligands by exponential enrichment (SELEX) has provided an alternate synthetic nucleotide, called an aptamer, that specifically binds with various biomarker molecules and cell membranes through cell-SELEX [15–17]. Firstly, aptamers were introduced in [16] for RNA ligands in contradiction of T4 DNA polymerase and Ellington *et al* (*in vitro* selection) [16]. The first biosensing application of aptamers was reported in 1996 as a fluorescence-labeled optical aptasensor for the detection of immunoglobulin G (IgG) [18].

Aptamers are single-stranded deoxyribonucleic acid (ssDNA) or single-stranded ribonucleic acid (ssRNA) that can selectively bind to the low molecular organic/inorganic/macromolecular substrates with high affinity compared to the binding of antibodies to antigens at lower concentrations (micromolar to the nanomolar range) [19, 20]. The synthesis of aptamers doesn't need any sophisticated model of target cells, but is based on the systematic evolution of ligands by the exponential enrichment (SELEX) procedure. This progression involves a random library of oligonucleotides consisting of linear nucleic acids (approx. 1015–1016). While the traditional *in vitro* selection process takes several days (one week to one month), recently automated methods provide a road from the substrate to the reagent within two to three days [21]. For example, an RNA-based aptamer transcribes the DNA library in an RNA pool by passing the library through a separating matrix containing target molecules. A few chains that have an affinity to bind with the target substrate get separated and others are washed out. These bound nucleic acid chains are processed by PCR amplification to get a mixture of active aptamers with different affinities. The process is repeated 8–15 times to yield aptamers with high affinity. The aptamers generate 3D structures, i.e. loops and hybridized phases using Watson–Crick base-pairing with their target molecules [22]. Aptamers are showing a high interest in the field of chromatography [23] and electrophoresis [24] as therapeutic and diagnostic agents [25], and as active materials for sensing and biosensing [26] due to their high selectivity and affinity. For biosensing applications aptamers can substitute antibodies in several contexts [26], i.e. (i) The *in vitro* selections enable the fabrication of aptamers' obligatory ligands for toxic molecules which are not available from the immune system. Aptamers with high binding affinity towards the substrate, i.e. small organic molecules, peptides, proteins, and viruses or cells at a very low concentration from nanomolar (10^{-9} M) to picomolar (10^{-12} M) [27, 28]. (ii) Chemical synthesis of aptamers produces highly unperturbed structures for obligatory ligands. These can be reproduced without any loss of integrity and discrimination [29]. (iii) Its chemical modifications with different labels or functional groups empower its tethering to transducers. The sensitivity of aptasensors can be improved by modification with nanomaterials, i.e. metal nanoparticles, quantum dots, graphene, carbon nanomaterials, and other nanocomposites [30]. (iv) The complex formation tendency of aptamers allows recognition of low molecular weight substrates. The remarkable property of conformational change after the complexation with the target biomarker make it suitable for utilization in biosensing applications [31]. (v) Specific adsorption and thermal stability add more advantages to using aptamers as the biosensing material. Since there are many advantages of aptamers over antibodies there is a major disadvantage associate with it; one needs highly pure conditions for their application due to their susceptibility towards nuclease activity. Several modifications on the 2′-position of the ribose ring or pyrimidine nucleotide make aptamers a nuclease-resistant moiety [32].

Since aptamers are biorecognition elements, aptamer-based biosensors show a significant advantage in clinical examinations in comparison with conventional techniques in terms of high selectivity and affinity to biomarkers, size, easy synthesis, stability, and chemical modification [29, 33]. Biosensors are made up of a transducer and a biological recognition element. Aptamers act as a biological recognition element, which is a biomolecule that can bind with specific target biomarkers. The associated transducer converts this bond to detectable and measurable signals. These properties of aptamer-containing biosensors (aptasensors) provide a quick analysis and immediate detection which can reimburse the confines of present clinical diagnostics [34, 35]. The development of aptasensor devices relies on every aspect, i.e. characterization of biorecognition probes with analytes, immobilization, anti-fouling surface formation, biosensor design, and fabrication with simple, sensitive, and cost-effective properties. The application of aptamers is a hopeful implement for the expansion of point-of-care (POC) biosensors in the detection of different types of cancer biomarkers [36].

3.1.1 Aptamer configuration

There are several types of structures, i.e. loops, hairpins, triplexes or quadruplexes, crystals, stems, and other 3D structures of aptamers that are reported to date. The loop formation in structures is the result of specific interactions between nucleic acids present on DNA aptamers. While a distinct multiple-loop aptamer structural arrangement has been reported for alpha-methylacyl-CoA racemase (AMACR) detection, a single loop configuration has been reported for PSA detection [37]. A double-stranded helical structure of aptamers is referred to as stem configuration. The name stem configuration is given due to its suitability to interact with the cancer stem cells. A combination of loop and stem structure is called a hairpin configuration. Several hairpin-configuration aptamers are reported for the free solution assay response for small molecules [38]. Guanine-rich aptamers are capable of forming four-stranded structures, referred to as quadraplex structures. Quadruplex structures of DNA aptamers were reported for thrombin, which stabilizes in the presence of cations, i.e. potassium, that acquires central positions on the quadrapoles [39]. A crystal structure was also reported for human thrombin. Different configurations of aptamers are confirmed by using different spectroscopic techniques i.e. x-ray crystallography, UV-vis spectroscopy, surface plasmon resonance [40], and nuclear magnetic resonance [41]. The chemical modification of aptamers is allowing for better immobilization strategies. It is easy to chemically modify the aptamers using amine, azide, thiol, or biotin groups [42].

3.2 Immobilization techniques for aptamers

There are several methods that have been employed to immobilize aptamers for the successful fabrication of biosensors. The aptamer of the biosensor captures the target analyte, like a cancer protein biomarker, to generate the measurable signals. In biosensor fabrication, the modification step is important to achieve selectivity, high sensitivity, lower detection limit, and reproducible results against the target biomarker. Aptamers are synthetically produced, work similarly to an antibody as a biorecognition element in biosensors, and successfully replace the antibody biorecognition agent [35]. Since they are synthetically produced, therefore, we can design the target-specific aptamer to achieve better functioning of the biosensor.

The main strategy behind the immobilization of aptamers on the modified electrode surface is physical adsorption, covalent attachment, chemisorption, and encapsulation or entrapment of the aptamer. They are immobilized on the electrode surface, which has been modified by the nanocomposite materials, self-assembly of monolayer (SAM), and polymer-based approach. Furthermore, the choice of immobilization strategy also depends on several factors such as the nature of the biorecognition molecule, the transducer, the interest of the target analyte, and the applicable condition of the aptasensor. A comparison of the aptamer immobilization techniques is listed in table 3.1. Aptamer-based biosensors have broad applications in the detection of biological molecules, such as protein biomarkers of cancer, cardiac disease, neurotransmitters, and other pathogens, as well as non-biological elements. Various methods of aptamer immobilization to construct the aptasensor is shown in figures 3.1(A)–(D) [43, 44]. Additionally, sandwich aptamers have also gathered attention since they offer high sensitivity and easy operation modules. In the sandwich assay, an aptamer including two or more recognition elements has been utilized, where one serves as capturing agent and the other as a probing agent [35, 43, 45]. Therefore aptasensor-based detection platforms have huge potential in biosensing applications. Nevertheless, nanotechnology

Table 3.1. Comparison of the aptamer immobilization methods [35, 50, 71].

Immobilization method	Type of interaction/bonding	Binding force	Surface	Advantage	Disadvantage
Electrostatic adsorption	Negatively charged aptamer binds to the positively charged electrode surface	Weak	—	Cost-effective, rapid, and simple	Low binding capacity, non-specific adsorption, low control of orientation like the randomness of aptamer causing instability such as changing the ionic strength of the buffer, pH
Physical adsorption	Non-covalent bindings such as hydrophobic, hydrogen bonding, van der Waals, and electrostatic interactions	Moderate	Thiol and amine-containing metal nanoparticles (AuNPs), silicon, glass	Slightly or no conformational change, easier method, rapid, low cost	Low control of orientation like the randomness of aptamer causing instability such as changing the ionic strength of the buffer, pH
Covalent linkage	The chemical bond between the capturing agent and electrode surface like EDC/NHS coupling between the COOH-functionalized electrode surface and the amine-terminated aptamer sequence	High	Graphene, graphene oxide, reduced graphene oxide, carbon dots, acid-pretreated CNTs	High stability, high degree of orientation control, ordered layer, and thickness of the electrode surface, high sensitivity	The costly, complex preparation method, requires prior modification of the probe and linker molecule, and an irreversible process
Chemisorption	Imply chemical bonding between the electrode surface and the probe	High	Graphene, graphene oxide, reduced graphene oxide, carbon dots, acid-pretreated CNTs	High stability, high degree of orientation control, ordered layer, and thickness of the electrode surface, high sensitivity	The costly, complex preparation method, requires prior modification of the probe and linker molecule, and an irreversible process

(Continued)

Table 3.1. (*Continued*)

Immobilization method	Type of interaction/bonding	Binding force	Surface	Advantage	Disadvantage
Affinity interaction	Interactions between the biotin group of aptamers and avidin or streptavidin	Moderate	Avidin or streptavidin-modified nanoparticles	Considerable orientation, well-orered layer, stable, high functionalization control	Costly biocompatible linkers and sticky ends modifications
Entrapment or encapsulation	Involve trapping of aptamer within a polymer	Weak	Gels, fibers, and micromolecules like pyrrole, chitosan, cellulose, dopamine, and acrylamide	High entrapments of aptamers, high stability against nuclease, good controlled polymer growth	Result in the leaching of aptamers and decease binding efficiency

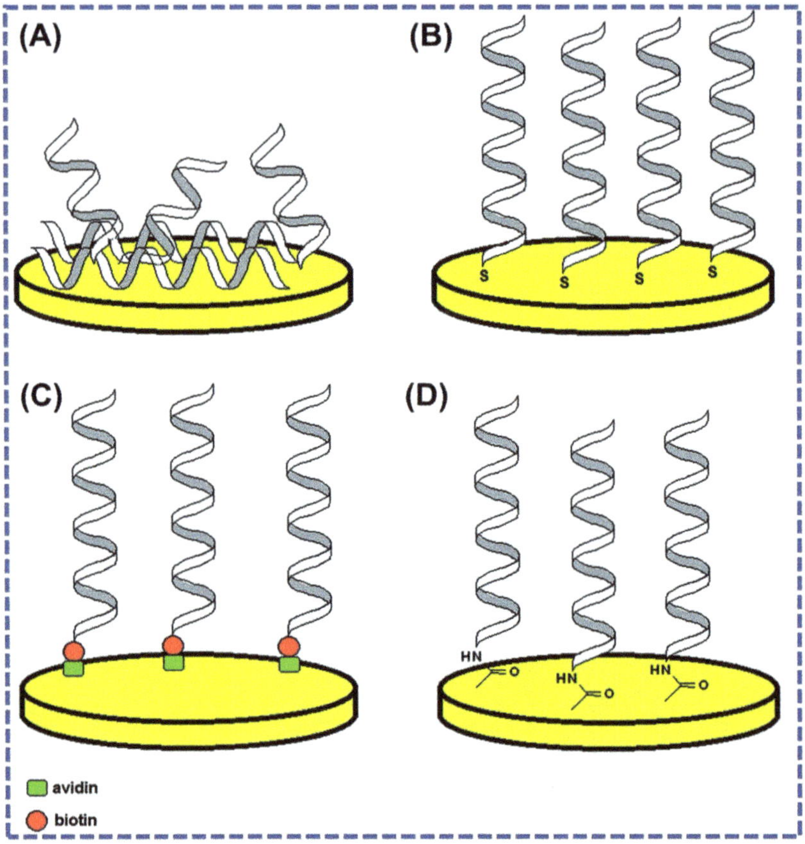

Figure 3.1. Methods of aptamer immobilization (A) physical adsorption, (B) thiol self-assembled monolayers, (C) avidin–biotin complex formation, and (D) surface activation with EDC/NHS. Reproduced with permission from [44]. Copyright (2016) Royal Society of Chemistry.

advancement further improves the aptasensor-based diagnostic application to generate high-throughput results.

3.2.1 Physical adsorption of aptamers

In the physical adsorption method, aptamers are adsorbed onto the electrode surface via weak interactions including hydrogen bonds, van der Waals forces, electrostatic forces of attraction, and hydrophilic and hydrophobic interactions. These immobilization strategies are simple, fast, and cost-effective. However, this strategy suffers from several disadvantages. The weaker interaction of the aptamer on the electrode surface could result in the removal of the aptamer. Therefore, the results from sample to sample may vary. Also, the confirmation of the aptamer could be disturbed or changed, which results in a low interaction of aptamer with the analyte.

Before the immobilization of the aptamer, there is the modification of the working electrode with suitable nanomaterials that support the attachments of the aptamer. Metal nanoparticles are nanomaterials that possess a large surface area and high stability to provide a suitable environment for the high loading of aptamers. However, before the immobilization of the aptamer, the metal nanoparticles need to be modified using the thiolated or aminated agent, which supports the covalent immobilization. Additionally, carbon nanomaterials (CNMs) such as graphene oxide (GO), graphene, reduced graphene oxide (rGO), carbon nanotubes (CNTs), and carbon dots (CDs) and their nanocomposites with metal nanoparticles have been also utilized for the fabrication of biosensors for the detection of cancer biomarkers. The oxygen-containing functionalities such as carboxylic acid, epoxy, hydroxy of GO, rGO, and CDs provide suitable binding sites for the immobilization of aptamers. However, the aptamers bind to the graphene surface via π-π interactions or other non-covalent interactions due to the unavailability of the functional group [46]. For instance, He *et al* developed a fluorescent aptasensor of GO for the detection of the Mucin 1 tumor biomarker. Herein, the Cy5 labeled aptamer was incubated with GO, where the specific aptamers bind on the GO surface via π–π interaction. Due to this π–π interaction, the Cy5 fluorophore close to the GO causes the quenching of fluorescence. When Mucin 1 is captured on the aptamers, they release the Cy5 and restore the fluorescence, which was a measure to estimate the detection limit for Mucin 1 concentration [47]. In another context, Yang *et al* developed an impedimetric aptasensor for the detection of prostate-specific antigen (PSA). Firstly they immobilized the ssDNA on the 3-mercapto-1-propanol functionalized AuNPs. Then, two methods (in-solution and on-chip) have been proposed for aptasensor fabrication and its application. In the on-chip method, the complementary DNA (cDNA) was directly immobilized on the ssDNA through hybridization. However, in the case of the in-solution method the cDNA bound to PSA was hybridized on the ssDNA to quantitatively detect the PSA. It was found that the in-solution strategy was more effective as compared to the on-chip method due to the better binding of antigens on the aptamer. Quantitatively it was found that the proposed aptasensor has a broad detection range with a lower limit of detection (LOD) of 0.25 ng ml^{-1}. The strategy for the DNA-directed immobilization aptamer sensors for PSA detection via on-chip and in-solution methods is illustrated in figures 3.2(A) and (B) [4].

3.2.2 Covalent immobilization method

Apart from the physical adsorption, aptamers can be covalently attached to the electrode surface through covalent bonds. In this bonding, the attachment of the aptamer has been done between the aptamer and cross-linker immobilized on the electrode surface through an amide linkage. For this purpose, several cross-linker agents such as EDC/NHS, N,N'-Dicyclohexylcarbodiimide/4-Dimethylaminopyridine (DCC/DMAP), and glutaraldehyde have frequently been utilized, forming carbodiimide bonds between the amine group of the aptamer and the carboxylic acid of the nanomaterial modified on the electrode surface. The covalent linkage of the aptamer provides a stable environment in the biosensor which enables highly sensitive, reproducible, and reliable results [35, 48–50]. For instance, Yang *et al* prepared an electrochemical aptasensor using GO to detect the alpha-feto protein (AFP). In this

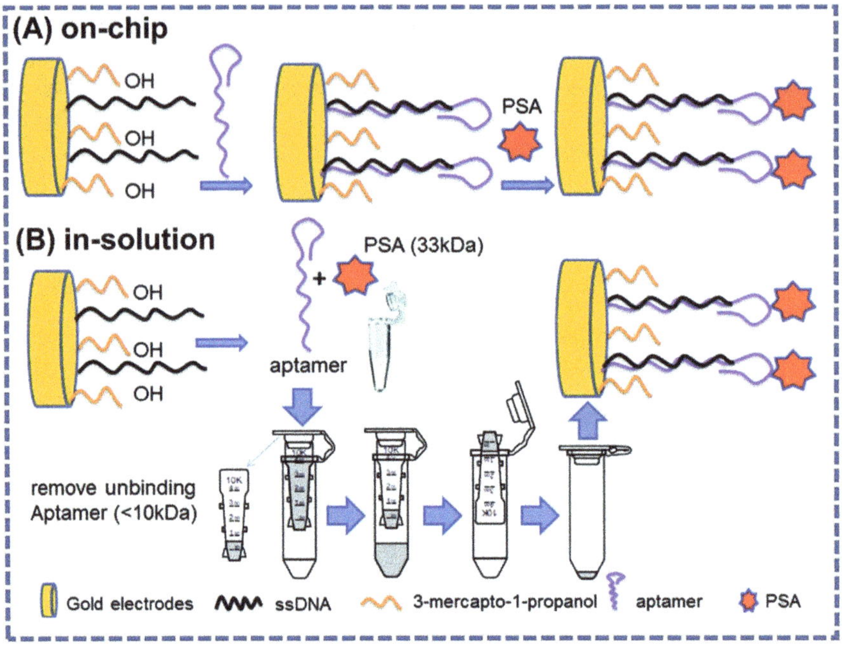

Figure 3.2. Strategy for the DNA-directed immobilization aptamer sensors for PSA detection: (A) on-chip and (B) in-solution method. Reproduced with permission from [4]. Copyright (2015) Royal Society of Chemistry.

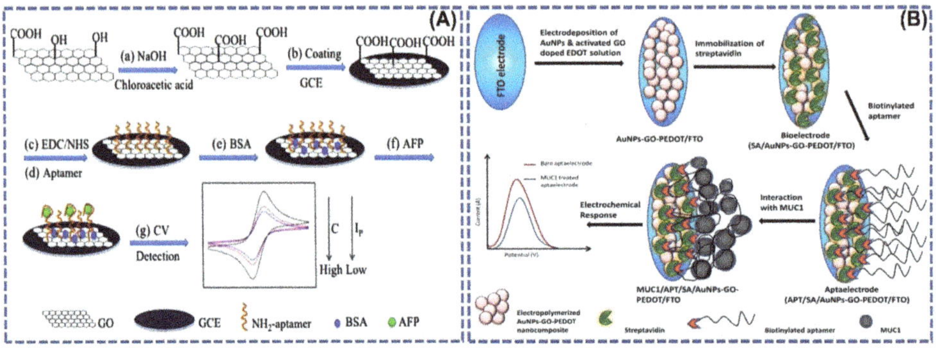

Figure 3.3. Schematic representation of the (A) proposed GO-based electrochemical aptasensor for AFP detection. Reproduced with permission from [51]. Copyright (2018) Elsevier. (B) development of APT/SA/AuNPs-GO-PEDOT coated FTO electrode for breast cancer detection. Reproduced with permission from [52]. Copyright (2018) Elsevier.

electrode fabrication, the aptamer against AFP was immobilized on the GO through a covalent attachment (figure 3.3(A)). Before the modification of the aptamer, the carboxylic acid functional group was activated through the EDC/NHS coupling agent which supports the covalent amide linkage between the amine group on the aptamers and the carboxylic group on the GO. The advantage of the covalent linkage is that it provides high stability of the sensor resulting in improved sensitivity and improved detection performance [51]. In another report, Mucin 1 was detected by Gupta *et al* using the GO-AuNPs-PEDOT nanocomposite-based electrochemical aptasensor. Herein, the authors modified the GO-AuNPs-PEDOT surface through streptavidin, where the amine group of streptavidin covalently binds to the EDC/NHS-activated COOH of GO (figure 3.3(B)). Subsequently, the biotinylated aptamer was immobilized on the modified surface through the streptavidin-biotin interaction. The developed aptasensor exhibits an effective detection platform for Mucin 1 and has a broad detection range and lower detection limit of 3.13 aM–31.25 nM and 0.031 fM, respectively [52].

A graphene-based label-free aptasensor was reported by Feng *et al* for the quantitative determination of HeLa cancer cells. Firstly, the authors modified the graphene using 3,4,9,10-perylene tetracarboxylic acid (PTCA) to generate the carboxylic acid functionalities, as well as to avoid the agglomeration and conjugated π-systems in graphene. After that, the AS1411 aptamers were covalently immobilized on the PTCA-graphene surface through carbodiimide bonding to form a stable aptasensor that detects at the lower concentration of 794 cells ml^{-1} (figure 3.4(A)). The advantage of this aptasensor is that after washing with water for 30 s, it will be reusable, reducing time consumption and the overall cost of the detection [53]. In a recent study, an AuNPs-decorated GO hybrid nanocomposite-based sandwich-type electrochemical aptasensor was reported by Saeed *et al* for the detection of dual biomarkers ERBBC2 and CD24 of breast cancer. Herein, the capture CD24 probe was covalently immobilized on the GO-AuNP-modified GCE in the presence of 6-mercaptohexanol and incubated for 3 h to fabricate an aptasensor. A similar strategy was taken to prepare another aptasensor by immobilization of the capture ERBB-2 probe on the GO-AuNPs/GCE

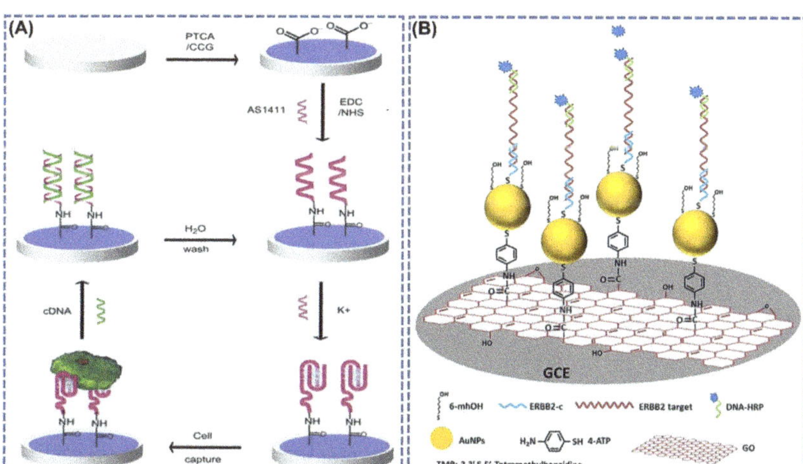

Figure 3.4. Schematic of the (A) reusable aptamer/graphene-based aptasensor. Reproduced with permission from [53]. Copyright (2011) Elsevier. (B) proposed sandwich-type DNA sensor, the prepared AuNPs-GO/GCE showing the hybridization of target DNA with the specific capture probe and HRP-labeled probe. Reproduced with permission from [54]. Copyright (2017) Elsevier.

(figure 3.4(B)). The strategy behind the detection of both biomarkers was that when the capture probe was hybridized with the target molecule on the electrode surface, they further hybridized with the HRP-labeled probe that examine the hybridization of the capture and target probe. On this basis, the change in current is the measure to calculate the detection of both biomarkers [54]. A hybrid nanocomposite of rhodium nanoparticles (RhNPs)-decorated reduced graphene oxide (rGO)-modified electrochemical aptasensor was developed by Sadeghi *et al* for sensitive detection of HER2-ECD in liquid biopsy. Herein, authors prepared the rGO and their nanocomposite with RhNPs via *in situ* electrochemical methods by reduction of GO and rhodium salt. Further, the nanocomposite surface was modified using 3-mercaptopropionic acid (MPA), which provides the carboxylic acid functionalities to support the direct immobilization of biomolecules. With the help of the EDC/NHS coupling agent, the anti-HER2 aptamers were covalently immobilized via amide linkage on the MPA-modified rGO-Rh nanocomposite. The fabricated aptasensor shows high stability, reproducibility, a broad detection range of 10 to 500 ng ml^{-1} and an excellent LOD of 0.667 ng ml^{-1} for HER2-ECD [55].

Shekari *et al* developed an aptasensor of AuNPs-modified three-dimensional graphene hydrogel (AuNPs-3DHG) for simultaneous detection of two breast cancer biomarker carcinoembryonic antigen (CEA) and carbohydrate antigen 15–3 (CA 15–3). Herein, the AuNPs-3DHG was drop cast on GCE and further electrochemically treated in presence of 3-mercaptopropionic acid (MPA) to generate the –COOH functionalities. Subsequently, the two aptamers respective to CEA and CA 15–3 were covalently immobilized using EDC/NHS cross-linker (figure 3.5(A)). The result in the aptasensor displays a remarkable detection limit which provides a promising platform for the detection of two BC biomarkers at the same time [56]. An impedimetric technique integrated microfluidic assay was reported by Nguyen

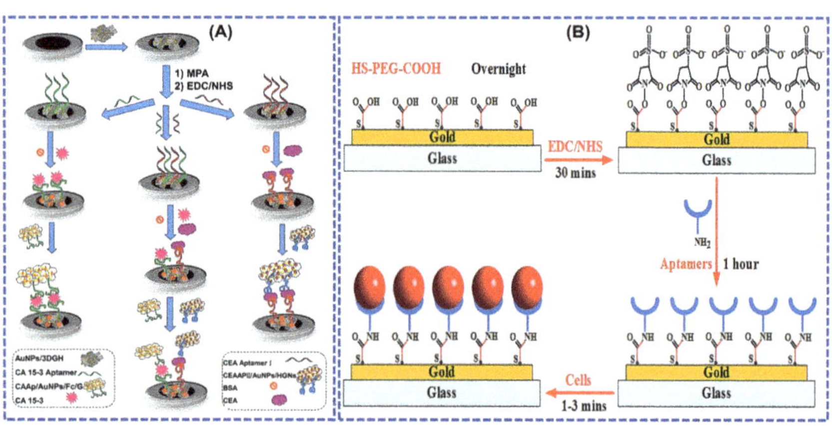

Figure 3.5. Schematic of the (A) several steps involved in the preparation of the sandwich-type aptasensor for the individual and simultaneous detection of CEA and CA 15–3 biomarkers. Reproduced with permission from [56]. Copyright (2021) Elsevier. (B) Aptamer immobilization procedure onto gold substrate for binding of target cells. Reproduced with permission from [57]. Copyright (2018) MDPI.

et al for the detection of A549 cell lines of lung cancer. A simple process was utilized to design the microfluidic assay. Firstly, they constructed the microchannels on the glass substrate and were modified by the thiol-PEG carboxylic acid functionalized AuNPs. Further, the aptamers were immobilized in these channels using the EDC/NHS (figure 3.5(B)). It was observed that when A549 cells are captured on the aptamer the capacitance of the sensors decreases. This decrease in capacitance is shown in the fashion of increasing the A549 cell. On this basis, they calculated that the aptasensor efficiently detected the lowest concentration of 1.5 $\times 10^4$ cells ml^{-1}. However, this further allows hope to develop a sensitive aptasensor that can efficiently detect the tumor cell [57]. In another report, Shekari *et al* detected the CEA through an impedimetric aptasensor based on a mesoporous silica-supported gold electrode. The silica was amine-functionalized, which was cross-linked using one end of the carbonyl group of glutaraldehyde. The other end of the carbonyl reacted with the amine group of the anti-CEA aptamer, which supports the covalent attachment of the aptamer on the electrode. They examined that the resulting aptasensor shows high selectivity, good reproducibility, and long stability [58]. Wan *et al* prepared a substrate for the isolation and detection of epidermal growth factor receptors (EGFR) cancer cells. Herein, the authors modified the glass surface using the PDMS and functionalized it with the APTES to enable the amine functionalities. These amino groups covalently immobilized the DNA on the modified PDMS. Further, the anti-EGFR RNA aptamer hybridized on the DNA surface for 1 h at 37 °C. The prepared aptamer platform selectively captures and isolates human glioblastoma (hGBM) cells against the over-expressed EGFR [59]. Since the covalent immobilization of aptamers is irreversible and provided a stable environment, therefore it overcomes the leaching problem of the biorecognition element of the biosensor. Hence, they significantly improve the sensitivity, shelf-life, and reproducibility of the aptasensor.

3.2.3 Chemisorption

In chemisorption, the aptamers are chemically bonded on the electrode surface, which offers high stability of the aptasensor. To work with this strategy, Dinani *et al* developed an aptasensor of a nanocomposite of Au-rGO with Fe_3O_4 for the detection of miRNA-128 as low as the fM concentration, where the aptamer was functionalized on the AuNPs via thiolated end of the aptamer. In this assay, the Fe_3O_4 nanoparticles remarkably improve the surface area, electron transfer rate, and catalytic activity. Hence, the overall working of the aptasensor is efficiently enhanced [60]. Similarly, Chung *et al* developed an electrochemical aptasensor to detect the KIT cancer biomarker in the serum sample. The sensor was fabricated by the chemisorption of the ferrocene (Fc) labeled aptamer on the surface of thiolated-AuNPs (figure 3.6(A)). Authors found that when KIT binds to the aptamer, they convert to a G-quadruplex structure where the Fc is closer to the electrode surface. However, in the absence of KIT, the Fc is away from the electrode surface. These changes in the position of Fc cause the alteration of the current response which was measured to estimate the KIT concentrations in patients' samples. The developed

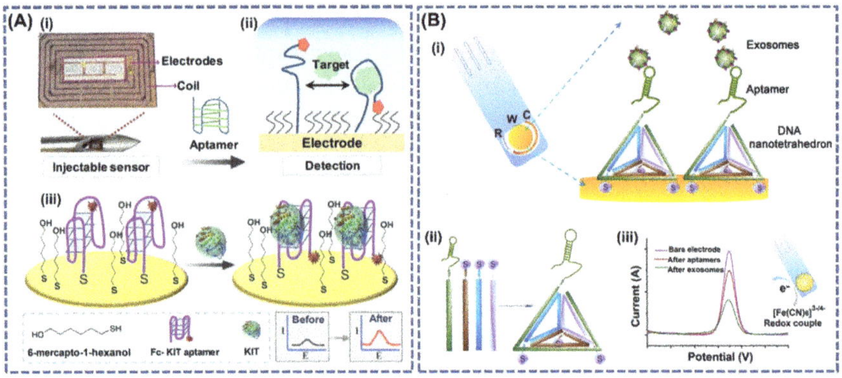

Figure 3.6. (A) Electrochemical KIT Aptasensor. (i) Vision of injectable sensor for continuous, *in vivo* cancer treatment monitoring. (ii) Conformation switching aptasensor concept. (iii) KIT aptamer with a Fc label in its unbound, unfolded state that modulates the Fc tag's position. Reproduced with permission from [61]. Copyright (2021) American Chemical Society. (B) Schematic illustration of the NTH-assisted electrochemical aptasensor. (i) Aptamer-containing NTHs were immobilized via three thiol groups onto the gold electrodes (ii) Facile self-assembly of DNA nanotetrahedra from four single-stranded DNA sequences. (iii) Redox signal changes after aptamer immobilization and after addition of exosomes. Reproduced with permission from [62]. Copyright (2017) American Chemical Society

aptasensor had a low LOD of 1.15 pg ml^{-1} in the detection range of 10 pg ml^{-1} to 100 ng ml^{-1} [61]. In a report by Wang *et al* the DNA nanotetrahedron-based aptasensor was developed for the detection of hepatocellular (HepG2) exosomes. The DNA nanotetrahedron was made from four single-strand sequences (three sequences are tris(2-carboxyethyl)phosphine pretreated 5′-thiolated and one is a 5′-aptamer-conjugated sequence) whereon the LZH8 aptamers chemically immobilized via Au-S bond (figure 3.6(B)). They found that the aptamers are highly oriented through this immobilization strategy, which significantly improves the selectivity for HepG2 exosomes over Hu1545 exosomes. Moreover, high orientation also enhanced the 100-times sensitivity of the aptasensor compared to the single-strand aptamer, where the DNA-based aptasensor exhibits a relatively 21.4% higher current response, which leads to better sensitivity of the aptasensor [62]. Similarly, Ou *et al* reported a dual aptamer-based sandwich electrochemical immunosensor for the detection of HER2 breast cancer biomarkers. Firstly, they prepared the aptamer-modified tetrahedra DNA immobilized on the gold electrode through an Au-S bond to make a probe-1 to capture the HER2. However, HRP functionalized Mn_3O_4/Pd@Pt was used as probe-2 to catalyze the hydroquinone with H_2O_2 after binding with the HER2 on probe-1. The developed immunosensor showed high selectivity and a lower LOD of 0.08 ng ml^{-1}. However, the sensor can hybridize with the cDNA-modified Pd@Pt/HRP making the dendrimer-like structure to further improve the signal responses [63]. In another report, Liu *et al* developed a sandwich assay of a lateral flow aptasensor for the detection of thrombin and platelet-derived growth factor-BB (PDGF-BB) simultaneously in serum samples up to the nanomolar concentrations. Firstly, they functionalized the two specific aptamers on the AuNPs through a thiol bond, which acts as a detection aptamer. Then after the aptamer-AuNPs were immobilized on the conjugate pad they selectively capture the thrombin and PDGF-BB. However, the test and control pad of the assay was modified by the streptavidin-biotinylated aptamer and streptavidin-biotinylated DNA, respectively. When a thrombin and PDGF-BB containing solution was dropped on the sample pad, it flowed on the strip and bound to the aptamers and further flowed on the test strip on the test zone. The red color that appeared on the test and control regions confirms the presence of both proteins. Since the color appears on the test strip, it is easy to analyze and visually interpret the results [64].

3.2.4 Self-assembled monolayer aptamers

A prostate-specific antigen (PSA) was detected by Alnaimi *et al* through the MWCNT-AuNPs nanocomposite-based aptasensor. Herein, the acid pre-treatment of MWCNT was done to generate the –COOH functional group and further modified with the AuNPs and deposited on the electrode surface. Subsequently, the self-assembled thiolated anti-PSA aptamer was covalently immobilized on the electrode through the binding between –COOH of MWCNT and –SH of the aptamer. However, before the immobilization, the denatured aptamer was heated to 95 °C to fold into the complex shape that supports the better binding on the electrode. Therefore, the stable and reproducible aptasensor was produced [65]. Ferreira *et al* developed an aptasensor for the detection of HER2 breast cancer biomarkers. The authors did a similar process to that described above for sensor fabrication. Firstly, aptamers were heated to unfold the structure and then the aptameric DNA solution with the 1-mercapto-6-hexanol (MCH) was placed on SPE where self-assembly of the monolayer (SAM) takes place to immobilize the aptamer. However, the fabrication of ternary SAM was done using a mixture of DNA and 1,6-hexanethiol (HDT). The impedimetric technique was utilized to detect the HER2 in PBS as well as diluted serum samples and also compared the working of both the SAM and ternary SAM aptasensor. The authors concluded that the ternary SAM shows high sensitivity and better detection ability as compared to the SAM. This is because of the ternary SAM which possesses anti-fouling property however, HDT act as a bridge that reduces the remaining space at the protein interaction position causing the increase of resistance of the electrochemical system. Hence, the overall sensitivity for ternary SAM get increases [66]. Recently, a label-free impedimetric aptasensor was reported by Wang *et al* for the quantitative estimation of CEA. The aptasensor was fabricated by the electrodeposition of AuNPs on the graphene SPE. Subsequently, the anti-CEA aptamers were immobilized on the AuNPs surface via the sulfhydryl self-assembly method to form the stable electrode. Since the working electrode was converted into a portable device, therefore they can serve as a point-of-care (PoC) sensing platform to detect the CEA in clinical samples [67]. Similarly, Zhu *et al* detected the SK-BR-3 breast cancer cell in a serum sample using a sandwich electrochemical aptasensor of modified AuNPs. Herein, the AuNPs were modified by self-assembled 2,5-bis(2-thienyl)-1H-pyrrole-1-(p-benzoic acid) (DPB) which supports the covalent immobilization of anti-HER2 detection aptamer for selective capturing of SK-BR-3. However, the capture aptamer was

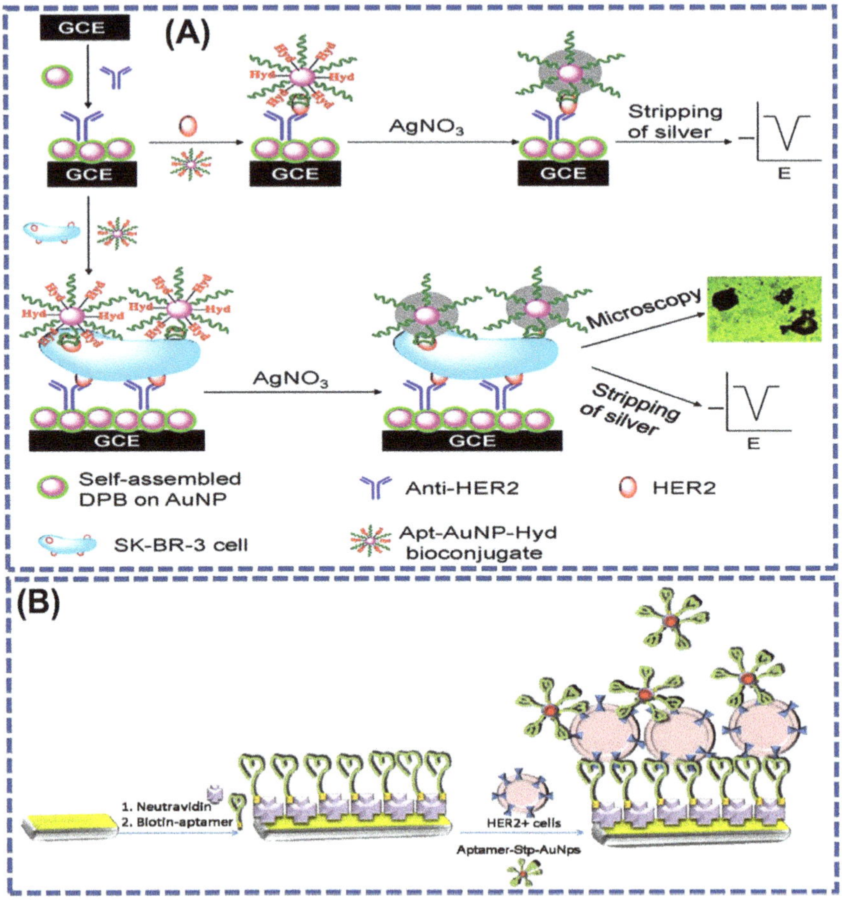

Figure 3.7. (A) Schematic representation of the immunosensor for detection of HER2 protein and HER2-overexpressing SK-BR-3 breast cancer cells. Reproduced with permission from [68]. Copyright (2013) American Chemical Society. (B) The scheme of the preparation of the aptasensor and binding of the cells at the aptamer surface. The gold nanoparticles modified by specific aptamers are used for the amplification of the cell detection. Reproduced with permission from [70]. Copyright (2019) MDPI.

immobilized on the AuNPs via a similar Au-S bond (figure 3.7(A)). When the target SK-BR-3 is captured between the anti-HER2 and aptamer it generates the measurable signal, which was estimated through stripping voltammetry. To further improve the working efficiency of the sensor by increasing signal intensity, they stained the target cell using AgNPs. They observed that the resulting aptasensor exhibits high selectivity and can differentiate between HER2 positive and negative cells [68].

3.2.5 Affinity interaction

Villalonga *et al* developed an electrochemical aptasensor using rGO-AuNPs nanocomposites for the detection of CEA. For the fabrication of the aptasensor, the thiolated and biotinylated anti-CEA aptamers had the hairpin-like structure immobilized on the surface of electrodeposited rGO-AuNPs and were then incubated at room temperature for 1.5 h to prepare the working electrode. When the CEA was captured on the aptamer, they caused the unfolding of the hairpin structure. Subsequently, the biotin binds to the streptavidin-conjugated HRP, which generates the amperometric signals to detect the CEA [69]. In another report, a thickness shear mode acoustics method (TSM) based aptasensor was reported by Poturnayová *et al* for the detection of SK-BR-3 cells up to the detection limit of 550 cells ml^{-1}. They fabricated the sandwich aptasensor on a quartz crystal surface, which was modified by the self-assembly of neutravidin followed by the immobilization of biotin-modified DNA aptamers. However, the second substrate was prepared by the modification of AuNPs using the biotinylated DNA aptamers (figure 3.7(B)). When the SK-BR-3 cell binds between both substrates, the resonant frequency was changed, which was a measure to estimate the detection of SK-BR-3. The proposed aptasensor shows high selectivity that can efficiently distinguish the SK-BR-3 from the MDA-MB-231 cell line [70].

3.3 Summary

Aptamer-based biosensor assay offers selective and sensitive detection of biomolecules including cancer biomarkers. Aptamers are synthesized through different synthetic methods, which results in the specific aptamer being able to selectively capture the target biomarker. Nevertheless, various methods are employed to immobilize the aptamers on the electrode surface to fabricate a biosensor. In the immobilization strategy, the strong attachment, structural orientation and hybridization of aptamers play a significant role in the biosensor, since the weak bonding and structural distortion could be altering the result. However, the sensitivity of the aptasensor can also be affected by the surface chemistry and detection method. In the recent scenario, aptasensors are currently in their nascent stage within the commercial landscape, warranting further research efforts to enhance their potential for broader clinical applications and to provide an improved diagnostic platform that can offer significant benefits.

Conflicts of interest

The authors declare no conflict of interest.

Acknowledgments

The authors sincerely thank Director, CSIR-Advanced Materials and Processes Research Institute (AMPRI) for his interest in this work. Pushpesh Ranjan and Shalu Yadav are grateful to Council of Scientific & Industrial Research (CSIR), India for Senior Research Fellowship. Mohd. Abubakar Sadique is thankful to Department of Science and Technology (DST)-Science and Engineering Research Board (SERB) for Junior Research Fellowship.

References

[1] World Health Organization 2022 Cancer (https://who.int/news-room/fact-sheets/detail/cancer) (Accessed: 20 March 2023)

[2] Chaffer C L and Weinberg R A 2011 A perspective on cancer cell metastasis *Science (1979)* **331** 1559–64

[3] Wu J, Fu Z, Yan F and Ju H 2007 Biomedical and clinical applications of immunoassays and immunosensors for tumor markers *TrAC, Trends Anal. Chem.* **26** 679–88

[4] Yang Z, Kasprzyk-Hordern B, Goggins S, Frost C G and Estrela P 2015 A novel immobilization strategy for electrochemical detection of cancer biomarkers: DNA-directed immobilization of aptamer sensors for sensitive detection of prostate specific antigens *Analyst* **140** 2628–33

[5] MacBeath G and Schreiber S L 2000 Printing proteins as microarrays for high-throughput function determination *Science (1979)* **289** 1760–3

[6] Wilson R, Cossins A R and Spiller D G 2006 Encoded microcarriers for high-throughput multiplexed detection *Angew. Chem. Int. Ed.* **45** 6104–17

[7] Liu J and Lu Y 2006 Fast colorimetric sensing of adenosine and cocaine based on a general sensor design involving aptamers and nanoparticles *Angew. Chem. Int. Ed.* **45** 90–4

[8] Zayats M, Huang Y, Gill R, Ma C and Willner I 2006 Label-free and reagentless aptamer-based sensors for small molecules *J. Am. Chem. Soc.* **128** 13666–7

[9] Wu Y, Zhou H, Wei W, Hua X, Wang L, Zhou Z and Liu S 2012 Signal amplification cytosensor for evaluation of drug-induced cancer cell apoptosis *Anal. Chem.* **84** 1894–9

[10] Yang C J, Jockusch S, Vicens M, Turro N J and Tan W 2005 Light-switching excimer probes for rapid protein monitoring in complex biological fluids *Proc. Natl Acad. Sci.* **102** 17278–83

[11] Wang X-L, Li F, Su Y-H, Sun X, Li X-B, Schluesener H J, Tang F and Xu S-Q 2004 Ultrasensitive detection of protein using an aptamer-based exonuclease protection assay *Anal. Chem.* **76** 5605–10

[12] Sohrabi H, Bolandi N, Hemmati A, Eyvazi S, Ghasemzadeh S, Baradaran B, Oroojalian F, Reza Majidi M, de la Guardia M and Mokhtarzadeh A 2022 State-of-the-art cancer biomarker detection by portable (Bio) sensing technology: a critical review *Microchem. J.* **177** 107248

[13] Fernandez L, Bustos R H, Zapata C, Garcia J, Jauregui E and Ashraf G M 2018 Immunogenicity in protein and peptide based-therapeutics: an overview *Curr. Protein Pept. Sci.* **19** 958–71

[14] Harding F A, Stickler M M, Razo J and DuBridge R 2010 The immunogenicity of humanized and fully human antibodies *MAbs* **2** 256–65

[15] Robertson D L and Joyce G F 1990 Selection *in vitro* of an RNA enzyme that specifically cleaves single-stranded DNA *Nature* **344** 467–8

[16] Tuerk C and Gold L 1990 Systematic evolution of ligands by exponential enrichment: RNA ligands to bacteriophage T4 DNA polymerase *Science (1979)* **249** 505–10

[17] Strehlitz B and Stoltenburg R 2009 Selex and its recent optimizations *Aptamers in Bioanalysis* (Wiley) 31–59

[18] Davis K A, Abrams B, Lin Y and Jayasena S D 1996 Use of a high affinity DNA ligand in flow cytometry *Nucleic Acids Res.* **24** 702–6

[19] Luzi E, Minunni M, Tombelli S and Mascini M 2003 New trends in affinity sensing: aptamers for ligand binding *TrAC, Trends Anal. Chem.* **22** 810–8

[20] Jenison R D, Gill S C, Pardi A and Polisky B 1994 High-resolution molecular discrimination by RNA *Science (1979)* **263** 1425–9

[21] Ellington A D and Szostak J W 1992 Selection *in vitro* of single-stranded DNA molecules that fold into specific ligand-binding structures *Nature* **355** 850–2

[22] Feigon J, Dieckmann T and Smith F W 1996 Aptamer structures from A to ζ *Chem. Biol.* **3** 611–7

[23] Michaud M, Jourdan E, Villet A, Ravel A, Grosset C and Peyrin E 2003 A DNA aptamer as a new target-specific chiral selector for HPLC *J. Am. Chem. Soc.* **125** 8672–9

[24] Mendonsa S D and Bowser M T 2003 In vitro evolution of functional DNA using capillary electrophoresis *J. Am. Chem. Soc.* **126** 20–1

[25] Brody E N and Gold L 2000 Aptamers as therapeutic and diagnostic agents *Rev. Mol. Biotechnol.* **74** 5–13

[26] Willner I and Zayats M 2007 Electronic aptamer-based sensors *Angew. Chem. Int. Ed.* **46** 6408–18

[27] Wilson D S and Szostak J W 1999 In vitro selection of functional nucleic acids *Annu. Rev. Biochem.* **68** 611–47

[28] Shamah S M, Healy J M and Cload S T 2008 Complex target SELEX *Acc. Chem. Res.* **41** 130–8

[29] Tombelli S, Minunni M and Mascini M 2005 Analytical applications of aptamers *Biosens. Bioelectron.* **20** 2424–34

[30] Jolly P, Formisano N and Estrela P 2015 DNA aptamer-based detection of prostate cancer *Chem. Pap.* **69** 77–89

[31] Willner I, Shlyahovsky B, Zayats M and Willner B 2008 DNAzymes for sensing, nanobiotechnology and logic gate applications *Chem. Soc. Rev.* **37** 1153–65

[32] Mairal T, Cengiz Özalp V, Lozano Sánchez P, Mir M, Katakis I and O'Sullivan C K 2008 Aptamers: molecular tools for analytical applications *Anal. Bioanal. Chem.* **390** 989–1007

[33] Lim Y C, Kouzani A Z and Duan W 2010 Aptasensors: a review *J. Biomed. Nanotechnol.* **6** 93–105

[34] Feng C, Dai S and Wang L 2014 Optical aptasensors for quantitative detection of small biomolecules: a review *Biosens. Bioelectron.* **59** 64–74

[35] Jolly P, Batistuti M R, Ustuner S, Mulato M, Arya S K and Estrela P 2017 *Nucleic Acid-Based Aptasensors for Cancer Diagnostics: An Insight into Immobilisation Strategies BT -Next Generation Point-of-care Biomedical Sensors Technologies for Cancer Diagnosis* ed P Chandra, Y N Tan and S P Singh (Springer) pp 205–31

[36] Yang D-K, Chen L-C, Lee M-Y, Hsu C-H and Chen C-S 2014 Selection of aptamers for fluorescent detection of alpha-methylacyl-CoA racemase by single-bead SELEX *Biosens. Bioelectron.* **62** 106–12

[37] Zhou G, Latchoumanin O, Bagdesar M, Hebbard L, Duan W, Liddle C, George J and Qiao L 2017 Aptamer-based therapeutic approaches to target cancer stem cells *Theranostics* **7** 3948–61

[38] Macaya R F, Schultze P, Smith F W, Roe J A and Feigon J 1993 Thrombin-binding DNA aptamer forms a unimolecular quadruplex structure in solution *Proc. Natl Acad. Sci.* **90** 3745–9

[39] Long S B, Long M B, White R R and Sullenger B A 2008 Crystal structure of an RNA aptamer bound to thrombin *RNA* **14** 2504–12

[40] Sakamoto T, Oguro A, Kawai G, Ohtsu T and Nakamura Y 2005 NMR structures of double loops of an RNA aptamer against mammalian initiation factor 4A *Nucleic Acids Res.* **33** 745–54

[41] Cavic B A and Thompson M 2002 Interfacial nucleic acid chemistry studied by acoustic shear wave propagation *Anal. Chim. Acta* **469** 101–13
[42] Centi S, Tombelli S, Minunni M and Mascini M 2007 Aptamer-based detection of plasma proteins by an electrochemical assay coupled to magnetic beads *Anal. Chem.* **79** 1466–73
[43] Hosseinzadeh L and Mazloum-Ardakani M 2020 *Advances in Aptasensor Technology*vol 99 (Elsevier)
[44] Jarczewska M, Górski Ł and Malinowska E 2016 Electrochemical aptamer-based biosensors as potential tools for clinical diagnostics *Anal. Methods* **8** 3861–77
[45] Zhang J and Cao Y 2018 *Aptasensors* (Elsevier)
[46] Sekhon S S, Kaur P, Kim Y H and Sekhon S S 2021 2D graphene oxide–aptamer conjugate materials for cancer diagnosis *NPJ 2D Mater. Appl.* **5** 21
[47] He Y, Lin Y, Tang H and Pang D 2012 A graphene oxide-based fluorescent aptasensor for the turn-on detection of epithelial tumor marker mucin 1 *Nanoscale* **4** 2054–9
[48] Ranjan P, Abubakar Sadique M, Yadav S and Khan R 2022 An electrochemical immunosensor based on gold-graphene oxide nanocomposites with ionic liquid for detecting the breast cancer CD44 biomarker *ACS Appl. Mater. Interfaces* **14** 20802–12
[49] Ranjan P, Yadav S, Abubakar Sadique M, Khan R and Kumar Srivastava A 2022 Ionic liquid-functionalized ZrO_2/reduced graphene oxide nanocomposites for carcinoembryonic antigen electrochemical detection *ACS Appl. Nano Mater.* **5** 14999–5010
[50] de Girolamo A, McKeague M, Pascale M, Cortese M and DeRosa M C 2018 Immobilization of aptamers on substrates *Aptamers for Analytical Applications* (Wiley) pp 85–126
[51] Yang S, Zhang F, Wang Z and Liang Q 2018 A graphene oxide-based label-free electrochemical aptasensor for the detection of alpha-fetoprotein *Biosens. Bioelectron.* **112** 186–92
[52] Gupta P, Bharti A, Kaur N, Singh S and Prabhakar N 2018 An electrochemical aptasensor based on gold nanoparticles and graphene oxide doped poly(3,4-ethylenedioxythiophene) nanocomposite for detection of MUC1 *J. Electroanal. Chem.* **813** 102–8
[53] Feng L, Chen Y, Ren J and Qu X 2011 Biomaterials A graphene functionalized electrochemical aptasensor for selective label-free detection of cancer cells *Biomaterials* **32** 2930–7
[54] Saeed A A, Sánchez J L A, O'Sullivan C K and Abbas M N 2017 DNA biosensors based on gold nanoparticles-modified graphene oxide for the detection of breast cancer biomarkers for early diagnosis *Bioelectrochemistry* **118** 91–9
[55] Sadeghi M, Kashanian S, Naghib S M and Arkan E 2022 A high-performance electrochemical aptasensor based on graphene-decorated rhodium nanoparticles to detect HER2-ECD oncomarker in liquid biopsy *Sci. Rep.* **12** 1–12
[56] Shekari Z, Zare H R and Falahati A 2021 Dual assaying of breast cancer biomarkers by using a sandwich–type electrochemical aptasensor based on a gold nanoparticles–3D graphene hydrogel nanocomposite and redox probes labeled aptamers *Sensors Actuators* B **332** 129515
[57] Nguyen N V, Yang C H, Liu C J, Kuo C H, Wu D C and Jen C P 2018 An aptamer-based capacitive sensing platform 98 for specific detection of lung carcinoma cells in the microfluidic chip *Biosensors (Basel)* **8** 98
[58] Shekari Z, Zare H R and Falahati A 2017 Developing an impedimetric aptasensor for selective label–free detection of CEA as a cancer biomarker based on gold nanoparticles loaded in functionalized mesoporous silica films *J. Electrochem. Soc.* **164** B739–45

[59] Wan Y, Mahmood M A I, Li N, Allen P B, Kim Y T, Bachoo R, Ellington A D and Iqbal S M 2012 Nanotextured substrates with immobilized aptamers for cancer cell isolation and cytology *Cancer* **118** 1145–54

[60] Dinani H S, Pourmadadi M, Yazdian F, Rashedi H, Ebrahimi S A S, Shayeh J S and Ghorbani M 2022 Fabrication of Au/Fe3O4/RGO based aptasensor for measurement of miRNA-128, a biomarker for acute lymphoblastic leukemia (ALL) *Eng. Life Sci.* **22** 519–34

[61] Chung S, Sicklick J K, Ray P and Hall D A 2021 Development of a Soluble KIT electrochemical aptasensor for cancer theranostics *ACS Sens.* **6** 1971–9

[62] Wang S *et al* 2017 Aptasensor with expanded nucleotide using DNA nanotetrahedra for electrochemical detection of cancerous exosomes *ACS Nano* **11** 3943–9

[63] Ou D, Sun D, Lin X, Liang Z, Zhong Y and Chen Z 2019 A dual-aptamer-based biosensor for specific detection of breast cancer biomarker HER2 via flower-like nanozymes and DNA nanostructures *J. Mater. Chem.* B **7** 3661–9

[64] Liu G, Gurung A S and Qiu W 2019 Lateral flow aptasensor for simultaneous detection of platelet-derived growth factor-BB (PDGF-BB) and thrombin *Molecules* **24** 756

[65] Alnaimi A, Al-Hamry A, Makableh Y, Adiraju A and Kanoun O 2022 Gold Nanoparticles-MWCNT based aptasensor for early diagnosis of prostate cancer *Biosensors (Basel)* **12** 1130

[66] Ferreira D C, Batistuti M R, Bachour B and Mulato M 2021 Aptasensor based on screen-printed electrode for breast cancer detection in undiluted human serum *Bioelectrochemistry* **137** 107586

[67] Wang Y, Chen L, Xuan T, Wang J and Wang X 2021 Label-free electrochemical impedance spectroscopy aptasensor for ultrasensitive detection of lung cancer biomarker carcinoembryonic antigen *Front. Chem.* **9** 721008

[68] Zhu Y, Chandra P and Shim Y B 2013 Ultrasensitive and selective electrochemical diagnosis of breast cancer based on a hydrazine-Au nanoparticle-aptamer bioconjugate *Anal. Chem.* **85** 1058–64

[69] Villalonga A, Vegas B, Paniagua G, Eguílaz M, Mayol B, Parrado C, Rivas G, Díez P and Villalonga R 2020 Amperometric aptasensor for carcinoembryonic antigen based on a reduced graphene oxide/gold nanoparticles modified electrode *J. Electroanal. Chem.* **877** 114511

[70] Poturnayová A, Dzubinová L, Buríková M, Bízik J and Hianik T 2019 Detection of breast cancer cells using acoustics aptasensor specific to HER2 receptors *Biosensors (Basel)* **9** 72

[71] Malecka K, Mikuła E and Ferapontova E E 2021 Design strategies for electrochemical aptasensors for cancer diagnostic devices *Sensors* **21** 736

Chapter 4

Rapid detection of circulating cancer cells point-of-care diagnostic using aptasensors

Shagun Gupta, Surbhi Sharma, Deepak Kala and Ankur Kaushal

Diagnosis and treatment of cancer relies on the early detection of circulating tumor cells present in the blood sample through simple and affordable methods. Current detection methods require high expertise in addition to knowledge and understanding of the equipment. A portable and cost-effective tool can be provided for point-of-care screening of these cells for the users to appropriately examine their health conditions. As biosensors are highly sensitive and selective analytical tools that provide a real-time and rapid detection with high accuracy, they can be exploited for detection purposes. Aptamer-based biosensors have also been proven to be an efficient technique with higher sensitivity and specificity. This book chapter summarizes various aptamer-based sensors for the detection of circulating tumor cells.

4.1 Introduction

Followed by the cardiovascular diseases, cancer is the second leading cause responsible for human deaths across the world. It is a non-communicable disease caused due to abnormal cell growth by mutation of human genes affecting the neighboring tissues or organs [1]. Performing an earlier cancer diagnosis is paramount. India has reported approximately 851 678 deaths due to cancer in 2020 including all age groups [2]. The primary indicators for tumor metastasis and diagnosis are the circulating cancer cells, which are challenging to detect precisely as they exist at extremely low levels in peripheral blood [3]. During the growth and formation of the primary tumor, cells are shed and circulate through the blood stream, are heterogeneous and can be detected via different physical and biological technologies [4]. Nowadays biosensors are playing an important role in the diagnostics. The biosensors used as an analytical device are known for precise detection of the target with minute concentration, and uses the recognition,

doi:10.1088/978-0-7503-5012-9ch4

transduction, and amplification principle. Biomolecular recognition takes place upon interaction of the analyte and recognition element producing a measurable signal which is amplified through a transducer [5]. So, in the development of sensors, aptamers have displayed high proficiency in the diagnosis due to their specific binding affinity to respective target biomarkers. Different aptamers like AS1411, Sgc8, VEGF165, and SYL3C TD05 have applications in the detection and capture of different cancer biomarkers and are chemically modified using chemical tags (quenchers, fluorescence probes, nanoparticles, electrochemical standards or enzymes) [6]. Contemporary advances in using aptasensors have been reported for the detection of various cancer cell types and their number or concentration. In comparison, other conventional methods are time consuming, expensive and require a skilled technician with good knowledge of the instruments. This chapter includes the various aptasensor platforms used in circulating tumor cell detection based on various optical and electrochemical techniques as a point-of-care analysis with rapid, cost-effective, accurate and real-time results.

4.1.1 Circulating tumor cells

Malignant tumors have the ability to turn metastatic and emerge with motility and invasiveness. When a single unit or cluster of cancer cells attains the ability to split from the primary tumor and relocate into the surrounding tissue, entering the blood circulation or lymphoid system, the metastatic trait of the tumor becomes apparent [7].

Escaping from their primary microenvironment, the circulating tumor cells (CTCs) might be challenged by the immunologic defense of the host. Even though the rate of released tumor cells is unknown in the patients, experimental models indicate that millions of tumor cells are continuously dispersed, though only very few may reach a far-off organ, persist in a dormant state or invade the immune system and grow into a metastatic tumor [7].

Various origins of cancer-derived materials, like circulating tumor cells or DNA and exosomes, are offered by peripheral blood, which may reflect the characteristics of the primary tumor. Hence, metastatic accumulates and liquid biopsies are ideally relevant to provide an assessment of the tumor [8]. Tumor cells can be used as real-time markers for the prediction of cancer progression and survival of the patient at an early stage as a higher number of CTCs decreases the time to relapse and increases risk of metastasis (table 4.1) [9]. The enrichment of these cells includes technologies depending on the properties that distinguish circulating cancer cells from the adjoining hematopoietic cells, including physical (size, charge, density deformability) and biological (invasion capacity, surface protein expression and viability) properties. Cytokines IL-6 and IL-8, which are derived from the tumor, act as attractants of CTCs and the actin cytoskeleton component fascin-1 and MMP1/ collagenase-1 helps CTCs to infiltrate into the mammary tumor [10]. Table 4.1 shows the various biomarkers related to different cancer types. Platforms for CTC detection must be rapid, repeatable, reliable, and cost-effective [11]. These platforms have advantages like higher sensitivity and specificity; biosensing platforms have

Table 4.1. Various cancer types and their biomarkers [12].

Type of cancer	Biomarker
Prostate cancer	PSA, PAP
Breast cancer	CA15-3. CA125, CA27,29, BRCA1, BRCA2, MUC-1, CEA, NY-BR-1, ING-1
Testicular cancer	alpha-fetoprotein, β-human chorionic gonadotropin, CAGE-1, ESO-1
Ovarian cancer	Cancer Antigen 125, alpha-fetoprotein, hCG, tumor antigen p53, CEA
Colon and pancreatic cancer	CEA, CA19-9, CA24-2, p53
Lung cancer	New York esophageal squamous cell carcinoma-1, CEA, CA19-9, squamous cell carcinoma, CYFRA21-1, NSE
Melanoma	Tyrosinase, New York esophageal squamous cell carcinoma-1
Liver cancer	AFP, CEA
Gastric carcinoma	CA72-4, CEA, CA19-9
Esophageal carcinoma	SCC
Trophoblastic	SCC, Hcg
Bladder cancer	BAT, FDP, HA-HAse, BLCA-4, CYFRA 21-1

been used for CTC detection and aptamers have been used as a promising affinity recognition ligand.

4.2 Aptasensors for the rapid detection of CTCs

Many studies have been performed regarding construction of aptamer-based optical and electrochemical biosensors for detection of the low level of tumor markers. They are released from circulating tumor cells, exosomes and apoptotic tumor cells in the blood and various body fluids on account of their broad potential as a diagnostic probe [13]. They were first explained in 1990 as a pristine class of receptor molecules. Aptamers are RNA oligonucleotides or single-stranded, short DNA bound to the targets with high affinity and selectivity while a three-dimensional interaction is assisted by an *in vitro* method of screening called SELEX (Systematic Evolution of Ligands by Exponential enrichment) [14]. The characteristics of aptamers that make them an ideal recognition element for biosensors include target binding affinity and specificity, their potential to bind to a broad range of targets, high purity and lower cost. They can be effortlessly modified with varying chemical tags (fluorescence probes, nanoparticles and electrochemical indicators) [15, 16]. Several aptamers against cancer biomarkers have been selected by SELEX including carcinoembryonic antigen, prostrate-specific antigen, platelet-procured growth factor, α-fetoprotein, and vascular endothelial growth factor (VEGF) [12]. Aptamer-based optical and electrochemical analytical tools have widely been invented and scrutinized as a diagnostic aid (figure 4.1).

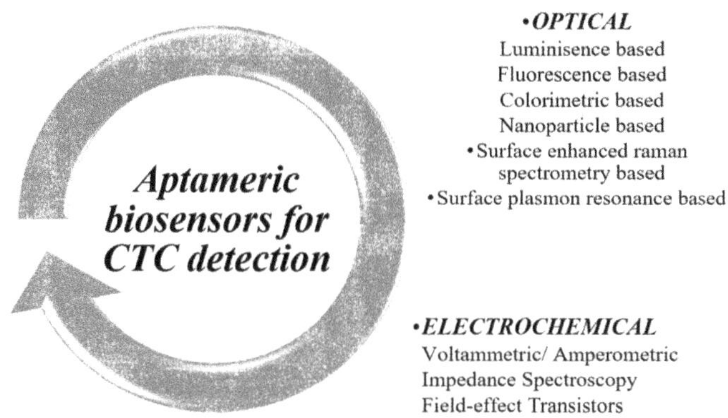

Figure 4.1. Types of optical aptasensors for circulating tumor cell detection.

4.2.1 Optical aptasensors

Optical aptasensors require a biorecognition element together with several signal transduction elements, and can be stratified on the basis of their light absorption or luminescence alterations resulting from interaction with different analytes [17]. Optical approaches have been extensively manipulated for real-time and direct examination of cancer-related biomolecules because of their of high sensitivity, simple operation, and prompt response, which is beneficial for the diagnosis of cancer [17]. Different types of aptasensors based on their optical properties are listed in figure 4.1 for the detection of CTCs.

4.2.1.1 Fluorescence-based aptasensors for detection of circulating cancer cells

Fluorescence is an optical approach implemented for aptasensors construction known for its high sensitivity, low-cost and operation simplicity [17]. Proposing organic fluorophores within conformationally varying regions of aptamers, the binding of the target is transduced in accordance with the change in the fluorophore's chemical environment, resulting in modulation of fluorescence characteristics such as intensity and anisotropy. Among various immunoassays, immunofluorescence assays are comprehensively used for location and quantitative information of proteins. This information can be collected by anticipating targeted antibody/antigen function with fluorophores (figure 4.2). Fluorescence-based aptasensors have a limitation of high limit of detection (hindered when concentrations are lower than 1 μg ml^{-1}) and low working efficiency compared to other detection techniques [18].

By labeling aptamers with fluorescent dyes, fluorescent probes can also be constructed. A microfluidic assay using fluorescence-labeled dye and a labeled aptamer cocktail for identification of circulating tumor cells was established by Zhao *et al* (2016), which demonstrated the synergistic effect with enhanced and differential capturing of circulating cancer cells for patients with non-small cell lung cancer (NSCLC) [19]. Quantum dots (QDs) have also been used as fluorophores for sensing circulating cancer cells. Min *et al* merged QDs' fluorescence with a magnetic bead

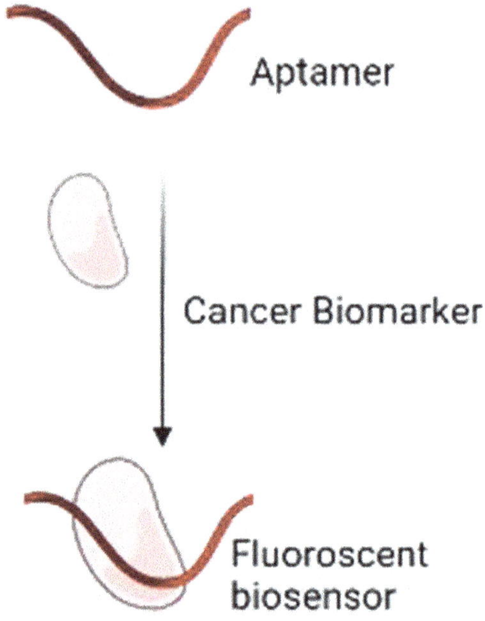

Figure 4.2. Basic principle of aptamer-based fluorescent sensors.

isolation assay and functionalized QDs with anti-epithelial cell adhesion molecule (EpCAM). The isolated QDs fluorescence intensity was measured via plate reader, allowing the quantification of captured circulating cancer cells with 70%–80% efficiency [20]. Zhou *et al* developed aptasensors for α-fetoprotein established on a Foster resonance energy transfer (FRET) where the signal element was the AFP aptamer labeled with CdTe quantum dots that were luminescent and served as a contributor, and the anti-AFP antibody functional AuNP was an upholder with a detection limit of 400 pg ml^{-1} [21]. Another experiment with highly efficient and accurate identification of numerous blood-circulating tumor cell types like breast cancer cells SKBR3, prostate lymph node carcinoma of the prostate and colon cancer cells SW-948 using penetrable graphene oxide membranes and aptamer modifications was developed showing a capture efficiency of about 95%. With each aptamer having a different fluorescent dye (S6, A9 and YJ-1) linked at the 5′ end for multicolor fluorescence imaging [22].

Another work performed by Zhang in 2015 demonstrated the advantages of utilizing a SELEX aptamer (BC-15) in the heterogenic biomarker detection of breast cancer tissue in humans. Human tumor cell line nuclei display a strong affinity towards BC-15 when pigmented with fluorescence and circulating tumor cells isolated from pancreatic cancer patients [23]. Zeng *et al* described a strategy based on a one-step fluorochrome quencher using the anti-CD30 RNA aptamer. When the probe based on the aptamer interacted with the desired target cell, it was assimilated and vehicled towards the lysosome, leading to its degradation, followed by quencher separation from the fluorochrome, thus emitting fluorescence. In a lymphocytic cancer patient's whole blood, circulating tumor cells were successfully identified with a little surrounding signal by the blood cells [24]. Wang *et al* developed a system comprised of an anti-EpCAM aptamer from a nanocatenane pseudo-DNA and HER2-coated MBs were employed for the isolation of CTCs. Ameliorated fluorescence signals for remarkably subtle CTC recognition in the presence of phi29 DNA polymerase, MB, and RCA (rolling circle amplification) primers system was created with an LOD of 10 CTCs ml^{-1} [25]. Cui *et al* described Fe_3O_4, graphene quantum dots, and nanosheets of molybdenum disulfide used to make a 'turn-on' magnetic fluorescent biosensor for devising photoluminescent graphene quantum dots (GQDs), which were escorted by an EpCAM aptamer and a magnetic agent for bio-imaging and embellishment of CTCs with a capture efficiency of 90% [26].

4.2.1.2 Chemiluminescence-based aptasensors for detection of CTCs

There is a phenomenon where light is emitted from a medium or matter that is a result of its previous excitation known as electrochemiluminescence or chemiluminescence. Chemiluminescence is the most sensitive optical approach [27]. Luminescent materials like nanoparticles, quantum dots, fluoropolymers, dyes and porphyrins are standardly trapped or encapsulated into matrices that are designed to accelerate the target interaction with sensing materials (figure 4.3) [28].

Cao *et al* developed a system in which the CTC-specific aptamer AS1411 modified magnetic nanoparticles for efficient identification and isolation from whole blood samples of CTCs was employed. Au@luminol nanoparticle—hybridized chain reaction (HCR) assemblage has multiple MUC1 aptamers particular to Michigan Cancer Foundation-7, and provides a response signal and peculiar recognition element too for sensing [29]. A detection system elicited from a single photon avalanche diode (SPAD) for an efficient chemiluminescence biosensor with high sensitivity and low noise was proposed with a detection efficiency higher than 55% at 425 nm. With the help of the aptamer surface, circulating biomarker proteins correlated with cancerous vascular endothelial growth factor's physiological levels were detected [30].

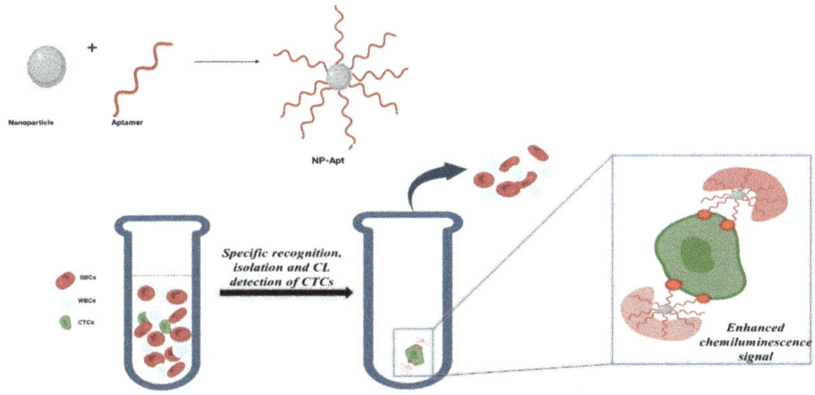

Figure 4.3. Basic principle of chemiluminescence-based aptasensors.

Choi *et al* developed a rapid 1,1′-oxalydiimidazole chemiluminescent-based aptasensor for the detection of prostate-specific antigen (PSA) in human serum, by immobilizing aptamers of DNA combined with a fluorescent dye (Cy3) on magnetic FeO_4 graphene oxide nanoparticles through π–π stacking [31]. Jolly *et al* reported two novel sandwich-based immunoassays for prostate cancer diagnosis where a DNA aptamer was used in place of the primary antibody and made it a aptamer-based ELISA-type chemiluminescence assay in a microfluidic device. By chemiluminescence, an aptamer-antibody assay or aptamer-lectin assay was used to quantify the levels of free PSA and its glycosylation [32]. A versatile and label-free chemiluminescence aptasensor depending on the luminol-hemin/G-quadruplex DNAzyme–H_2O_2 system and g-C_3N_4NS for sensitive detection of various biomarkers like carcinoembryonic antigen (CEA) was developed with a detection limit of 63 pg ml^{-1} [33].

4.2.1.3 Colorimetric aptasensors for detection of CTCs

Colorimetric-based detection is the simplest and most convenient mode of sensing developed for aptasensors. Triggered by the target analytes, the signal of color change can also be seen by the naked eye and the sources for the aptasensors contain nanomaterials (mainly gold), enzymes and enzyme mimics like HRP-mimicking DNAzyme.

A CEA visualization assay was prepared depending upon target-specific recognition, colorimetric reaction and aptamer-based self-catalysis of the DNAzyme. Using a capture probe with one aptamer and another as a reporter probe with G-quadruplex-hemin DNAzyme, the assay ranged from 0.1 to 8.0 ng ml^{-1} determined CEA. Hydrogen peroxide-concilated oxidation of 3,3′,5,5′-tetramethylbenzidine resulted in the change of color and an increase in absorption intensity at 450 nm with the detection limit of 0.06 ng ml^{-1} [34]. Zhu *et al* in 2010 gave a unique technique for detecting human leukemic lymphoblasts (CCRF-CEM). Use of a DNAzyme that is peroxidase-active as the sensing element and an aptamer of the tumor cell was indentured as an element for recognition to produce catalysis-induced colorimetric signals [35]. Li *et al* in 2017 put forward a method to detect circulating tumor DNA aided with the designed hairpin capture probes consisting of two main parts, a specific target recognition element and a signal amplification element. Five oligonucleotides (H1, H2, Initiator, L1 and L2) were designed to contain hairpin structures with stability and scarcely hybridized at room temperature to each other. Introducing an initiator into the apparatus disturbed the stability of H1 and H2 by hybridization of H1 and initiator, which triggered a chain reaction. In the hybridized chain reaction product, the homopyrimidine parts of L1 and L2 cognized the prime groove of homopyrimidine-homopurine dsDNA, thus forming the triplex of DNA by HCR products and asymmetric split G-rich parts of L1 and L2 gathered to form a G-quadruplex structure [36].

A highly sensitive and specific colorimetric method of detection was invented with the help of a capture probe (VEGF aptamer-modified magnetic beads) and signal probe (MUC1 aptamer-modified PtAuNP). The color alterations caused by the chemical action of PtAuNP in the direction of TMB in the presence of H_2O_2 with a detection limit 10 cells ml^{-1} in serum and phosphate buffer solution can be seen by the naked eye [37]. The modified and unmodified nanomaterials for colorimetric aptasensing can also be utilized for analytical purposes. For example, stabilization of unmodified gold nanoparticles can be done using single-stranded DNA and be adsorbed onto the AuNPs' surface. This will prevent the aggregation of AuNPs in salt but upon conversion of the aptamer into target-aptamer complex, it can be released from AuNPs and salt addition will lead to aggregation of AuNPs [38]. Alternately, functionalized AuNPs (Apt-AuNPs) have been used to fabricate colorimetric aptasensors that are sensitive and have a high surface area to volume ratio and are utilized in science of surface functionalization.

4.2.1.4 Surface plasmon resonance-based aptasensors for detection of CTCs

SPR-based assays are broadly used due to label-free and kinetic studies examining properties giving highly sensitive, direct and real-time target detection [39]. This optical sensing platform has the light-guiding structure comprised of a multimode plastic fiber and a planer layer of gold for immobilization of recognition elements as a plasmon guide, as shown in figure 4.4 [40]. It is precisely suited for the confirmation in biological fluids due to the liquid's refractive index range in contact with the platform, which is right for the measurement in an aqueous medium (1.33–1.42) [41].

Hong *et al* demonstrated an *in vitro* sensor biomarker which is set up on an analysis system comprised of immuno-silver nanomarbles and nanoscattering spectrum imaging by employing localized surface plasmon resonance (LSPR). The sensing substrate was fabricated utilizing the nanoparticle through the adsorption method, and highly monodisperse silver nanomarbles (SNMs) with high quality images were also prepared. For the detection of epithelial cell adhesion molecules (EpCAMs), which are manifested on cancer cells, the surface of the silver nano-marble was conjugated with an anti-EpCAM aptamer resulting in sensitive and

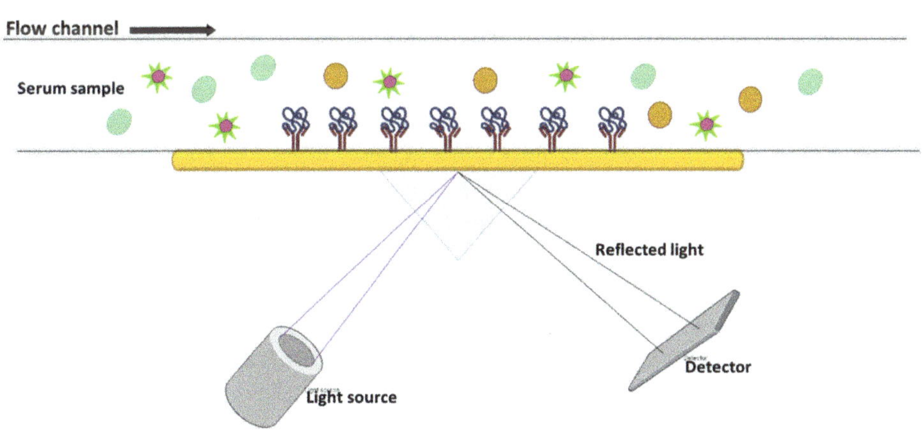

Figure 4.4. Basic principle of SPR-based aptasensors.

efficacious EpCAMs detection at the femto-molar and single-cell level, with a detection limit of 67fM [42]. For spotting vascular endothelial growth factor (VEGF), SPR-based aptasensors were developed. The system consists of two aspects; the functional layer, which allowed the signal transduction based on DNA aptamers, and a light-guiding structure based on plastic optical fibre (POF) with a planar gold layer as a sensing region, suitable for bioreceptor implementation with an LOD of 3nM [43]. Li *et al* described a novel approach for the diagnosis of human breast carcinoma MCF-7 cells using Mucin-1 protein (MUC-1) as a recognition element functionalized on gold nanorods (GNRs) with a detection limit of 100 cells ml^{-1} [44]. In the work of Loyez *et al*, an all-fibre plasmonic aptasensor featuring multiple narrowband resonance in the near-infrared wavelength range was developed for the detection of circulating breast cancer cells. Aptamers against mammaglobin-A were immobilized on the surface of the sensor. A limit of detection of 49 cells ml^{-1} was obtained, while the supplementary use of gold nanoparticles (functionalized) allowed a two-fold amplification of the response of the biosensor, achieving a detection limit of 10 cells ml^{-1} with quick reaction time [45].

Jia *et al* in 2016 described the practice of peptide linker histidine (His)-tagged arginine-glycine-aspartic acid to capture cancer cells when bound to integrin and amplification of the surface plasmon resonance signal after NiO nanoparticle binding via the His-tag on the peptide. The association between the human mucin (MUC-1) and a MUC-selective aptamer-modified gold surface, the breast cancer cells were captured exhibiting a 20-fold enhancement of the SPR signal at the detection limit of 136 cells ml^{-1}. The biosensor was able to discriminate between the breast cancer cell line MCF-7 and normal islet beta cells [46]. Lobry *et al* in 2020 developed an aptasensor using plasmonic-tilted fiber Bragg gratings as a sensing tool for the detection of Human Epidermal Growth Factor Receptor-2 (HER2) protein. A single polarization fiber (allowing inline P-polarization state needed for SPR excitation) was utilized as a biosensor substrate while the separation was based on tracking a spectral feature. Using anti-HER2 antibodies, the amplification of the detection was achieved [47]. A dual gold nanoparticle-assisted signal amplification to enhance the signal was used for detection of exosomes via an SPR-based aptasensor with a detection limit of 5×10^3. Guided hybridization attachment of AuNPs as a result of electronic coupling between gold film and gold nanoparticles and the coupling effect in plasmonic nanostructures helped in amplification of dual nanoparticles. The gold film surface was blocked using 11-Mercaoto-1-undecanol and gold nanoparticle non-specific adsorption onto the surface plasmon resonance chip surface was suppressed, resulting in the resumption of the SPR sensor. The SPR sensor was capable of differentiating exosomes discharged by MCF-7 breast cancer cells and KCF-10A normal breast cells [48].

4.2.1.5 Surface-enhanced Raman scattering based aptasensors for detection of CTCs

Surface-enhanced Raman spectroscopy (SERS) is an ultrasensitive vibrational spectroscopy tool for characterization in the field of nanoscience. It is used in cancer-related applications as a device for the optical imaging and detection due to its strong signal intensity, photostability, biocompatibility and amalgamating ability. The excitation of localized SPR at the nanostructured metal surface with light-activated induction of boosting of Raman scattering via the molecules detected near the metal surface (figure 4.5). This results in a remarkably sensitive plasmon-enhanced spectroscopic mechanism.

Wang *et al* in 2020 proposed a method based on SERS for the determination and examination of exosomes (SKBR3, T84 & LNCaP) using gold shell magnetic nanobeads modified by aptamers as a capturing substrate by cognizing the generic surface protein CD63. Breast cancer, prostate cancer and colorectal cancer patients were investigated for the practical implementation of the method by taking blood samples [49]. A SERS-colorimetric dual mode aptasensor was presented by Li *et al* in 2018 for the detection of human Mucin-1 (MUC1) with a detection limit reaching to 0.1 U ml^{-1}. the combination of these two techniques increased the sensitivity, dependency and efficiency of MUC1 detection. For separating MUC1 from the biological complex medium, the magnetic nanobeads functionalized with the MUC1-specific aptamer as a capturing substrate were used [50].

Liang *et al* in 2018 fabricated aptamer-charged SERS probes for the masking of MCF-7 cancer cells. Two nucleic acid aptamers, AS1411 and MUC1, and two control oligonucleotides, C-con and T-con, were attached on a gold surface for target-specific recognition, successfully targeting MCF-7 cells with a limit of detection up to five cancer cells [51]. An on-chip design incorporating SERS with size-based microfluidic cell isolation for *in situ* profiling of circulating cancer cells was proposed by Zhang *et al* to achieve significant purity and capture rate of CTCs. Use of spectrally orthogonal SERS probes, the phenotypic information of captured circulating cancer cells was obtained using the revised classic least-square algorithm on the basis of their composite spectral signatures. Cells from different human breast

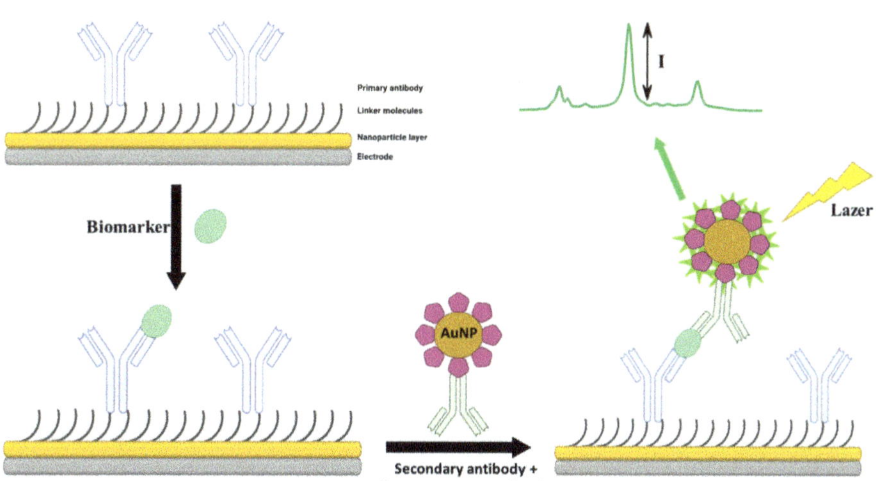

Figure 4.5. Basic principle of SERS-based aptasensors.

cancer subtypes upon combining with categorization algorithm PLS-DA were classified with high sensitivity and selectivity [52].

There are however some drawbacks in detection techniques based on SERS for CTCs, leading to unfulfilled results in detection or characterization of the analyte. An initial enrichment step is required for capturing CTCs in whole blood, making the process more complicated for detection. Multidimensional characterization and accuracy of the analyte cannot be attained by information with regard to vibration from the spectrum alone.

4.2.1.6 Nanomaterial-based optical aptasensors for detection of CTCs (nanoparticles)

In the neoteric CTC detection techniques, nanomaterials such as quantum dots, gold nanoparticles, magnetic nanoparticles, dendrimers/stimuli-responsive polymers and graphenes/graphene oxides have played an influential role [53]. Nanomaterial-based aptasensors can be combined with colorimetric as well as electrochemical detection techniques, making them a promising tool for higher sensitivity and selectivity for the desired tumor cell detection. Nanomaterials, due to their high ratio of surface area to volume, provide more area for elevated interaction between the analyte and the materials, thus enhancing the capturing capacity of the rare cancer cells present in blood serum (figure 4.6) [54].

Wang *et al* investigated in 2017 investigated the proficiency of ssDNA, which enhanced the native peroxidase-like activity of nanosheets made from graphitic carbon nitride (g-C_3N_4) against a CD63 surface biomarker produced by a breast cancer cell line. The catalytic activity of peroxidase accelerated the oxidation of 3,3′,5,5′-tetramethylbenzidine, producing a noticeable blue color [55]. Nima *et al* presented in 2014 a technique for increased molecular and spectral specificity by manipulating silver–gold nanorods for the diagnosis of cancer. Four Raman-active molecules (4MBA, PATP, PNTP, 4MSTP) and four antibodies that are breast cancer marker specific (Anti-EpCAM, Anti-CD44, Anti-Keratin and Anti-IGF-1 Receptor beta) with silver–gold nanorods were functionalized with CD45 leukocyte-specific marker [56]. Iodide-responsive copper–gold nanoparticles in combination with an iodide-catalyzed H_2O_2–3,3,5,5-tetramethylbenzidine reaction system was presented as a colorimetric analysis for the detection of tumor cells. Aptamer Sgc8c was used as a recognition tool for analysis of CCRF-CEM to prepare the probe [57]. Shayesteh *et al* in 2020 developed a colorimetric aptasensor to track down prostate-

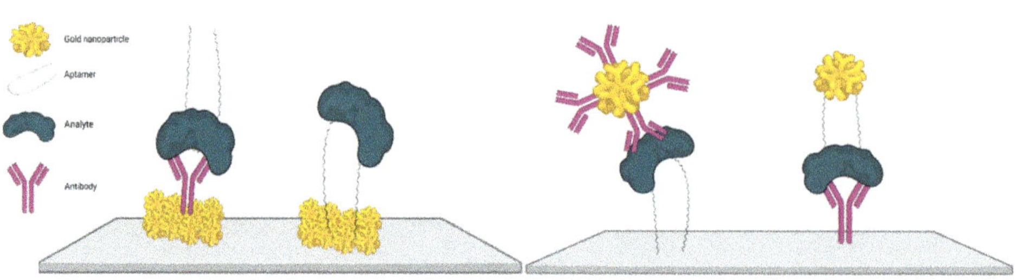

Figure 4.6. Basic principle of nanomaterial-based aptasensors.

specific antigen (PSA). Using aptamer non-thiolated poly-adenine DNA, gold nanoparticles were functionalized via DNA base adsorption. Adsorption on the gold nanoparticles intercepts the aggregation of polyA Apt and poly-diallyl-dimethyl ammonium chloride. The addition of PSA induces the 3D secondary structure formation producing an optical signal accompanied by a color change from red to blue. PSA concentration ranged from 0.1 to 100 ng ml^{-1} with LOD 20 pg ml^{-1} [58].

He *et al* constructed in 2012 an aptasensor for Mucin-1 detection by utilizing graphene oxide as a quencher, suppressing the fluorescence of single-stranded dye-labeled Mucin-1 aptamer. When Mucin-1 is absent, the adsorption results in efficient suppressing of dye-fluorescence. The recovery of fluorescence is due the weaker binding of Mucin-1 and the aptamer complex to graphene oxide. The detection limit obtained was found to be 28 Nm. The sensitivity of the graphene oxide-based aptasensor to Mucin-1 in blood serum and buffer was highly efficient [59]. For the sensitive detection of human hepatocellular carcinoma SMMC-7721 cells, Xie *et al* reported an aptasensor based on fluorescence using graphene oxide due to its quenching ability [60]. A semiconductor quantum dot-based multifunctional nanoparticle probe was developed by Gao *et al* in 2004, designed with encapsulating luminescent quantum dots (tri-n-octylphosphine oxide capped) along with an ABC triblock copolymer (consisting of polybutylacrylate, a polyethylacrylate and a polymethacrylate segment), which was linked to ligands using tumor-targeting and drug delivery [61].

4.3 Electrochemical aptasensors

The electrochemical biosensor comprises an identification system that selectively interacts with the target analyte and turns the interaction into a particular signal [62]. Electrochemical transducers consist of amperometric, conductometric, impedimetric or potentiometric principles [63]. Nucleic acids are also used as recognition elements where a single strand of oligonucleotides is fixed on to the electrode and target DNA hybridization takes place, producing an electrochemical signal. Electrochemical aptasensors provide high compatibility with fabrication technologies, high selectivity and sensitivity, miniaturization with low-cost, rapid, real-time analysis and nominal power requirements [64].

An electrochemical aptasensor based on graphite electrodes, which was modified with gold nanoparticles and also covered with graphitized mesoporous carbon nanoparticles as a sensing platform, was reported for the detection of human prostate-specific antigen with signal amplification of biotin-avidin system. Liu *et al* detected concentrations as low as 0.25 ng ml^{-1} to 200 ng ml^{-1} [65].

The circulating cancer cells are challenging to detect as they are present in minute concentrations. Using aptasensors for the detection of these cells have successfully overcome the barrier by detecting the concentrations as low as 4–5 cells ml^{-1}. The optical and electrochemical analysis, due to their higher specificity, sensitivity and rapid real-time results, has been proven to be compelling and offers a wide range of possibilities for the future development of the aptasensors for on-site CTC detection [66].

4.4 Conclusion

The evolutions in the field of biosensor technology put forward the ability to discover next-generation tools for diagnostics and medicine. Biosensors are entering almost every aspect of healthcare and establishing an utmost input in the development of plenty of products that are incredibly powerful. Aptamers in prognosis are playing a major part in the development of on-site or point-of-care devices for the on-the-spot detection of circulating tumor cells at juvenile stages with more fidelity and less time. These sensors overcome the drawbacks and limitation of the traditional methods. Mingling nanotechnology with biosensors subsequently will revolutionize the field of diagnostics by delivering cost-effective nanodevices that will offer real-time monitoring potential with respect to patient's health and the therapy in accordance to their genetic and diseased profile.

References

[1] Garcion E, Naveilhan P, Berger F and Wion D 2009 Cancer stem cells: beyond Koch's postulates *Cancer Lett.* **278** 3–8

[2] International Agency for Research in Cancer *Global Cancer Observatory* (Accessed: 3 February 2020)

[3] Shen C, Liu S, Li X and Yang M 2019 Electrochemical detection of circulating tumour cells based on DNA generated electrochemical current and rolling circle amplification *Anal. Chem.* **91** 11614–9

[4] Alix-Panabières C, Schwarzenbach H and Pantel K 2012 Circulating tumour cells and circulating tumour DNA *Annu. Rev. Med.* **63** 199–215

[5] Liu D, Wang J, Wu L, Huang Y, Zhang Y, Zhu M, Wang Y, Zhu Z and Yang C 2020 Trends in miniaturized biosensors for point-of-care testing *TrAC, Trends Anal. Chem.* **122** 115701

[6] Kordasht H K and Hasanzadeh M 2020 Aptamer based recognition of cancer cells: recent progress and challenges in bioanalysis *Talanta* **220** 121436

[7] Joosse S A, Gorges T M and Pantel K 2015 Biology, detection, and clinical implications of circulating tumour cells *EMBO Mol. Med.* **7** 1–11

[8] Pantel K and Speicher M R 2016 The biology of circulating tumour cells *Oncogene* **35** 1216–24

[9] Plaks V, Koopman C D and Werb Z 2013 Circulating tumour cells *Science* **341** 1186–8

[10] Sundling K E and Lowe A C 2019 Circulating tumour cells: overview and opportunities in cytology *Adv. Anat. Pathol.* **26** 56–63

[11] Kim M-Y, Oskarsson T, Acharyya S, Nguyen D X, Zhang X H-F, Norton L and Massagué J 2009 Tumour self-seeding by circulating cancer cells *Cell* **139** 1315–26

[12] Kou X, Zhang X, Shao X, Jiang C and Ning L 2020 Recent advances in optical aptasensor technology for amplification strategies in cancer diagnostics *Anal. Bioanal.Chem.* **412** 6691–705

[13] Vandghanooni S, Sanaat Z, Farahzadi R, Eskandani M, Omidian H and Omidi Y 2021 Recent progress in the development of aptasensors for cancer diagnosis: focusing on aptamers against cancer biomarkers *Microchem. J.* **170** 106640

[14] Feng C, Dai S and Wang L 2014 Optical aptasensors for quantitative detection of small biomolecules: a review *Biosens. Bioelectron.* **59** 64–74

[15] Hassan E M, Willmore W G and DeRosa M C 2016 Aptamers: promising tools for the detection of circulating tumour cells *Nucleic. Acid. Ther.* **26** 335–47
[16] Yang K, Hu Y, Dong N, Zhu G, Zhu T and Jiang N 2017 A novel SERS-based magnetic aptasensor for prostate specific antigen assay with high sensitivity *Biosens. Bioelectron.* **94** 286–91
[17] Zahra Q, Ali Khan Q and Luo Z 2021 Advances in optical aptasensors for early detection and diagnosis of various cancer types *Front. Oncol.* **11** 632165
[18] Liu J, Li S and Bhethanabotla V R 2018 Integrating metal-enhanced fluorescence and surface acoustic waves for sensitive and rapid quantification of cancer biomarkers from real matrices *ACS Sens.* **3** 222–9
[19] Zhao L *et al* 2016 Enhanced and differential capture of circulating tumour cells from lung cancer patients by microfluidic assays using aptamer cocktail *Small* **12** 1072–81
[20] Min H, Jo S-M and Kim H-S 2015 Efficient capture and simple quantification of circulating tumour cells using quantum dots and magnetic beads *Small* **11** 2536–42
[21] Zhou L, Ji F, Zhang T, Wang F, Li Y, Yu Z, Jin X and Ruan B 2019 An fluorescent aptasensor for sensitive detection of tumour marker based on the FRET of a sandwich structured QDs-AFP-AuNPs *Talanta* **197** 444–50
[22] Viraka N, Priya B, Kanchanapally R, Pramanik A, Sinha S S, Chavva S R, Hamme A and Ray P C 2015 Aptamer-conjugated graphene oxide membranes for highly efficient capture and accurate identification of multiple types of circulating tumour cells *Bioconjugate Chem.* **26** 235–42
[23] Zhang J, Li S, Liu F, Zhou L, Shao N and Zhao X 2015 SELEX aptamer used as a probe to detect circulating tumour cells in peripheral blood of pancreatic cancer patients *PLoS One* **10** e0121920
[24] Zeng Z, Tung C-H and Zu Y 2014 A cancer cell-activatable aptamer-reporter system for one-step assay of circulating tumour cells *Mol. Ther. Nucleic. Acids* **3** e184
[25] Wang J, Dong H-Y, Zhou Y, Han L-Y, Zhang T, Lin M, Wang C, Xu H, Wu Z-S and Jia L 2018 Immunomagnetic antibody plus aptamer pseudo-DNA nanocatenane followed by rolling circle amplication for highly-sensitive CTC detection *Biosens. Bioelectron.* **122** 239–46
[26] Cui F, Ji J, Sun J, Wang J, Wang H, Zhang Y, Ding H, Lu Y, Xu D and Sun X 2019 A novel magnetic fluorescent biosensor based on graphene quantum dots for rapid, efficient, and sensitive separation and detection of circulating tumour cells *Anal. Bioanal.Chem.* **411** 985–95
[27] Safarpour H, Dehghani S, Nosrati R, Zebardast N, Alibolandi M, Mokhtarzadeh A and Ramezani M 2020 Optical and electrochemical-based nano-aptasensing approaches for the detection of circulating tumour cells (CTCs) *Biosens. Bioelectron.* **148** 111833
[28] Zahra Q U A, Khan Q A and Luo Z 2021 Advances in optical aptasensors for early detection and diagnosis of various cancer types *Front. Oncol.* **11** 632165–5
[29] Cao H-X, Liu P-F, Wang L, Liu Z-J, Ye S-Y and Liang G-X 2020 Nonenzymatic chemiluminescence detection of circulating tumour cells in blood based on Au@ luminol nanoparticles, hybridization chain reaction and magnetic isolation *Sensors Actuators* B **318** 128287
[30] Pasquardini L *et al* 2015 SPAD aptasensor for the detection of circulating protein biomarkers *Biosens. Bioelectron.* **68** 500–7
[31] Choi H K and Lee J H 2013 Role of magnetic Fe_3O_4 graphene oxide in chemiluminescent aptasensors capable of sensing tumour markers in human serum *Anal. Methods* **5** 6964–8

[32] Jolly P, Damborsky P, Madaboosi N, Soares R R G, Chu V, Conde J P, Katrlik J and Estrela P 2016 DNA aptamer-based sandwich microfluidic assays for dual quantification and multi-glycan profiling of cancer biomarkers *Biosens. Bioelectron.* **79** 313–9
[33] Lin K L, Yang T, Zou H Y, Li Y F and Huang C Z 2019 Graphitic C3N4 nanosheet and hemin/G-quadruplex DNAzyme-based label-free chemiluminescence aptasensing for biomarkers *Talanta* **192** 400–6
[34] Zou M and Wang S 2017 An aptamer-based self-catalytic colorimetric assay for carcinoembryonic antigen *Bull. Korean Chem. Soc.* **38** 1143–8
[35] Zhu X, Cao Y, Liang Z and Li G 2010 Aptamer-based and DNAzyme-linked colorimetric detection of cancer cells *Protein Cell* **1** 842–6
[36] Li R, Zou L, Luo Y, Zhang M and Ling L 2017 Ultrasensitive colorimetric detection of circulating tumour DNA using hybridization chain reaction and the pivot of triplex DNA *Sci. Rep.* **7** 1–10
[37] Wang K, Fan D, Liu Y and Wang E 2015 Highly sensitive and specific colorimetric detection of cancer cells via dual-aptamer target binding strategy *Biosens. Bioelectron.* **73** 1–6
[38] Mo T *et al* 2022 Aptamer-based biosensors and application in tumour theranostics *Cancer Sci.* **113** 7
[39] Zahra Q U, Khan Q A and Luo Z 2021 Advances in optical aptasensors for early detection and diagnosis of various cancer types *Front. Oncol.* **11** 632165–5
[40] Cennamo N, Pesavento M, Lunelli L, Vanzetti L, Pederzolli C, Zeni L and Pasquardini L 2015 An easy way to realize SPR aptasensor: a multimode plastic optical fiber platform for cancer biomarkers detection *Talanta* **140** 88–95
[41] Jorgenson R C and Yee S S 1993 A fiber-optic chemical sensor based on surface plasmon resonance *Sensors Actuators* B **12** 213–20
[42] Hong Y, Lee E, Ku M, Suh J-S, Yoon D S and Yang J 2016 Femto-molar detection of cancer marker-protein based on immuno-nanoplasmonics at single-nanoparticle scale *Nanotechnology* **27** 185103
[43] Cennamo N, Pesavento M, Lunelli L, Vanzetti L, Pederzolli C, Zeni L and Pasquardini L 2015 An easy way to realize SPR aptasensor: a multimode plastic optical fiber platform for cancer biomarkers detection *Talanta* **140** 88–95
[44] Li Y, Zhang Y, Zhao M, Zhou Q, Wang L, Wang H, Wang X and Zhan L 2016 A simple aptamer-functionalized gold nanorods based biosensor for the sensitive detection of MCF-7 breast cancer cells *Chem. Commun.* **52** 3959–61
[45] Loyez M, Hassan E M, Lobry M, Liu F, Caucheteur C, Wattiez R, DeRosa M C, Willmore W G and Albert J 2020 Rapid detection of circulating breast cancer cells using a multiresonant optical fiber aptasensor with plasmonic amplification *ACS Sens.* **5** 454–63
[46] Jia S, Li P, Koh K and Chen H 2016 A cytosensor based on NiO nanoparticle-enhanced surface plasmon resonance for detection of the breast cancer cell line MCF-7 *Microchim. Acta* **183** 683–8
[47] Lobry M, Loyez M, Chah K, Hassan E M, Goormaghtigh E, DeRosa M C, Wattiez R and Caucheteur C 2020 HER2 biosensing through SPR-envelope tracking in plasmonic optical fiber gratings *Biomed. Opt. Express* **11** 4862–71
[48] Wang Q, Zou L, Yang X, Liu X, Nie W, Zheng Y, Cheng Q and Wang K 2019 Direct quantification of cancerous exosomes via surface plasmon resonance with dual gold nanoparticle-assisted signal amplification *Biosens. Bioelectron.* **135** 129–36

[49] Li N, Zong S, Zhang Y, Wang Z, Wang Y, Zhu K, Yang K, Wang Z, Chen B and Cui Y 2020 A SERS-colorimetric dual-mode aptasensor for the detection of cancer biomarker MUC1 *Anal. Bioanal.Chem.* **412** 5707–18
[50] Wang Z, Zong S, Wang Y, Li N, Li L, Lu J, Wang Z, Chen B and Cui Y 2018 Screening and multiple detection of cancer exosomes using an SERS-based method *Nanoscale* **10** 9053–62
[51] Liang D, Jin Q, Yan N, Feng J, Wang J and Tang X 2018 SERS nanoprobes in biologically Raman silent region for tumour cell imaging and *in vivo* tumour spectral detection in mice *Advanced Biosystems* **2** 1800100
[52] Zhang Y, Wang Z, Wu L, Zong S, Yun B and Cui Y 2018 Combining multiplex SERS nanovectors and multivariate analysis for *in situ* profiling of circulating tumour cell phenotype using a microfluidic chip *Small* **14** 1704433
[53] Myung J H, Tam K A, Park S-J, Cha A and Hong S 2016 Recent advances in nano-technology-based detection and separation of circulating tumour cells *Wiley Interdiscip. Rev. Nanomed. Nanobiotechnol.* **8** 223–39
[54] Wang Y-M, Liu J-W, Adkins G B, Shen W, Trinh M P, Duan L-Y, Jiang J-H and Zhong W 2017 Enhancement of the intrinsic peroxidase-like activity of graphitic carbon nitride nanosheets by ssDNAs and its application for detection of exosomes *Anal. Chem.* **89** 12327–33
[55] Li W, Wang H, Zhao Z, Gao H, Liu C, Zhu L, Wang C and Yang Y 2019 Emerging nanotechnologies for liquid biopsy: The detection of circulating tumour cells and extracellular vesicles *Adv. Mater.* **31** 1805344
[56] Nima Z A *et al* 2014 Circulating tumour cell identification by functionalized silver-gold nanorods with multicolor, super-enhanced SERS and photothermal resonances *Sci. Rep.* **4** 1–8
[57] Ye X, Shi H, He X, Wang K, He D, Yan L, Xu F, Lei Y, Tang J and Yu Y 2015 Iodide-responsive Cu–Au nanoparticle-based colorimetric platform for ultrasensitive detection of target cancer cells *Anal. Chem.* **87** 7141–7
[58] Shayesteh O H and Ghavami R 2020 A novel label-free colorimetric aptasensor for sensitive determination of PSA biomarker using gold nanoparticles and a cationic polymer in human serum *Spectrochim. Acta* A **226** 117644
[59] He Y, Lin Y, Tang H and Pang D 2012 A graphene oxide-based fluorescent aptasensor for the turn-on detection of epithelial tumour marker mucin 1 *Nanoscale* **4** 2054–9
[60] Xie Q, Tan Y, Guo Q, Wang K, Yuan B, Wan J and Zhao X 2014 A fluorescent aptasensor for sensitive detection of human hepatocellular carcinoma SMMC-7721 cells based on graphene oxide *Anal. Methods* **6** 6809–14
[61] Gao X, Cui Y, Levenson R M, Chung L W K and Nie S 2004 *In vivo* cancer targeting and imaging with semiconductor quantum dots *Nat. Biotechnol.* **22** 969–76
[62] Zhang Z, Li Q, Du X and Liu M 2020 Application of electrochemical biosensors in tumour cell detection *Thorac. Cancer* **11** 840–50
[63] Sassolas A, Blum L J and Leca-Bouvier B D 2009 Electrochemical aptasensors *Electroanalysis* **21** 1237–50
[64] Hianik T and Wang J 2009 Electrochemical aptasensors—recent achievements and perspectives *Electroanalysis* **21** 1223–35
[65] Liu B, Lu L, Hua E, Jiang S and Xie G 2012 Detection of the human prostate-specific antigen using an aptasensor with gold nanoparticles encapsulated by graphitized mesoporous carbon *Microchim. Acta* **178** 163–70

[66] Wang J, Dong H Y, Zhou Y, Han L Y, Zhang T, Lin M, Wang C, Xu H, Wu Z S and Jia L 2018 Immunomagnetic antibody plus aptamer pseudo-DNA nanocatenane followed by rolling circle amplication for highly-sensitive CTC detection *Biosens. Bioelectron.* **122** 239–46

Chapter 5

Aptamer-based bioassays using proteins/biomarkers: a critical role of cancer point-of-care testing

Pushpesh Ranjan, Lal Singh Banjara, Shalu Yadav, Mohd Abubakar Sadique, Raju Khan and Rudramani Tiwari

Aptamer-based biosensors have been widely utilized for the diagnostic and therapeutic of cancer biomarkers due to their superior characteristics. They show high sensitivity, selectivity, stability, and flexibility, hence potentially employed as point-of-care testing (POCT). Moreover, the chemical modifications and flexible conformations make them suitable probes for the fabrication of high-throughput aptasensors. In this chapter, we have discussed the various nanomaterial-based electrochemical, optical, lateral flow, and microfluidic aptasensors that have been utilized for the rapid and real-time POCT of cancer biomarkers in patients' samples for diagnostic application.

5.1 Introduction

Aptamers are a class of biomolecules that possess high affinity and specificity for selective target molecules, similar to antibodies. They have shown great potential in various areas such as sensing, biosensing, drug discovery, and therapeutics. One of the most promising applications of aptamers is their use in the development of bioassays for the detection and quantification of different diseases, including cancer. Cancer is one of the leading causes of death worldwide, and early detection is crucial for improving patient outcomes [1, 2]. Aptamer-based bioassays offer several advantages over traditional diagnostic methods, such as immunoassays for cancer detection. The high specificity and sensitivity of aptamers towards target molecules enables the development of highly sensitive and specific diagnostic tests that can detect cancer at an early stage. Apart from high specificity and sensitivity,

doi:10.1088/978-0-7503-5012-9ch5

aptamer-based bioassays also offer a rapid turnaround time, often in less than an hour, making them ideal for point-of-care testing (POCT). Additionally, aptamer-based bioassays can be cost-effective as the cost of producing aptamers is relatively low compared to other diagnostic methods [3, 4].

Cancer POCT has emerged as a promising approach for the early detection of cancer and improving patient outcomes. Aptamer-based bioassays offer several advantages over traditional POCT methods, allowing for early and accurate diagnosis of the disease, monitoring of disease progression or treatment response, and personalized therapy. Numerous studies have been conducted to explore the use of aptamer-based bioassays for POCT of cancer [5, 6]. For instance, one study developed an aptamer-based bioassay for the detection of prostate-specific antigen (PSA), a prostate cancer biomarker. The assay was able to detect PSA at concentrations in the fg ml^{-1} or lower, which is much lower than the clinical threshold for prostate cancer diagnosis [7, 8]. Another study developed an aptamer-based biosensor for the detection of circulating tumor cells (CTCs) in the blood of cancer patients. The aptamer-based biosensor was able to detect CTCs with high specificity and sensitivity [9–11]. In conclusion, aptamer-based bioassays offer several advantages over traditional diagnostic methods for the detection of cancer, including high specificity and sensitivity, rapid turnaround time, and potential cost-effectiveness. The use of aptamer-based bioassays in POCT of cancer has the potential to improve patient outcomes through early and accurate diagnosis, monitoring of disease progression or treatment response, and personalized therapy.

5.2 Importance of biomarkers on the POCT of cancer

Cancer is the leading health concern worldwide due to its high mortality. Cancer is the second highest death-causing disease after cardiovascular. According to the World Health Organization (WHO) and other cancer research institutions, there are more than 100 types of cancer that cause millions of deaths, and a high socio-economic burden. It is predicted that one in six people dies due to cancer, however, it depends upon cancer type and geographical region [12, 13]. To reduce cancerous death, early diagnosis significantly benefits timely treatment and time-to-time health check-ups, which remarkably improve the survival of cancer patients. Therefore, for the early detection of cancer, a high-sensitivity, selective, and accurate diagnostics platform is highly essential [14, 15]. There are several conventional techniques utilizing molecular analysis through the scanning, or biopsy process. However, they are time-consuming, expensive, and labor-extensive. Additionally, the biomarker-based early diagnosis using biosensors is highly utilized in this scenario which detected the protein/exosome biomarkers associated with cancer. The protein biomarker(s) indicates the existence of either a specific cancer or multiple cancers, which is detected in different types of real patients' samples such as saliva, blood, serum, urine, sweat, and other biological samples. Therefore, protein biomarker detection is highly relevant for knowing the occurrence of cancer disease and its early detection, prognosis, and timely treatment [16, 17].

5.3 Probes in POC aptasensing of cancer

POCT is most commonly utilized for the diagnosis of different diseases such as viruses, glucose, pregnancy, etc, on an extensive level. In the testing device, the working electrode is fabricated using different probes, i.e. aptamer, antibody, enzyme, DNA, RNA, etc, which enable the qualitative, semi-quantitative, or quantitative outcome after the capture of their respective molecules in real patients' samples. Among these, the aptamer and antibodies gain high consideration and are the most commonly used probe for the designing of POCT devices for specific biomarker detection [18, 19]. Antibodies are biological molecules derived from the *in-vivo* condition. However, aptamers are synthetic compounds chemically prepared in *in situ* laboratory conditions. Antibodies are environmentally sensitive and they can easily degrade, which adversely affects the working of the biosensor. However, aptamers show several advantages over antibodies as a probe for working electrode modification. Aptamers are cost-effective, stable, smaller in size, and can rapidly and easily be synthesized and modified. Besides, the enzyme-based probes also gain considerable attention in the analysis of cancerous markers which support the electrocatalysis sandwich assay as a label-biosensors. From that perspective, the aptamer-based diagnostic device is the better alternative for the detection of cancer proteins or surface biomarkers [19, 20]. They can efficiently detect the ultra-low concentration of target molecules in biological fluids. Nevertheless, the flexible conformations of aptamers easily capture the target biomarker and provide highly sensitive and reliable results which advance the development of high-throughput POC devices. Besides that, the aptamer-based biosensor is in the primary stage but continuously growing. However, the aptamer-based POC device can play a significant role in the healthcare diagnostic market and could be a better alternative to antibodies or enzyme-based biosensors. Moreover, the low price of aptamers can also support the fabrication of the cost-effective device, which benefits the diagnosis at a very low price and serve as on-site POCT for healthcare applications [18, 21, 22].

5.4 Aptamer-based POCT of cancer

Based on the various advantages of aptamers, they can be potentially utilized in diagnostic and therapeutic applications. They serve as improved POCT platforms for clinical application for cancer and other disease biomarkers. The early detection of cancer biomarkers using the electrochemical, optical, microfluidic, and lateral flow aptasensor is widely acceptable. In the electrochemical aptasensor, the detection is based on the electrochemical response, i.e. current, potential, and impedance after the binding of the target biomarker on the aptamers which is immobilized on the electrode surface. Similarly, the optical and lateral flow aptasensor outcome the colorimetric or optical signals, which can be easily interpreted and detected even with the naked eye. Moreover, a microfluidic device integrated with an electrochemical or optical technique offers a single and/or multiplex detection platform in a short time (in seconds to minutes). Along with this, the single usability, disposability, and requirement of low-volume of clinical samples (in μl) in microfluidic devices further advances their applicability. In this section, we will discuss the various aptamer-based biosensors which are utilized for the early detection of cancer biomarkers and can serve as a POC detection technique [6, 18, 23, 24]. Some of the aptamer-based detection platforms for cancer biomarkers are listed in table 5.1.

5.5 Electrochemical POC aptasensing

An electrochemical aptasensor is a promising platform for the detection of cancer biomarkers. The detection principle is based on the electrochemical current, impedance, or potential after the binding of the aptamer to the specific biomarker. They have several advantages, such as high sensitivity, lower detection limit, selectivity, rapid analysis, cost-effectiveness, and miniaturized. Therefore, they offer high-throughput POC sensing of a cancer biomarker in clinical samples [25–29]. For instance, Haya *et al* developed an electroactive polymer-based electrochemical aptasensor to detect Mucin-1 (MUC1), a breast cancer biomarker in body fluid. Herein, authors electrochemically grew the two polymers 3,4-ethylenedioxythiophene (EDOT) and 2,2-(3,4-dihydro-2H-thieno[3,4-b][1,4]dioxepine-3,3-diyl)diacetic acid (ProDOT$(COOH)_2$) on the indium tin oxide (ITO) surface. Further, acid functionalization has been introduced to immobilize the selective aptamers against MUC1 through covalent linkage. They examined that the ratio of both polymers remarkably influenced the detection performance, where 1:2 of EDOT/ProDOT $(COOH)_2$ showed high efficiency for this aptasensor. The developed aptasensor has shown superior sensitivity and a very low limit of detection (LOD) of 369 fg ml^{-1}. However, the limited stability of about 6 days may limit their long-term storage for MUC1 detection purposes [30]. In another context, An *et al* reported an electrochemical aptasensor based on copper-catalyzed click chemistry for the quantitative estimation of the CD63 exosome in serum. They immobilized the aptamers on a glassy carbon electrode (GCE) to capture the targeted exosome and 4-oxo-2-nonenal alkyne (alkynyl-4-ONE) compound. Further, the azide-functionalized DNA probes were attached to the exosome by click chemistry for the hybridization process through a DNA hybridization chain reaction (HCR), which was introduced for signal amplification and labeled with horseradish peroxidase (HRP). In this process, the labeled HRP catalyzed the hydrogen peroxide (H_2O_2) and o-phenylenediamine (OPD) into 2,3-diaminophenazine (DAP), where DAP concentration was estimated to quantify the CD63 concentration [31]. Very recently, Zhang *et al* developed a label-free dual signal aptasensor based on an antimonene quantum dot (SB) and zeolitic imidazolate framework-67 (ZIF-67) for sensitive detection of two breast cancer biomarkers, human epidermal growth factor receptor-2 (HER2) and estrogen receptor (ER). In this aptasensor, the aptamers were adsorbed on the ZIF-67 porous surface through the SB. Subsequently, methylene blue (MB) and 3,3′,5,5′-tetramethylbenzidine (TMB) were encapsulated to generate the dual signal responses. When the target HER2 and ER were captured on the aptamers, they were released from the electrode surface where the signal of the TMB and MB appeared. The electrochemical detection shown the aptasensor was highly efficient for both biomarkers' detection. Apart from this, fluorescence is also used to detect HER2 and ER in the

Table 5.1. List of aptamer-based detection platforms for cancer biomarkers.

Nanocomposites	Technique	Biomarker	Cancer	Sample	LOD	References
EDOT/ProDOT$(COOH)_2$	Electrochemical	MUC1	Breast	—	369 fg ml^{-1}	[30]
OPD-DAP	Electrochemical	CD63	—	Serum	96 particles μl^{-1}	[31]
Apt@Sb@MB@ZIF-67/ Apt@Sb@TMB@ZIF-67	Electrochemical/ Fluorescence	HER2 and ER	—	Serum	3.4 fg ml^{-1} (HER2) 6.9 fg ml^{-1} (ER)	[32]
$NaYF_4$:Yb,Er UCNPs@ CdTe nanocrystals	Electrochemical	CEA	—	—	4.8 pg ml^{-1}	[33]
Graphene-PEDOT:PSS	Electrochemical	CEA		Serum,	1.06 ng ml^{-1}	[34]
MoS_2/SiO_2	Electrochemical	PSA, Sarcosine	Prostate	Serum	2.5, 14.4 fg ml^{-1}	[35]
	Electrochemical	MCF-7	Breast	Serum	7 cells ml^{-1}	[10]
PET-Au-graphene	Electrochemical	PDGF-BB	—	—	0.65 pM	[36]
PBA-boronate	Electrochemical	AFP	—	—	0.037 ng ml^{-1}	[37]
Boronic acid	Electrochemical	AFP	—	Serum	0.32 pg ml^{-1}	[38]
CRISPR-Cas12a	Optical	PSA	Prostate	—	4.0 pg ml^{-1}	[41]
DNA-FNP	Optical	PSA, CEA	—	Serum	1.0 pg ml^{-1} (PSA and CEA both)	[42]
$NaYF_4$:Yb,Er	Optical	CA125	Ovarian	Serum	9.0×10^{-3} U ml^{-1}	[46]
AuNPs	LFA	PDGF-BB	Liver	Serum, 10 min	1.0 nM	[47]
Streptavidin-AuNPs	LFA	Osteopontin		Serum, 5 min	10 ng ml^{-1}	[48]
CdTe QDs	Optical	MUC1, A549	Lung	Blood	0.15 fg ml^{-1} 3.0 cells ml^{-1}	[49]
Au nanocluster	Optical	MUC1	—	—	221 cells ml^{-1}	[50]
AuNPs-Au nanosheet	Optical	MCF-7	Breast	Fetal bovine serum	5×10^3 exosomes ml^{-1}	[51]
POCT alkaline-earth sulfide nanodots	Optical	VEGF and sIL-6R	—	—	—	[52]

(*Continued*)

Table 5.1. (*Continued*)

Nanocomposites	Technique	Biomarker	Cancer	Sample	LOD	References
PDA	Optical	CD63	—	10 min	7.7×10^3 particle ml^{-1}	[53]
NH_2-GO-THI-AuNP	Microfluidic	EGFR	—	Serum	5 pg ml^{-1}	[58]
NH_2-G-THI-AuNPs	Microfluidic	CEA	Lung	Serum	10 pg ml^{-1}	[59]
NH_2-G-THI-AuNPs and PB-PEDOT-AuNPs	Microfluidic	CEA NSE	Lung	Serum	2, 10 pg ml^{-1}	[60]
CNT-MXene Nanosheet	Microfluidic	CEA	—	Serum	2.88 pg ml^{-1}	[61]
Au/SPE	Microfluidic	A549 cells	Lung	Serum	14 cells ml^{-1}	[62]
Au film	Microfluidic	PSA	Prostate	—	0.01 ng ml^{-1}	[63]
MoS_2-NS-GNP-CHT	Microfluidic	CD63 and EpCAM mRNA	Breast	Plasma	17 exosomes μl^{-1}	[64]
Magnetic beads	Microfluidic	CD63	Liver	Serum	4.39×10^3 particles ml^{-1}	[65]
Agarose	Microfluidic	CD63, CD81	—	Serum	10^3 exosomes	[66]

supernatant. Dual detection has advantages in that it effectively overcome the experimental interference and can be self-calibrated to give a better sensing platform [32]. Qiu *et al* proposed a ratiometric photoelectrochemical aptasensor based on $NaYF_4$:Yb,Er @CdTe nanocrystals for the detection of carcinoembryonic antigens (CEA) on the 3D-printed portable device. Authors fabricated the two-working electrode on a single strip, where two aptamers, aptamer1 (WE1) and capture DNA (WE2) were covalently immobilized and subsequently capture DNA was hybridized using the CEA aptamer labeled-AuNPs. The signal-off and signal-on occured on WE1 and WE2, respectively, based on exciton–plasmon interactions (WE2) and steric hindrance effect (WE1) phenomena, which quantitatively examined the determination of CEA in the concentration range of 10.0 pg ml^{-1} to 5.0 ng ml^{-1}. The ratiometric determination improves the anti-interference capability and reduces the background instability, which improves the sensitivity and detection limit of the aptasensor. In addition, the 3D printing of the aptasensor may reduce the overall cost of the aptasensor and its portable nature can offer the POC sensing of CEA. The representation of a 3D-printed device, and fabrication and the detection of CEA is shown in figures 5.1(A) and (B) [33].

Successively, Yen *et al* detected the CEA in serum samples on the paper-based impedimetric aptasensor. Herein, they fabricated the aptasensor by modifications of paper strips using graphene and poly (3,4-ethylenedioxythiophene) (PEDOT): poly (styrene sulfonate) (PSS). Successively, the aptamers were immobilized on a modified strip through the cross-linker and detected the CEA as low as 0.45 ng ml^{-1} in PBS and 1.06 ng ml^{-1} in serum, which is lower than the clinical cut-off value. Moreover, they show excellent reproducibility and significant selectivity over other

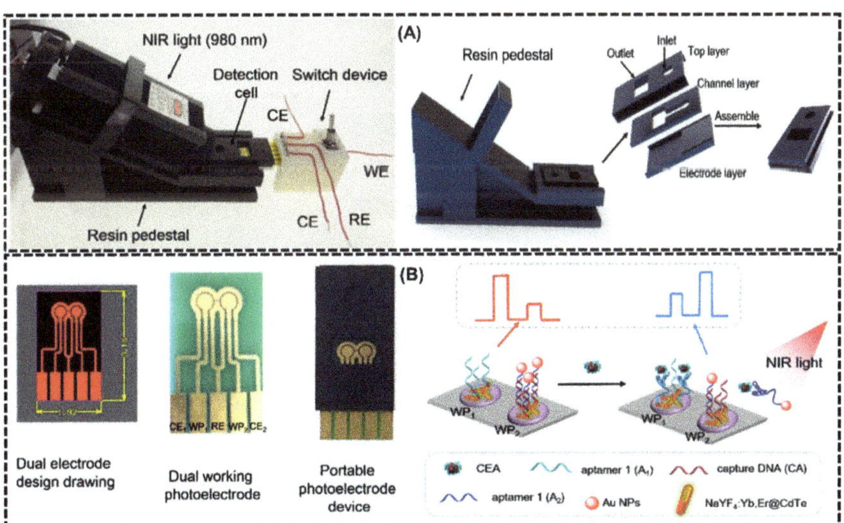

Figure 5.1. (A) Picture of the 3D printing device. (B) Structure of the spatial-resolved dual-working photoelectrodes and fabrication of the upconversion-mediated ratiometric PEC aptasensor for CEA detection. Reproduced with permission from [33]. Copyright (2019) American Chemical Society.

biological interference. Nevertheless, this disposable aptasensor provided the POCT of cancer biomarkers [34]. Very recently, Yan *et al* simultaneously detected the two biomarkers of prostate cancer, i.e. prostate-specific antigen (PSA) and sarcosine in serum. Herein, they utilize the flower-like structured molybdenum disulfide (MoS_2) to immobilize the capture aptamers and DNA hybridization capacity. However, silicon dioxide (SiO_2) was used to tag the DNA probes, which significantly amplified the signal intensity of the sensing system to improve the working efficiency of the aptasensor. In this case, the detection of two biomarkers at the same time can provide high accuracy of the detection result. Moreover, the one-step detection in a very low-volume (~12.0 μl) serum sample can provide a rapid detection platform. Figure 5.2 [35].

In a recent study, Khoshroo *et al* proposed the detection of an MCF-7 breast cancer cell line in serum on a paper-based electrochemical aptasensor with a low LOD of 7 cells ml^{-1}. The aptasensor was developed through the modification of paper strips using AuNPs followed by the immobilization of the aptamers respective to MCF-7. The DPV technique was utilized for the rapid detection of MCF-7 as compared to the control sample, where it provided a cost-effective, and robust

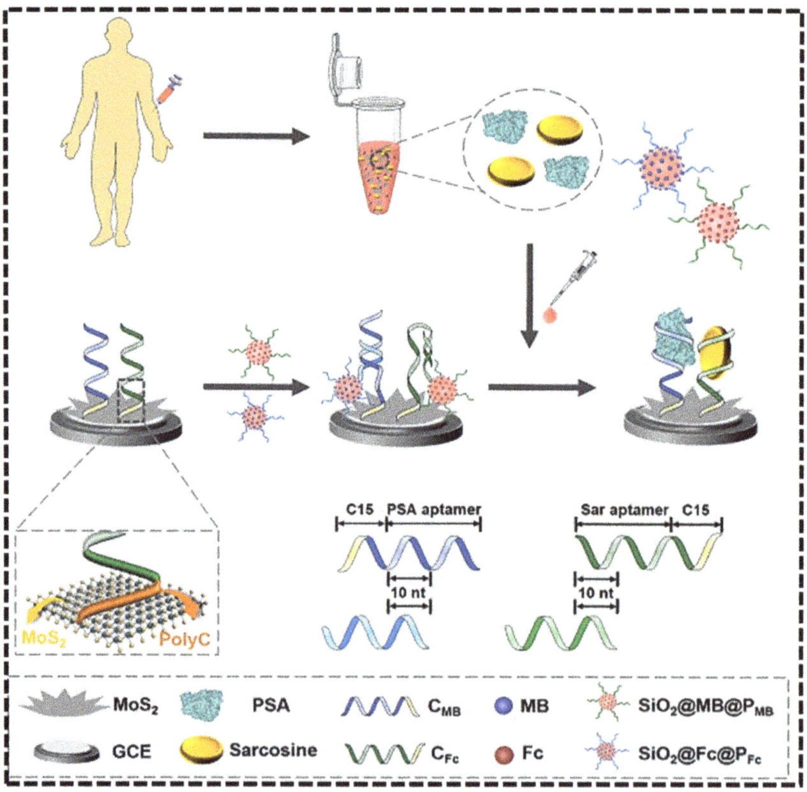

Figure 5.2. MoS_2 nanostructured and nano-signal amplification-based electrochemical aptasensor for sensitive detection of prostate cancer. Reproduced with permission from [35]. Copyright (2022) Elsevier.

sensing platform [10]. In another context, Forouzanfar *et al* developed a graphene-based label-free electrochemical aptasensor for the detection of platelet-derived growth factor-BB (PDGF-BB) cancer biomarkers. They fabricated a gold-covered polyethylene terephthalate (PET/Au) electrode and modified it using the bipolar electrochemically exfoliated graphene sheet (figure 5.3(A)). The electrochemical process allows the exfoliation, reduction, and deposition of graphene sheets simultaneously. The high-conducting graphene sheet improves the conductivity of the assay and also supports the high immobilization of aptamers which remarkably enhances the lower detection efficiency of the aptasensor which achieved the LOD of 0.65 pM [36]. Very recently, Hu *et al* developed a boron-based POC electrochemical aptasensor for the detection of α-fetoprotein (AFP), a glycoprotein in serum. The aptamer captures the AFP, which binds to the ferrocene-labeled phenylboronic acid (PBA) via the cis-diol oligosaccharide sites of AFP (figure 5.3(B)). Since the AFP has a large number of binding sites, therefore the attachment of high ferrocene improves the signal amplification that provides a sensitive detection platform and reduces false results [37]. Similarly, these authors detected the AFP as low as 0.32 pg ml^{-1} through the electrochemical-based atom transfer radical polymerization (ATRP) strategy. In this assay, the DNA aptamers of the electrode were bound to the AFP. Further, the boronic acid conjugated with cis-diol sites of the AFP via ATRP reaction. Subsequently, the ferrocene-labeled long-chain polymer binds to the electrochemically ATRP, where high polymerizations provide a large number of ferrocenes, which effectively improves the detection performance. Since these detection strategies are sensitive, simple, robust, and disposable, they offer cost-effective POC early sensing of AFP and could be also for other cancer biomarkers [38].

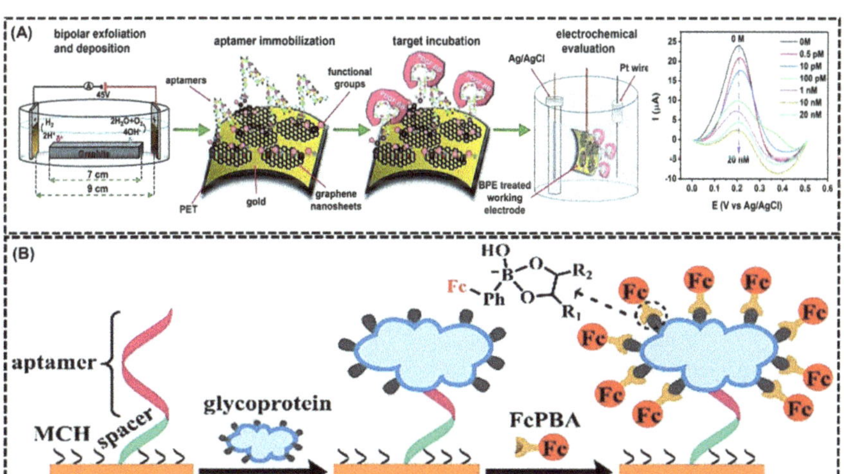

Figure 5.3. Schematic illustration of (A) bipolar exfoliation cell and deposition for development of PET/Au/rGOApt PDGF-BB aptasensors. Reproduced with permission from [36]. Copyright (2021) Royal Society of Chemistry. (B) A boronate affinity-based electrochemical aptasensor for point-of-care glycoprotein detection. Reproduced with permission from [37]. Copyright (2022) American Chemical Society.

5.6 Optical POC aptasensing

Optical aptasensors most often utilize biosensing platforms for the detection of cancer biomarkers due to numerous advantages. The reliable result, simple operation, cost-effectiveness, and straightforward result interpretation make them highly suitable in cancer diagnostics. In this aptasensor, they exhibit optical signals after binding to the cancer marker. However, in many cases, the colorimetric signals offer an easy-to-use detection platform. They can categorize based on transducer such as surface plasmon resonance (SPR), chemiluminescence, surface-enhanced Raman spectroscopy (SERS), colorimetric, and fluorescence [9, 24, 39, 40]. For instance, Taghdisi *et al* developed a DNA and CRISPR-Cas12a-based fluorescent aptasensor platform for quantitative estimation of PSA in serum having an LOD of 4.0 pg ml^{-1}. In this method, the DNA was transformed into the cruciform structure when capturing the PSA and further the pico green (PG) was added as a fluorophore to generate the fluorescent signals. In this sensing strategy, if the PSA was absent in the serum, the CRISPR-Cas12a digested the DNA structure, which caused the lower emission of fluorescence signals in the presence of PG [41]. A multiplex aptasensor platform was reported by Pei *et al* for the simultaneous detection of PSA and CEA. Herein, the authors synthesized the DNA-modified magnetic beads (DNA-MBs) (figure 5.4(A)) and further modified them with aptamers. Subsequently, they reacted with the DNA-functionalized nanoparticles. The modified MBs are separated through the magnet where functionalized nanoparticles are rehybridized, which is examined through microscopic imaging (figure 5.4(B)) [42].

In the optical assay, carbon dots show remarkable properties that are highly suitable for the fabrications of biosensors. The high fluorescence, luminescence activity, photostability, and broad range of absorption and emission wavelengths make them promising materials for optical sensing [43–45]. Zhang and co-workers proposed a luminescence resonance energy transfer (LRET)-based optical

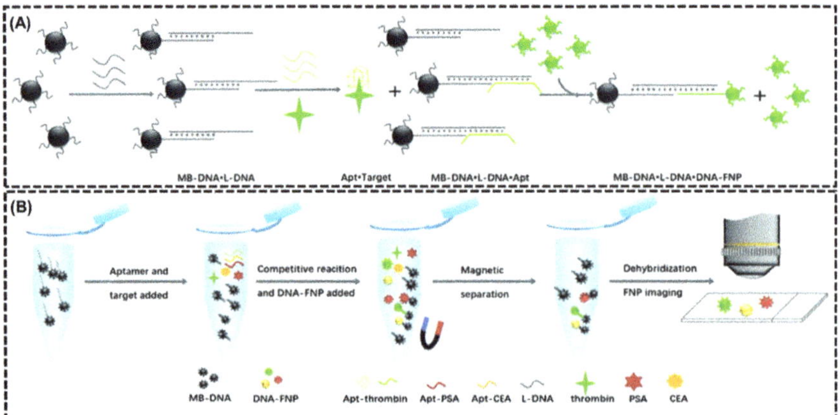

Figure 5.4. Schematic representation of the (A) aptasensor for cancer biomarker detection by fluorescent nanoparticle counting using thrombin as an example and (B) the workflow for multiplexed detection. Reproduced with permission from [42]. Copyright (2020) Royal Society of Chemistry.

aptasensor of carbon dots (CDs) and $NaYF_4$:Yb,Er upconversion nanoparticles (UNPs) for the detection of carbohydrate antigen 125 (CA125), an ovarian cancer biomarker. The probe was designed as CDs attached to the aptamer-functionalized UNPs through π–π interactions, where CDs absorbed the energy from UNPs and quenched their luminescence. However, when the target CA125 binds to this probe, they block the binding of CDs and recover the luminescence intensity. This luminescence recovery is proportional to the concentration of CA125. On this basis, they quantitatively calculated the detection limit of 9.0×10^{-3} U ml^{-1} [46]. Liu *et al* reported a colorimetric visualization-based lateral flow aptasensor (LFA) for the detection of platelet-derived growth factor-BB (PDGF-BB) in serum samples within 10 min. The LFA strips were fabricated by the modification of the conjugate pad by thiolated aptamer-functionalized AuNPs, which serves as a detection aptamer. However, the test zone was modified by biotinylated aptamer which works as a capture aptamer. The target PDGF-BB was captured between these detections and capture aptamers to form a sandwich assembly that exhibited the color band on the LFA strip. Nevertheless, they also detected the thrombin marker on the same strip, which has a significant role in vital functions of the body. Dual-marker detection can provide a better diagnostics platform [47]. Similarly, an LFA was developed by Mukama *et al* for the detection of osteopontin (OPN) cancer biomarkers associated with several cancers such as breast, lung, liver, colon, and oral. The authors fabricated the LFA through the modifications of the nitrocellulose membrane in several steps, in which the conjugation pad of the assay was modified by streptavidin-conjugated AuNPs. Subsequently, the anti-OPN antibody and complementary ssDNA were immobilized on the test and control line (figures 5.5(A) and (B)). In the detection process, the OPN antigen in the clinical sample was captured by a biotinylated aptamer, which was placed on a conjugation pad. Then they capture modified AuNPs and flowed them on the strip. On the test line, they appear as red color signals that were observed by the naked eye and indicated the presence of OPN. Through this assay, the samples were tested within 5 min either through qualitative or semi-quantitative methods. Since the application of LFA is easy and rapid, therefore they can easily observe and sense target molecules (figure 5.5(C)) [48].

Recently, Chen *et al* reported the quantum dot-based fluorescent aptasensing platform for the detection of MUC1 and A549 cells for lung cancer. They utilized enzyme-free amplification techniques such as catalyzed hairpin assembly (CHA) and hybrid chain reaction (HCR) with cadmium telluride (CdTe) QDs in the presence of C–Ag^{+}–C containing a hairpin structure. The fluorescence and visual methods provide the sensitive detection platform for both markers (figure 5.6), which was confirmed by the quantitative estimation in 51 clinical patients' samples. However, this method can easily differentiate the 1.0 fg ml^{-1} (MUC1) and 100 cells ml^{-1} (A549) through visual detection [49].

Very recently, Sanati *et al* detected the MUC1 using the gold nanocluster (GNC)-based aptasensor on a hand-held smartphone device. The fluorescent assay was constructed by the modification of polyurethane (PU) by graphene oxide (GO). After the modification, the surface area increases to 8.45 times and also enhances the

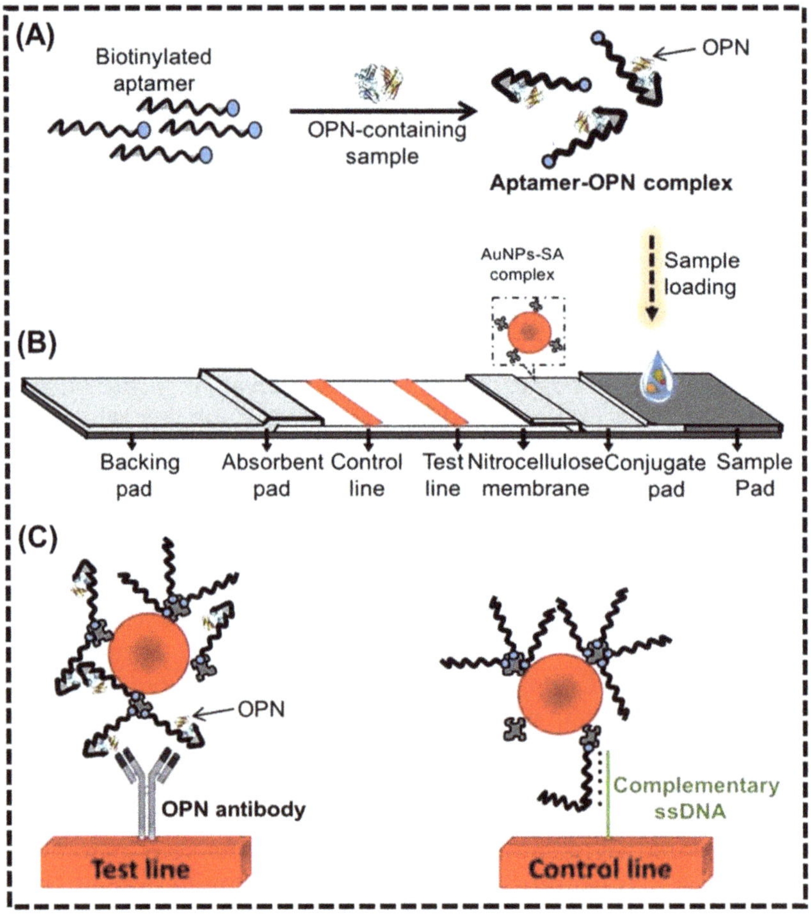

Figure 5.5. Illustrative scheme of the OPN LFA. (A) The synthesis of biotinylated aptamer was incubated with OPN to obtain a stable aptamer-OPN complex and applied to the sample pad. (B) The LFA assembly. (C) The sensing mechanism of the LFA on the test and control line. Reproduced with permission from [48]. Copyright (2020) Elsevier.

wettability. Further, the MUC1-aptamer-modified GNC was immobilized on the modified PU sheet. After capturing the MUC1, they generated the fluorescence signal, which was estimated through the smartphone linear to the red color intensity which detected as low as 221 cells ml^{-1} of MUC1. Apart from this, the high sensitivity and selectivity towards positive-control (MCF-7, and HT-29) and negative-control (HEK293, and L929) cell lines exhibited a reliable platform for MUC1 detection [50]. In another report, an SPR optical aptasensor was utilized by Wang *et al* to detect the MCF-7 exosome of breast cancer in a bovine serum albumin (BSA) solution. The SPR sensor was made by dual nanoparticles (Au film and AuNPs) via hybridization to attach through electronic coupling. Since AuNPs display excellent SPR effects, therefore the sensitive estimation of exosomes was done. They found that this assay exhibits high sensitivity and a 10^4-fold better

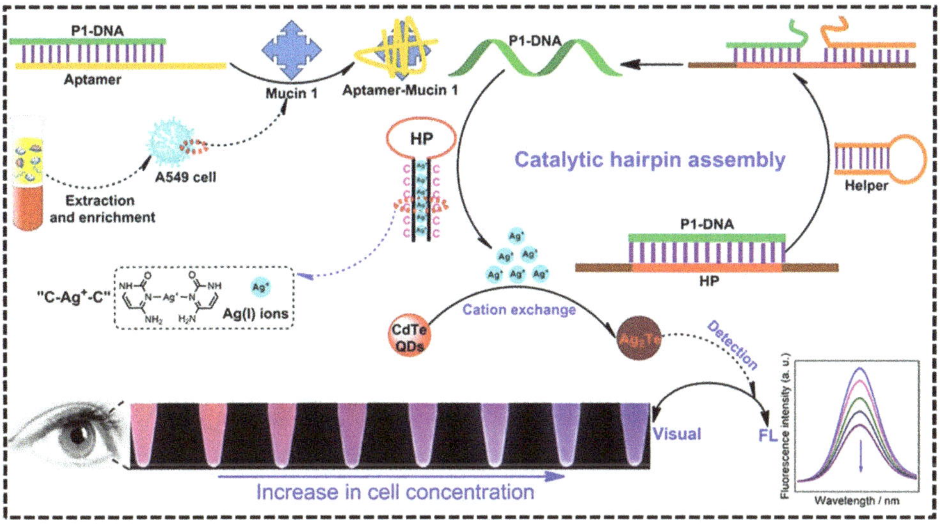

Figure 5.6. Schematic diagram of the homogeneous analysis of MUC1 and A549 cells in lung cancer patients. Reproduced with permission from [49]. Copyright (2021) American Chemical Society.

detection limit compared to the conventional ELISA kit. Moreover, they can easily distinguish the MCF-7 in the presence of the control cell line MCF-10A [51]. Very recently, Zhu *et al* developed a dual-amplification strategy and colorimetric signal monitoring-based POC ratiometric fluorescence assay for the detection of two markers, vascular endothelial growth factor (VEGF) and soluble interleukin-6 receptors (sIL-6R). Herein, authors utilized the ~10 nm size alkaline-earth sulfide nanodots (ASNDs) for sensor fabrication. The ASNDs excited by NIR-light exhibit tuneable emissive light that can successively replace the UV–vis-based fluorescent assay. They found that after capturing VEGF and sIL-6R, the ratiometric signal of red–green–blue (RGB) increases continuously. On this basis, they explained that the quantitative estimation of VEGF and sIL-6R through a ratiometric signal is significantly better than the estimation of a single RGB signal (figures 5.7(A) and (B)) [52].

Xu and co-workers did the detection of CD63 cancer biomarkers on the colorimetric aptasensor platform, which had an LOD of 7.7×10^3 particle ml^{-1}, a 3.5-fold better detection limit than the conventional dot-blot strategy. In this detection system, the latex beads (aldehyde/sulfate latex) captured the target CD63 exosome and surface marker, whereas the aldehyde group captured the exosome via aldimine condensation. Further, the surface marker conjugated to aptamers that are attached to streptavidin modified HRP. The HRP triggered the enzyme catalysis reaction where they polymerize the colorless dopamine (DA) into a colored polydopamine (PDA) in an H_2O_2 solution. In this process, the PDA is deposited on the surface of exosome markers through the sulfhydryl, hydroxy, and amine functionalities of the exosome (figure 5.8). They observed that HRP significantly improved the catalytic reaction. Moreover, the concentration of exosomes also increases the deposition of PDA. As a result, the polymerization

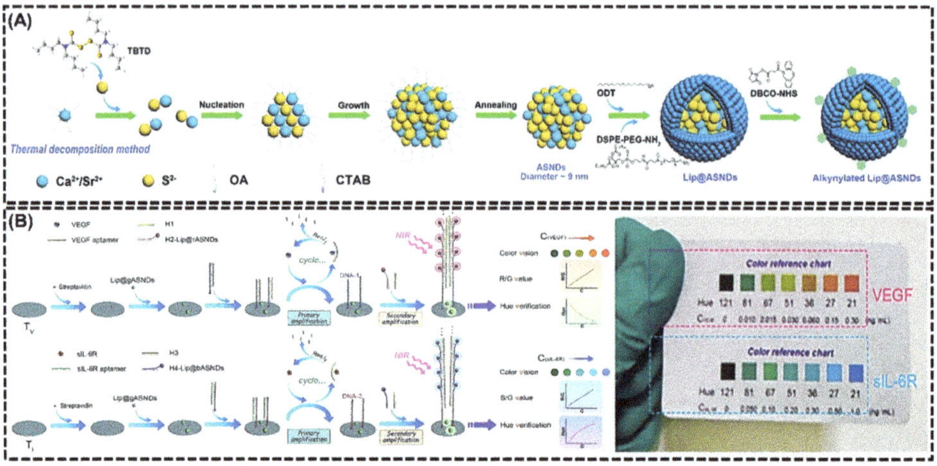

Figure 5.7. Schematic of the synthesis of alkynylated NIR-excited alkaline-earth sulfide nanodots. (B) A dual-amplification strategy and colorimetric signal-based assay for the detection of VEGF and sIL-6R. Reproduced with permission from [52]. Copyright (2022) American Chemical Society.

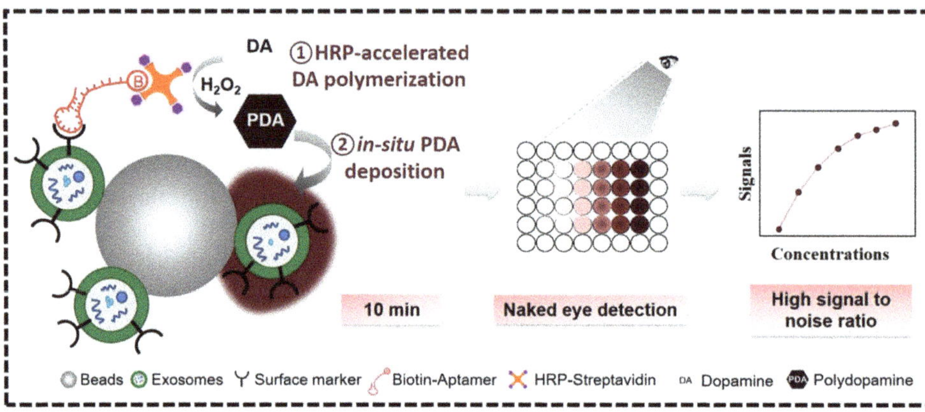

Figure 5.8. Schematic illustration of the proposed aptasensor with HRP-accelerated dopamine polymerization and deposition for exosome detection. Reproduced with permission from [53]. Copyright (2020) Elsevier.

process of DA also increases. Therefore, the high PDA significantly improves the colorimetric signal, which enhances the sensitivity of the assay [53].

5.7 Microfluidics/lab-on-a-chip POC aptasensing

Microfluidic devices deal with the detection of target analytes in a very low volume of sample – in the range of nano- to microliter. They possess several advantages over the conventional POC device, such as rapid detection, a disposable chip, multiplex detection, and the requirement of a single drop of sample. An aptamer-based microfluidic chips consists of micro-channels that functionalize with the target-specific aptamers. They bind to the target biomarker and generate quantifiable signals based on the electrochemical or optical transducer. Additionally, multiple tasks such as sample separation, mixing, and detection have been performed on a single device, which reduces the time-consuming process and offers a better diagnostic platform [54, 55]. In a recent scenario, a paper-based microfluidic device combined with the paper strip offered a reliable POCT platform. They facilitate easy operation and rapid detection, and can enable on-site testing in the resource-limited area [56, 57]. For instance, a paper-based microfluidics aptasensor integrated with an electrochemical technique was fabricated by Wang *et al* to detect the epidermal growth factor receptor (EGFR) in serum. They modified the paper strip using the nanocomposites of amino-functionalized graphene (NH_2-GO), thionine, and AuNPs (NH_2-GO-THI-AuNPs). Subsequently, the anti-EGFR aptamer was immobilized through an Au–S bond to provide the selective capturing of EGFR. The electrochemical examination revealed that the aptasensor has a broad detection limit of 0.05–200 ng ml^{-1}, LOD of 5.0 pg ml^{-1}, and a high sensitivity to the conventional ELISA kit. Since the microfluidic paper strip is disposable, low-cost, user-friendly, and easy to fabricate, they could potentially be utilized for the POCT of cancer biomarkers [58]. Similarly, this group also fabricated a similar aptasensor for the detection of CEA using the NH_2-G-THI-AuNPs nanocomposites synthesized through the hydrothermal method, where GO reduces into rGO. The reduction improves the electrochemical conductivity and forms a stable nanocomposite, which significantly enhances the detection ability of the aptasensor [59]. In addition to this, they also fabricated a similar microfluidic aptasensor for the simultaneous detection of neuron-specific enolase (NSE) and CEA in real patients' samples as shown in figure 5.9. The paper strip was constructed through the screen-printing and wax--printing method, which allows for the filtration and autoinjection of samples. Herein, for the detection of NSE and CEA, they employed the two different nanocomposites, Prussian blue-poly (3,4-ethylenedioxythiophene)-AuNPs (PB-PEDOT-AuNPs) and NH_2-G-THI-AuNPs nanocomposites, to modify the paper strip. Subsequently, the PB-PEDOT-AuNPs were modified by an anti-NSE aptamer while the NH_2-G-THI-AuNPs were modified by the anti-CEA aptamer for selective capture of the respective markers. The electrochemiluminescence (ECL) technique was used to detect the NSE and CEA up to the pg ml^{-1} level with high selectivity and sensitivity [60]. Very recently, Zhao *et al* also detected the CEA using a similar aptasensor of an electrochemical technique-integrated microfluidic device. In this system, the highly conductive MXene and carbon nanotube (MXene-CNT) nanocomposites and anti-CEA aptamers were employed to construct the aptasensor. The high conductivity of both nanomaterials remarkably improves the sensitivity of the assay. However, the quick detection in serum samples, lower LOD, and considerable selectivity advance the assay in POCT of cancer disease [61]. Similarly, Khaksari *et al* developed an electrochemical aptasensor-based microfluidics device for the quantitative detection of A549 lung cancer cells in human serum samples. The microfluidic chip contains a gold-modified screen-printed electrode, which was modified by the covalent immobilization of thiolated-IDA aptamers. The conformational variations of aptamer structure in the real samples offer the sensitive detection of A549 cells. The electrochemical current decreases with the A549 cells, which is

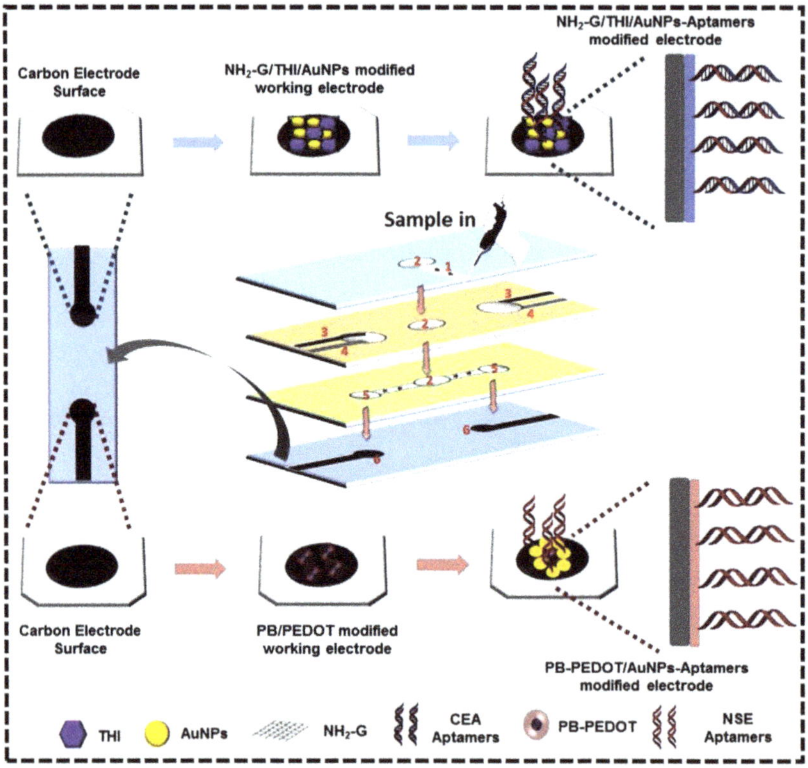

Figure 5.9. Schematics of the fabrication and modification process of the multi-parameter electrochemical paper-based aptasensor. Reproduced with permission from [60]. Copyright (2019) Elsevier.

calculated to quantify the detection limit. Since the whole detection process was automatic and control is programmable, they make the detection processes easier and with high accuracy [62].

Very recently, a SERS-integrated microfluidics assay was developed by Lu *et al* to detect PSA at levels as low as 0.01 ng ml^{-1}. The microfluidic chip was fabricated by the deposition of a gold film on a nanocone on a glass slide covered by PDMS. A SERS active material was conjugated to generate the SERS signal and also provide the binding of the aptamer to form an immunocomplex in the microfluidic chip. The SERS signal offers the highly sensitive detection of PSA. Nevertheless, they also detected thrombin at the same time. The dual detection on a single assay provides better diagnostic results [63]. An exosome against breast cancer was detected by Kashefi-Kheyrabadi *et al* using an electrochemical-based detachable microfluidic assay. They employed the MoS_2-nanosheets-graphene nanoplatelets-chitosan (MoS_2-NS-GNP-CHT) nanocomposites to modify the electrode surface. Subsequently, a layer of AuNPs was deposited through the electroplating method to improve the current responses as well as the stability of the sensor. Further, the respective aptamers were immobilized on the modified sensor surface. For detection, the plasma sample was placed on the 3D-printed housing inlet connected to the microfluidic device, where they capture the exosome on the aptamers and generated the redox signals. On this basis, they detected up to 17 exosomes in a 1 μl sample. The advantage of the assay is that after detection the aptasensor was detached from the housing inlet, the exosomal parts were harvested, and later the RT-PCR was performed for molecular study [64]. In a report by Xu *et al* they detected CD63, an exosome of liver cancer, within 3.5 h on the portable aptasensor of a microfluidic assay combined with the electrochemical technique. On this chip, the isolation and detection were simultaneously taking place, which reduces the time-consuming process. The magnetic bead enables the high-level capturing of CD63, which enhances the sensitivity. However, to further improve the efficiency of the aptasensor, they designed the chip into a Y shape, where there is no need for any surface modifications and allows anisotropic flow for better exosome capturing (figure 5.10(A)). In this process, when the CD63 aptamer was captured on ssDNA they formed a hairpin structure. However, after binding to the CD63 exosome, they formed a G-quadruplex in the presence of hemin by opening the hairpin structure. They promote the electro-catalyzed reaction to generate the electrochemical signals to quantify the CD63 as illustrated in figure 5.10(B) [65]. Similarly, the cancerous exosomes were detected by Qian and co-workers using the agarose-based microfluidic chip. Since the exosome concentrations could be low in real patients' samples, therefore the detection of the exosome is challenging. In this perspective, they applied the catalyzed hairpin assembly (CHA) approach for sensitive detection at very lower concentrations within 2.5 h in the extremely low ~1.0 μl of the clinical

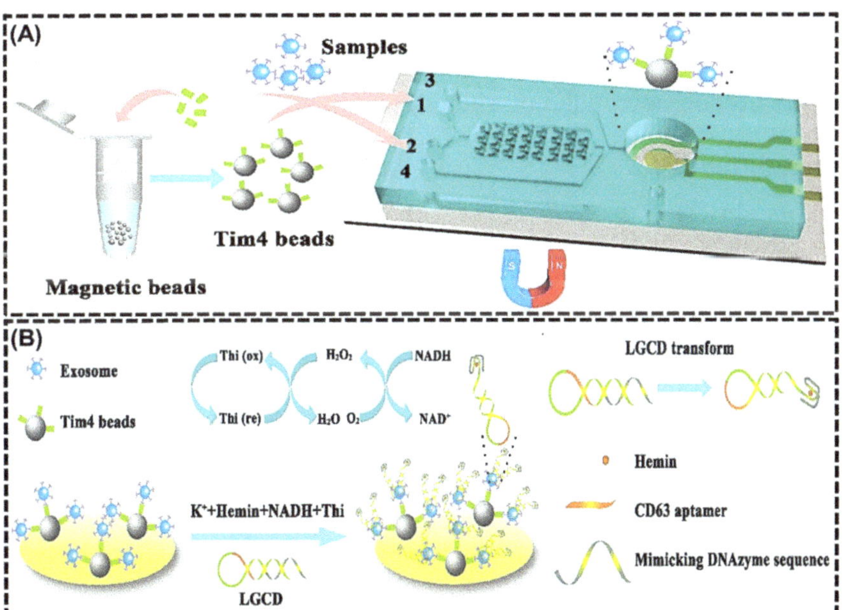

Figure 5.10. Schematic diagram of the (A) ExoPCD-chip which offers integrated exosome isolation and analysis platform. (B) the electrochemical sensor on the surface of the ITO electrode. Reproduced with permission from [65]. Copyright (2018) American Chemical Society.

samples. Nevertheless, the aptasensor displays high selectivity that can distinguish the target exosomes from the healthy ones [66].

5.8 Summary

At the current extent, the aptamer-based biosensor is potentially utilized for the diagnosis of cancer biomarkers. They can serve as an alternative to antibody-based biosensors with superior properties. Antibody-based biosensors offer high sensitivity and selectivity; however, the limited stability of biosensors, time-consuming preparation (several months), and high cost of antibodies limits their application in the fabrication of biosensors on the large scale. On the other side, aptamers possess several advantages over antibodies, such as low cost, ease of synthesis (within a day to a week), and modifications. Apart from this, nanotechnology also plays a significant role in nano-aptasensor fabrication. Different types of nanomaterials, i.e. conductive and fluorescent, offer a suitable surface for the aptamer immobilization to target the selective molecule and emit quantifiable signals based on the transducers [67]. In this scenario, aptasensors are rapidly growing and they could be a better alternative in POC diagnostics. To further technological advancement, the aptasensor can be translated into portable devices and successfully connected to algorithmic devices such as artificial intelligence, machine learning, and the Internet of medical things, which offers superior and rapid diagnostic and smart management of cancer [68–70]. Nevertheless, numerous aptamer-based technologies are translating from laboratory to market, which will be benefitting the home-based detection of cancer [71].

Confliction of interest

The authors declare no conflict of interest.

Acknowledgments

The authors sincerely thank Director, CSIR-Advanced Materials and Processes Research Institute (AMPRI) for his interest in this work. Pushpesh Ranjan and Shalu Yadav are grateful to Council of Scientific & Industrial Research (CSIR), India for Senior Research Fellowship. Mohd. Abubakar Sadique is thankful to Department of Science and Technology (DST)-Science and Engineering Research Board (SERB) for Junior Research Fellowship.

References

[1] Zhou W, Jimmy Huang P J, Ding J and Liu J 2014 Aptamer-based biosensors for biomedical diagnostics *Analyst* **139** 2627–40

[2] Keefe A D, Pai S and Ellington A 2010 Aptamers as therapeutics *Nat. Rev. Drug Discov.* **9** 537–50

[3] Etzioni R, Urban N, Ramsey S, McIntosh M, Schwartz S, Reid B, Radich J, Anderson G and Hartwell L 2003 The case for early detection *Nat. Rev. Cancer* **3** 243–52

[4] Han J, Gao L, Wang J and Wang J 2020 Application and development of aptamer in cancer: from clinical diagnosis to cancer therapy *J Cancer* **11** 6902–15

[5] Mehmood S, Khan A Z, Bilal M, Sohail A and Iqbal H M N 2019 Aptamer-based biosensors: a novel toolkit for early diagnosis of cancer *Mater. Today Chem.* **12** 353–60

[6] Dhiman A, Kalra P, Bansal V, Bruno J G and Sharma T K 2017 Aptamer-based point-of-care diagnostic platforms *Sensors Actuators* B **246** 535–53

[7] Farshchi F and Hasanzadeh M 2020 Nanomaterial based aptasensing of prostate specific antigen (PSA): recent progress and challenges in efficient diagnosis of prostate cancer using biomedicine *Biomed. Pharmacother.* **132** 110878

[8] Hassani S, Salek Maghsoudi A, Rezaei Akmal M, Rahmani S R, Sarihi P, Ganjali M R, Norouzi P and Abdollahi M 2020 A sensitive aptamer-based biosensor for electrochemical quantification of PSA as a specific diagnostic marker of prostate cancer *J. Pharm. Pharm. Sci.* **23** 243–58

[9] Safarpour H, Dehghani S, Nosrati R, Zebardast N, Alibolandi M, Mokhtarzadeh A and Ramezani M 2020 Optical and electrochemical-based nano-aptasensing approaches for the detection of circulating tumor cells (CTCs) *Biosens. Bioelectron.* **148** 111833

[10] Khoshroo A, Fattahi A and Hosseinzadeh L 2022 Development of paper-based aptasensor for circulating tumor cells detection in the breast cancer *J. Electroanal. Chem.* **910** 116182

[11] Zamay A S, Zamay G S, Kolovskaya O S, Zamay T N and Berezovski M V 2017 Aptamer-based methods for detection of circulating tumor cells and their potential for personalized diagnostics *Adv. Exp. Med. Biol.* **994** 67–81

[12] Siegel R L, Miller K D, Wagle N S and Jemal A 2023 Cancer statistics, 2023 *CA Cancer J. Clin.* **73** 17–48

[13] World Health Organization 2022 Cancer (https://who.int/news-room/fact-sheets/detail/cancer) (Accessed: 30 March 2023)

[14] Ranjan P *et al* 2020 Biosensor-based diagnostic approaches for various cellular biomarkers of breast cancer: a comprehensive review *Anal. Biochem.* **610** 113996

[15] Parihar A, Ranjan P, Sanghi S K, Srivastava A K and Khan R 2020 Point-of-care biosensor-based diagnosis of COVID-19 holds promise to combat current and future pandemics *ACS Appl. Bio Mater.* **3** 7326–43

[16] Solhi E and Hasanzadeh M 2020 Critical role of biosensing on the efficient monitoring of cancer proteins/biomarkers using label-free aptamer based bioassay *Biomed. Pharmacother.* **132** 110849

[17] Parihar A, Jain S, Parihar D S, Ranjan P and Khan R 2022 Biomarkers associated with different types of cancer as a potential candidate for early diagnosis of oncological disorders Biosensor *Based Advanced Cancer Diagnosis* (Academic) ch 3 pp 47–57

[18] Gopinath S C B, Lakshmipriya T, Chen Y, Phang W M and Hashim U 2016 Aptamer-based 'point-of-care testing' *Biotechnol. Adv.* **34** 198–208

[19] Citartan M and Tang T H 2019 Recent developments of aptasensors expedient for point-of-care (POC) diagnostics *Talanta* **199** 556–66

[20] Liu L S, Wang F, Ge Y and Lo P K 2020 Recent developments in aptasensors for diagnostic applications *ACS Appl. Mater. Interfaces* **13** 9329–58

[21] Hu X, Zhang D, Zeng Z, Huang L, Lin X and Hong S 2022 Aptamer-based probes for cancer diagnostics and treatment *Life* **12** 1937

[22] Maimaitiyiming Y, Hong D F, Yang C and Naranmandura H 2019 Novel insights into the role of aptamers in the fight against cancer *J. Cancer Res. Clin. Oncol.* **145** 797–810

[23] Varty K, Brien C O and Ignaszak A 2021 Breast cancer aptamers : current sensing targets, available aptamers, and their evaluation for clinical use in diagnostics *Cancers* **13** 3984

[24] Vandghanooni S, Sanaat Z, Farahzadi R, Eskandani M, Omidian H and Omidi Y 2021 Recent progress in the development of aptasensors for cancer diagnosis: focusing on aptamers against cancer biomarkers *Microchem. J.* **170** 106640
[25] Omage J I *et al* 2022 Cancer diagnostics and early detection using electrochemical aptasensors *Micromachines* **13** 1–28
[26] Díaz-Fernández A, Lorenzo-Gómez R, Miranda-Castro R, de-los-Santos-Álvarez N and Lobo-Castañón M J 2020 Electrochemical aptasensors for cancer diagnosis in biological fluids—a review *Anal. Chim. Acta* **1124** 1–19
[27] Ranjan P, Abubakar Sadique M, Yadav S and Khan R 2022 An electrochemical immunosensor based on gold-graphene oxide nanocomposites with ionic liquid for detecting the breast cancer CD44 biomarker *ACS Appl. Mater. Interfaces* **14** 20802–12
[28] Ranjan P, Yadav S, Abubakar Sadique M, Khan R and Kumar Srivastava A 2022 Ionic liquid-functionalized ZrO_2/reduced graphene oxide nanocomposites for carcinoembryonic antigen electrochemical detection *ACS Appl. Nano Mater.* **5** 14999–5010
[29] Ranjan P and Khan R 2022 Electrochemical immunosensor for early detection of β-Amyloid Alzheimer's disease biomarker based on aligned carbon nanotubes gold nanocomposites *Biosensors* **12** 1059
[30] Haya G, Runsewe D O, Otakpor M U, Pohlman G E, Towne A, Betancourt T and Irvin J A 2023 Functionalized thiophene-based aptasensors for the electrochemical detection of Mucin-1 *ACS Appl. Polym. Mater.* **5** 1208–18
[31] An Y, Jin T, Zhu Y, Zhang F and He P 2019 An ultrasensitive electrochemical aptasensor for the determination of tumor exosomes based on click chemistry *Biosens. Bioelectron.* **142** 111503
[32] Zhang Y, Li N, Xu Y, Lu P, Qi N, Yang M, Hou C and Huo D 2022 An ultrasensitive dual-signal aptasensor based on functionalized Sb@ZIF-67 nanocomposites for simultaneously detect multiple biomarkers *Biosens. Bioelectron.* **214** 114508
[33] Qiu Z, Shu J, Liu J and Tang D 2019 Dual-channel photoelectrochemical ratiometric aptasensor with up-converting nanocrystals using spatial-resolved technique on homemade 3D printed device *Anal. Chem.* **91** 1260–8
[34] Yen Y K, Chao C H and Yeh Y S 2020 A graphene-PEDOT:PSS modified paper-based aptasensor for electrochemical impedance spectroscopy detection of tumor marker *Sensors (Switzerland)* **20** 1372
[35] Yan R, Lu N, Han S, Lu Z, Xiao Y, Zhao Z and Zhang M 2022 Simultaneous detection of dual biomarkers using hierarchical MoS_2 nanostructuring and nano-signal amplification-based electrochemical aptasensor toward accurate diagnosis of prostate cancer *Biosens. Bioelectron.* **197** 2022–4
[36] Forouzanfar S, Khakpour I, Alam F, Pala N and Wang C 2021 Novel application of electrochemical bipolar exfoliated graphene for highly sensitive disposable label-free cancer biomarker aptasensors *Nanoscale Adv.* **3** 5948–58
[37] Hu Q *et al* 2022 Boronate affinity-based electrochemical aptasensor for point-of-care glycoprotein detection *Anal. Chem.* **94** 10206–12
[38] Hu Q, Cao X, Li S, Liang Y, Luo Y, Feng W, Han D and Niu L 2022 Electrochemically controlled atom transfer radical polymerization for electrochemical aptasensing of tumor biomarkers *Anal. Chem.* **94** 13516–21
[39] Zahra Q U, Khan Q A and Luo Z 2021 Advances in optical aptasensors for early detection and diagnosis of various cancer types *Front. Oncol* **11** 1–7

[40] Kou X, Zhang X, Shao X, Jiang C and Ning L 2020 Recent advances in optical aptasensor technology for amplification strategies in cancer diagnostics *Anal. Bioanal. Chem.* **412** 6691–705

[41] Taghdisi S M *et al* 2022 A highly sensitive fluorescent aptasensor for detection of prostate specific antigen based on the integration of a DNA structure and CRISPR-Cas12a *Anal. Chim. Acta* **1219** 340031

[42] Pei X, Wu X, Xiong J, Wang G, Tao G, Ma Y and Li N 2020 Competitive aptasensor for the ultrasensitive multiplexed detection of cancer biomarkers by fluorescent nanoparticle counting *Analyst* **145** 3612–9

[43] Yadav S, Sadique M A, Ranjan P, Sathish N and Khan R 2022 Carbon dots for the fabrication of biosensors *Carbon Dots* (IOP Publishing) pp 8–10

[44] Ranjan P, Khan R, Gogoi S, Murali S, Sadique Mohd A, Yadav S and Khan A 2022 Carbon dots—an overview ed R Khan, S Murali and S Gogoi *Carbon Dots in Agricultural Systems* (Academic) ch 1 pp 1–19

[45] Ranjan P, Khan R, Yadav S, Sadique Mohd A, Murali S and Ban M K 2022 Physical and chemical properties of carbon dots ed R Khan, S Murali and S Gogoi *Carbon Dots in Agricultural Systems* (Academic) ch 5 pp 117–33

[46] Zhang X, Wang Y, Deng H, Xiong X, Zhang H, Liang T and Li C 2021 An aptamer biosensor for CA125 quantification in human serum based on upconversion luminescence resonance energy transfer *Microchem. J.* **161** 105761

[47] Liu G, Gurung A S and Qiu W 2019 Lateral flow aptasensor for simultaneous detection of platelet-derived growth factor-BB (PDGF-BB) and thrombin *Molecules* **24** 756

[48] Mukama O, Wu W, Wu J, Lu X, Liu Y, Liu Y, Liu J and Zeng L 2020 A highly sensitive and specific lateral flow aptasensor for the detection of human osteopontin *Talanta* **210** 120624

[49] Chen P *et al* 2021 Homogeneous visual and fluorescence detection of circulating tumor cells in clinical samples via selective recognition reaction and enzyme-free amplification *ACS Nano* **15** 11634–43

[50] Sanati A *et al* 2023 Smartphone-assisted lab-in-a-tube device using gold nanocluster-based aptasensor for detection of MUC1-overexpressed tumor cells *Anal. Chim. Acta* **1252** 341017

[51] Wang Q, Zou L, Yang X, Liu X, Nie W, Zheng Y, Cheng Q and Wang K 2019 Direct quantification of cancerous exosomes via surface plasmon resonance with dual gold nanoparticle-assisted signal amplification *Biosens. Bioelectron.* **135** 129–36

[52] Zhu Y, Wang J, Xie H, Fu C, Zhou J, Liu H, Zeng P and Sun Y 2022 Double signal amplification strategy for dual-analyte fluorescent aptasensors for visualizing cancer biomarker proteins *Anal. Chem.* **94** 10451–61

[53] Xu L, Chopdat R, Li D and Al-Jamal K T 2020 Development of a simple, sensitive and selective colorimetric aptasensor for the detection of cancer-derived exosomes *Biosens. Bioelectron.* **169** 112576

[54] Khan R, Dhand C, Sanghi S K, Salammal S T and Mishra A B P 2022 *Commercialization of Microfluidic Point-of-Care Diagnostic Devices* (CRC Press)

[55] Parihar A, Parihar D S, Ranjan P and Raju K 2022 *Role of Microfluidics-Based Point-of-Care Testing (POCT) for Clinical Applications* (CRC Press)

[56] Yetisen A K, Akram M S and Lowe C R 2013 paper-based microfluidic point-of-care diagnostic devices *Lab Chip* **13** 2210–51

[57] Ming T *et al* 2020 Paper-based microfluidic aptasensors *Biosens. Bioelectron.* **170** 112649

[58] Wang Y *et al* 2020 Low sample volume origami-paper-based graphene-modified aptasensors for label-free electrochemical detection of cancer biomarker-EGFR *Microsyst. Nanoeng.* **6** 32
[59] Wang Y, Xu H, Luo J, Liu J, Wang L, Fan Y, Yan S, Yang Y and Cai X 2016 A novel label-free microfluidic paper-based immunosensor for highly sensitive electrochemical detection of carcinoembryonic antigen *Biosens. Bioelectron.* **83** 319–26
[60] Wang Y, Luo J, Liu J, Sun S, Xiong Y, Ma Y, Yan S, Yang Y, Yin H and Cai X 2019 Label-free microfluidic paper-based electrochemical aptasensor for ultrasensitive and simultaneous multiplexed detection of cancer biomarkers *Biosens. Bioelectron.* **136** 84–90
[61] Zhao P, Zheng J, Liang Y, Tian F, Peng L, Huo D and Hou C 2021 Functionalized carbon nanotube-decorated MXene nanosheet-enabled microfluidic electrochemical aptasensor for carcinoembryonic antigen determination *ACS Sustain. Chem. Eng.* **9** 15386–93
[62] Khaksari S, Ameri A R, Taghdisi S M, Sabet M, Ghaani Bami S M J, Abnous K and Mousavi Shaegh S A 2023 A microfluidic electrochemical aptasensor for highly sensitive and selective detection of A549 cells as integrin α6β4-containing cell model via IDA aptamers *Talanta* **252** 123781
[63] Lu Y, Zhan C, Yu L, Yu Y, Jia H, Chen X, Zhang D and Gao R 2023 Multifunctional nanocone array as solid immunoassay plate and SERS substrate for the early diagnosis of prostate cancer on microfluidic chip *Sensors Actuators* B **376** 133046
[64] Kashefi-Kheyrabadi L, Kim J, Chakravarty S, Park S, Gwak H, Kim S I, Mohammadniaei M, Lee M H, Hyun K A and Jung H I 2020 Detachable microfluidic device implemented with electrochemical aptasensor (DeMEA) for sequential analysis of cancerous exosomes *Biosens. Bioelectron.* **169** 112622
[65] Xu H, Liao C, Zuo P, Liu Z and Ye B C 2018 Magnetic-based microfluidic device for On-chip isolation and detection of tumor-derived exosomes *Anal. Chem.* **90** 13451–8
[66] Qian C, Xiao Y, Wang J, Li Y, Li S, Wei B, Du W, Feng X, Chen P and Liu B F 2021 Rapid exosomes concentration and *in situ* detection of exosomal microRNA on agarose-based microfluidic chip *Sensors Actuators* B **333** 129559
[67] Kumar N, Sorna G, Raju Khan V, Ranjan P, Abubakar Sadique M, Yadav S, Singhal A, Mishra A and Murali S 2021 Efficiency of nanomaterials for electrochemical diagnostics based point-of-care detection of non-invasive oral cancer biomarkers *Adv. Mater. Lett.* **12** 1–20
[68] Parihar A, Yadav S, Sadique M A, Ranjan P, Kumar N, Singhal A, Khare V, Khan R, Natarajan S and Srivastava A K 2023 Internet-of-medical-things integrated point-of-care biosensing devices for infectious diseases: toward better preparedness for futuristic pandemics *Bioeng. Transl. Med.* 1–28
[69] Amethiya Y, Pipariya P, Patel S and Shah M 2022 Comparative analysis of breast cancer detection using machine learning and biosensors *Intell. Med.* **2** 69–81
[70] Wu S *et al* 2022 Application of artificial intelligence in clinical diagnosis and treatment: an overview of systematic reviews *Intell. Med.* **2** 88–96
[71] Ranjan P, Singhal A, Sadique M A, Yadav S, Parihar A and Khan R 2021 Scope of biosensors, commercial aspects, and miniaturized devices for point-of-care testing from lab to clinics applications *Biosensor Based Advanced Cancer Diagnostics: From Lab to Clinics* (Elsevier) pp 395–410

Chapter 6

Cancer diagnostics the synthesis and selection of aptamers for diagnostic applications

Rudramani Tiwari, Pushpesh Ranjan, Shalu Yadav, Mohd Abubakar Sadique, Raju Khan, S Krishnamoorthi, Ajay Kumar Meena and Subhash Chandra Verma

Aptamers are three-dimensional structures synthetically prepared from nucleic acid (RNA or DNA) through the Systematic Evolution of Ligands by Exponential Enrichment (SELEX) method. Aptamers offer a broad range of applications including cancer diagnostics and therapeutics. For the target application, the preparation and selection steps are important and determine the effectiveness of the aptamer. Also, the nature of the interaction, binding affinity, and structural conformations are important parameters for the development and screening of aptamers. In this regard, several modified SELEX methods are involved in the synthesis of target-specific aptamers very efficiently. However, a few challenges which directly influence their working efficiencies, such as poor sensitivity, selectivity, stability, and toxicity, need to be rectified before the aptamer selection. This chapter accounts for the SELEX and different modified methods for the synthesis and selection of aptamers for the diagnosis of cancer biomarkers.

6.1 Introduction

Aptamers are three-dimensional (3D) single-strand nucleic acid (RNA or DNA) oligonucleotides obtained from the Systematic Evolution of Ligands by Exponential Enrichment (SELEX) method. They are thermally and chemically stable and used for broad applications including in biological sciences for the detection of specific biomarkers with high selectivity and specificity. The aptamers are synthesized *in vitro* through the random library of 10^{12}–10^{16} different RNA/DNA oligonucleotides in the required synthetic conditions [1, 2]. In the SELEX synthesis process, first is the selection step where the targeted molecules are added in the defined conditions such as pH, buffer composition, incubation time, the concentration ratio of library and targeted molecules, and temperature to the library for binding, partition,

doi:10.1088/978-0-7503-5012-9ch6

separation, and elution. In the second step, the amplification process takes place where the oligonucleotides are used as templates and are amplified through PCR and/or RT-PCR. In the last step, the conditioning step, the aptamers are characterized by sequencing and then their specific binding efficiency is evaluated for the target of the high-affinity aptamers for selective detection of interest of analytes. In the SELEX method, 6–20 rounds take place for the synthesis of specific aptamers [3–5].

After the synthesis of aptamers, post-SELEX modifications are necessary to improve the enzymatic and chemical stability as well as the binding affinity towards the target analytes. However, they can also be modified with different functionalities such as carboxyl, amino, biotin, thiol, etc, to further broaden their applications, such as bioimaging, targeted drug delivery, etc. Apart from this, there have been several modified SELEX processes employed to enhance the accuracy and shorten the time for aptamer synthesis and selection [3, 4, 6]. Aptamers have the ability to form different 3D structures, such as G-quadruplex, loop, stem, hairpins (stem-loop), etc (figure 6.1(A)), which provide the high-affinity interaction towards the target molecules via hydrogen bonding, hydrophilic and hydrophobic interactions, π–π interactions, and van der Waals forces to form a complex such as an aptamer-antigen complex (figure 6.1(B)) [4, 5, 7, 8].

Over the years, the SELEX method has undergone fast development, which has led to the selection processes such as cell-SELEX, capillary electrophoresis (CE)-SELEX, microfluidics-SELEX for the screening of biological molecules including cancer biomarkers [9–11].

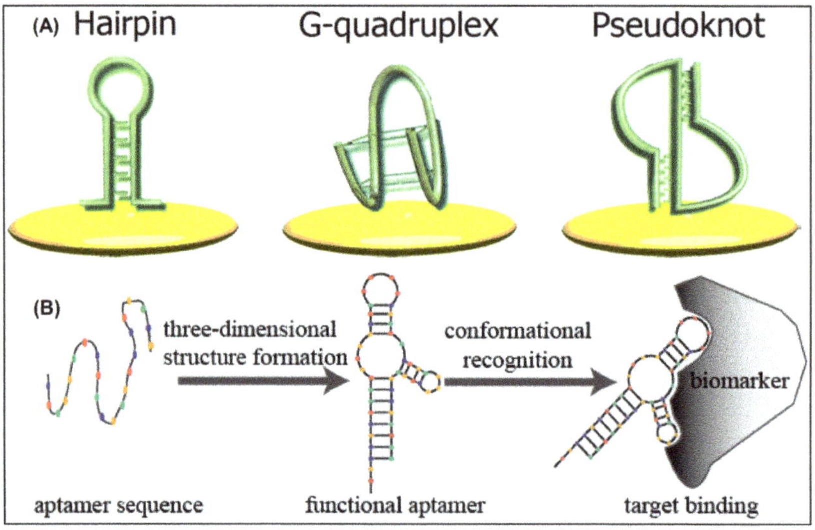

Figure 6.1. Schematic illustration of the (A) different conformations of aptamers. Reproduced with permission from [7]. Copyright (2016) American Chemical Society. (B) Aptamer conformational recognition of targets to form an aptamer–target complex. Reproduced with permission from [5]. Copyright (2018) MDPI.

6.2 Post-SELEX modifications

After successful screening and separation of desired sequences, their optimizations are required in terms of length, size, stability, cost, and clearance based on the clinical aspect. While aptamers are stable *in vitro*, they show susceptibility towards nucleases and get degraded by enzymatic activity under *in vivo* conditions. Additionally, nucleic acids showing weak interactions i.e. hydrogen bonding, van der Waals forces, including π–π stacking, and electrostatic interaction via phosphate groups, etc, ensure fast filtration with a small circulation time. The use of short SELEX (<50 nucleotide) reduces the effective selection due to less complexity, and synthesis of long SELEX (>50 nucleotide) is difficult and costly [12–14]. To avoid this problem long SELEX sequences get selected followed by length standardization to obtain particular functional sequences that improve the aptamer's properties in terms of *in vivo* biological persistence and stability. Due to the availability of only four base pairs, it is tough to modify the functional groups; for versatile functional group modification the LOOPER method and aptamer cyclization were also reported [15]. The rotational truncation approach is also useful for achieving the synthesis of predicted sequences with better binding ability based on information resulting from the 3D structure prediction and computational docking modeling for the target's structure [12]. For example, modification in ssDNA-ssRNA-based aptamer selection employed the 2′-ribose of the pyrimidines with 2′-fluoro and 2′-amino groups, for enhancing the nuclease resistance. Modification by post-selection chemical synthesis is also applicable by the capping at the oligonucleotide 30-terminus, by the 2′-position of (deoxy) ribose residues, C5-position of pyrimidines, by an epoxy group of (deoxy) ribose residues, by locked nucleic acids (LNAs), xeno-nucleic acids (XNAs), by introducing 2′-O-metyl purines, phosphorothioates, α-phosphate groups, and unnatural base pairs [15–20]. Other alternatives, i.e. spiegelmers, are reported that have L-ribose instead of D-ribose on their structures to provide physiochemical stability of artificial oligonucleotides from various nucleases enzymes. The low-molecular mass aptamers are susceptible to renal filtration, and modifications made by aptamer conjugation with cholesterol, proteins, nanomaterials, liposomes, polymers, etc, are applicable to restrict/reduce the renal filtration without making structural or functional changes. For example, length modification of the aptamer by attaching polyethylene glycol (PEG) is reported, which allows cost-effective short aptamer length elongation [5, 12, 21]. All the mentioned modification methods that are employed post-SELEX affect the selectivity and affinity towards target molecules, and simultaneously undesired chemical toxicity, immunogenicity, and side effects are also possible. Therefore affinity and effects monitoring is necessary after each modification [22, 23].

6.3 Principle of the classic SELEX method

The aptamers from the library of enormous nonbinding sequences are done using a process known as systematic evolution of ligands by exponential enrichment (SELEX). In this process, several cycles of separation, amplification, purification of bound sequences, and polymerase chain reaction (PCR) are employed to develop aptamers with high affinity. Conventional SELEX purification usually requires 8–12 cycles of selection onto the solid supports using affinity chromatography or nitrocellulose filtration for efficient separation from non-bonded targets [24, 25]. The RNA or DNA has been used for the sequencing of aptamers to design the 3D-structured aptamers for screening of the target molecule. However, DNA makes for an easier screening process since it is more stable than RNA. In the current scenario, both RNA and DNA are widely utilized for the synthesis of aptamers to target biological and non-biological molecules, such as cancer biomarkers and organic compounds. Since aptamers are small molecules, they are easy to synthesize within a few hours to a week in better reproducibility from batch-to-batch samples. Therefore, they make a cost-effective screening platform for target molecules [15, 22, 26]. In this section, the various types of SELEX methods employed in the aptamers field are discussed in detail.

6.3.1 Magnetic-bead-SELEX method

A different strategy includes a magnetic field for complex separation from the reaction mixture by using magnetic beads as a solid support for the immobilization of aptamers or targets, and is called magnetic-bead SELEX. In this approach, capture molecule-coated magnetic beads are modified by aptamers and incubated with the target molecule's mixture. During incubation, the surface structure of the magnetic bead gets changed due to interchanges of target molecules. Separation and amplification of released aptamers are done via magnetic separation and PCR, respectively. The affinity and specificity of the aptamer can be increased by the association of negative SELEX with magnetic-bead SELEX [11]. This approach alters the modification of the natural structure of the target molecules, which may affect the selection of high-affinity aptamers. However, this method increases the range of targets due to the immobilization of several small molecules on the magnetic bead surface. Simultaneously the free aptamers and complexes appreciate facile separation to save time and energy during selection. Since this method requires a comparatively large amount of reaction mixture and the presence of beads affects the selection of aptamers, some additional protocols, for example negative selection, and higher stringency washing conditions including changing the amount, duration, etc, are attached with this procedure to increase affinity and better selection [15, 23]. For example, biotoxin screening by magnetic bead-based aptamers is very sensitive even for a small number of targets and enhances the sensitivity of the electrochemiluminescence assay [27].

Method extension via higher stringency conditions allows poor extents of DNA binding but a large number of sequences with greater affinity. For the quantification process confocal microscopy was used, and for specificity and affinity evaluation flow cytometry and surface plasmon resonance (SPR) technologies were used. The advantages associated with this method are the need for low mixture volumes (50–100 μl), direct PCR amplification of the magnetic bead surfaces, and transferring the magnetic beads under a magnetic field. The drawback associated with this method is the blockage in the microchannels due to the aggregation of beads [28].

The aptamers with a dissociation constant in nanomolar concentration can be done by using discovered magnetic-assisted rapid aptamer selection (MARAS) technique. The use of negative selection with MARAS allows the completion of the process in a very small time without repeating the selection cycles [20].

6.3.2 Cell-SELEX method

It is challenging to get high-purity recombinant human proteins, i.e. transmembrane and intracellular, with their native conformation. Several researchers have shown that aptamers selected in contradiction of purified proteins might fail to identify the targets in their native conformation [15, 23, 29]. To overcome these issues a new method was introduced named cell-SELEX, which uses the whole cell as its target. Using the whole cell as a target provides a native state of recombination during the screening process under physiological states, which enhances the possibility of successful screening of aptamers. The cell-SELEX method is similar to the conventional SELEX, which follows steps of incubation, separation, and amplification, but with some specific conditions, i.e. using negative selection for separation(figure 6.2), and the use of specific cell types as target molecules instead of purified proteins, to improve the specificity and selectivity. Since natural cells are used as unknown target molecules here new cell biomarkers are discovered and aptamers are attached to the cell surface, which results in no need for any solid support [4, 29].

Firstly, Morris *et al* introduced in 1998 human red blood cell membrane preparations (RBC ghosts) as target cells to isolate aptamers for different cell

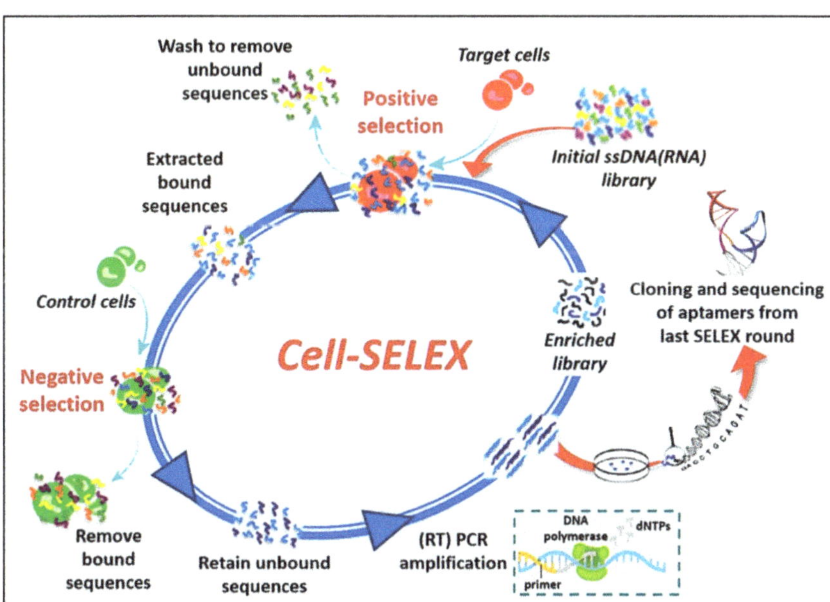

Figure 6.2. Schematic depiction of the cell-SELEX process. Reproduced with permission from [4]. Copyright (2017) MDPI.

membrane targets [12] and developed a protocol for whole living cell-SELEX (whole cell-SELEX). In the selection process for a known target or recognizing a specific cell phenotype, whole cell-SELEX protocols can be adopted while avoiding the simultaneous enrichment of unwanted targets containing aptamers. Cell-SELEX introduces negative selection before the positive selection in each cycle of screening, which allows the separation of sequences against desired targets. Many aptamers based on known targets are isolated using positive selection in cell-SELEX strategies, i.e. transforming growth factor-β type receptors (TGFβRIII. TGFβRII and TGF-β2) [12].

There are several protocols reported for different types of aptamer selection, for example, several anti-integrin alpha V (ITGAV) aptamers are isolated using a specific protocol known as 'Isogenic cell-SELEX' (Icell SELEX). A hybrid-SELEX or crossover-SELEX protocol is reported for successful enhancement and screening of the aptamers for Tenascin-C (TNC), anti-transferrin receptor (TfR), and G-protein-coupled cholecystokinin B receptor (CCKBR) [30]. Another variant of cell-SELEX named 'differential cell-SELEX' had been developed to recognize a specific phenotype instead of a specific target. This method offers the selection of multiple discriminative targets even if they are not previously known. Aptamers based on this approach are reported for T-cell acute lymphocytic leukemia (ALL) cells from B-cell lymphoma cells and small-cell lung cancer versus large-cell lung cancer. Significantly this method discriminates between cell types with diverse characteristics, i.e. tumorigenesis and metastatic potential [31–33].

In order to enhance the performance of some nanomaterials, i.e. single-walled carbon nanotubes (SWCNTs), graphene oxide SELEX (GO-SELEX) [15, 34–36] is introduced as a loading media for aptamer screening purposes. In this process with the introduction of targets, aptamers with high affinity for targets are released from the loading media, and the rest of the non-specific fragments remain on the SWCNTs or GO, and results screened aptamers with high specificity and affinity towards target molecules. Apart from the advantages of the cell-SELEX method, they still have a few limitations: (i) a non-specific binding of aptamer and cells that resist effective enrichment of particular sequences. (ii) The complex surface constituents and membrane proteins create difficulty in the identification of targets and the discovery of biomarkers. (iii) Presence of negative charges on nucleic acids and the cell surface repel each other, which causes difficulties for aptamers to bind on the cell surface. To overcome these issues several modifications are introduced with cell-SELEX, i.e. ligand-guided selection (LIGS), fluorescence-activated cell sorting (FACS), a microfluidic-based system, cell internalization-SELEX, and 3D Cell-SELEX for screening aptamer binding cells [37–39], microfluidic devices, high-throughput sequencing techniques, and flow cytometry for saving time and energy. Among the above-discussed modified cell-SELEX methods, some fascinating methods are briefly described below.

6.3.2.1 Fluorescence-activated cell sorting-SELEX (FACS-SELEX)

An extended protocol of cell-SELEX with fluorescence-activated cell sorting (FACS-SELEX) allows the selection of aptamers via targeting a definite cell subpopulation. This protocol introduces fluorescence-active aptamer library incubation with target cells, a cell-sorting device for screening and separation of aptamers as bounded or unbounded cells subpopulations. After that separation of bounded aptamers, they are amplified. This protocol eliminates the dead cell population with two additional advantages. First, it reduces the experimental steps via combining both positive and negative selection in a single cycle. Second, this protocol allows the monitoring of the selection process during the cycle. The FACS-SELEX protocol has been reported for the selection of an aptamer named EP166 in contradiction of the transmembrane protein EpCAM, which is generally present on the surface of most adenocarcinomas and cancer stem cells [12, 40, 41].

6.3.2.2 Cell internalization-SELEX

This is another extension of cell-SELEX protocol designed for the specific diseased cells of secondary reagents. A rapid internalization was observed during the binding of aptamers, which permitted the cell-specific internalization of active therapeutic substances, i.e. microRNAs, radionuclides, toxins, viruses, enzymes, nanoparticles, small interfering RNAs (siRNAs), anti-microRNAs and anti-cancer therapeutics [12, 42]. Since the process obeyed the internalization step it has been known as cell internalization-SELEX. This protocol enhances efficiency and minimizes therapeutic toxicity by elucidating the secondary reagents of target cells. These properties of cell internalization-SELEX allow the selection of fast internalizing aptamers with eliminating the poor internalizing sequences. For example, this protocol has been introduced for a transmembrane receptor (HER2) over-expressed in breast cancer and linked with a poor diagnosis [43].

6.3.2.3 Ligand-guided selection-SELEX (LIGS-SELEX)

For selection of aptamers against the known target, a new protocol known as ligand-guided selection (LIGS-SELEX) has been introduced. This protocol uses a high-affinity secondary binder with aptamers for the chosen target, i.e. a monoclonal antibody, which competes with and displaces the bound aptamers for their isolation. This method has already been used for aptamer selection against IgM and CD3 markers on B-cell lymphoma and T-cell leukemia, respectively [37, 38, 44].

6.3.3 Capillary electrophoresis-SELEX (CE-SELEX) method

Recently a new homogenous, high-resolution, and more efficient separation technique based on capillary electrophoresis (CE) has been introduced for SELEX, known as CE-SELEX. This technique uses only 1–4 cycles and allows the binding and separation in free solution systems for hindrance-free interactions of aptamers. CE-SELEX is a development of the homogenous method that allows the incubation of random libraries with the target molecule and the selection of aptamers against free target molecules [24, 45]. The solution mixture in CE-SELEX contains free aptamers, free target molecules, and target-aptamer complexes. This solution mixture is injected into a capillary column and separated under high voltage to get high-purity aptamers (figure 6.3) [46, 47]. In the presence of external voltage on

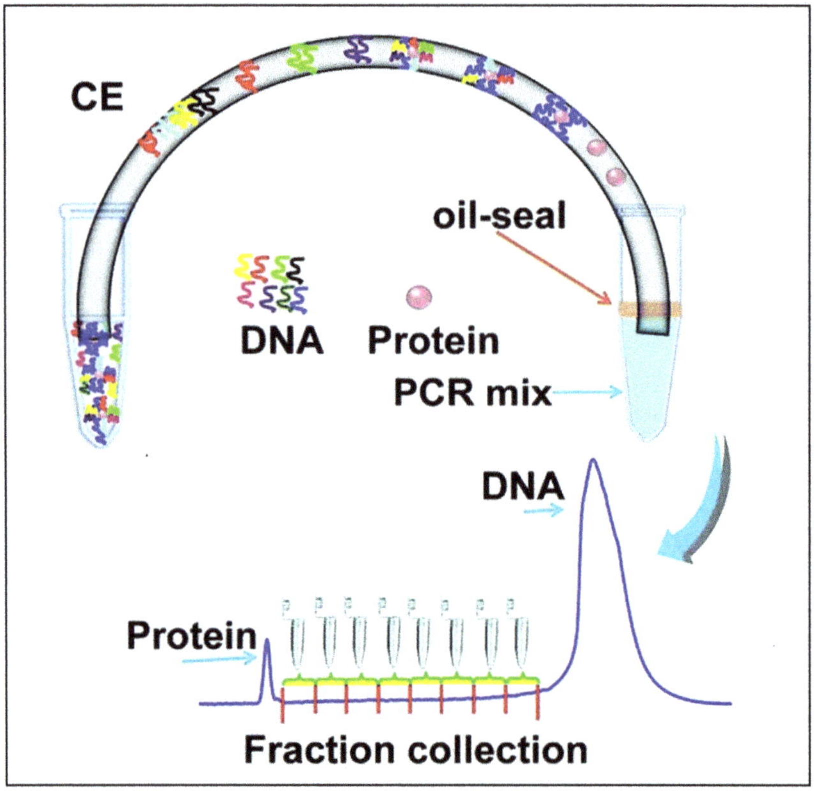

Figure 6.3. Schematic representation of FCE-SELEX selection for aptamers. Reproduced with permission from [47]. Copyright (2015) Royal Society of Chemistry.

the capillary, the separation of constituents of the solution mixture depends upon the different migration rates caused by different charge-mass ratios. CE-SELEX describes the affinity between target molecules and free aptamer due to the different concentrations of free ssDNA, free target molecules, and target molecule-ssDNA complexes. For example, alpha-fetoprotein and HE4 (ovarian cancer biomarker) [15] had been screened by CE-SELEX and electrophoretic peaks for target molecule-ssDNA complexes appear when these have sufficient affinity.

Besides these parameters, the low mobility between the free aptamer and the small-size target molecule–aptamer complex generates difficulty in separation, which presents major applications of CE-SELEX for larger target molecules. Previous studies reflect that CE-SELEX requires aptamers with large mobility shifts upon binding and are suitable only for large target molecules [29, 43]. Despite that, current studies report aptamers for a few small molecular targets, which are separated by using CE-SELEX: N-methyl mesoporphyrin (MW—580 g mol^{-1}) (figure 6.4) [24] and neuropeptide Y (4272 Da), which are too small compared to DNA (25 kDa). For small target molecules mobility of the complex and nonbinding sequences are showing minute changes, which result in partial separation of the desired complex. However, if a small amount of the pure complex gets separated,

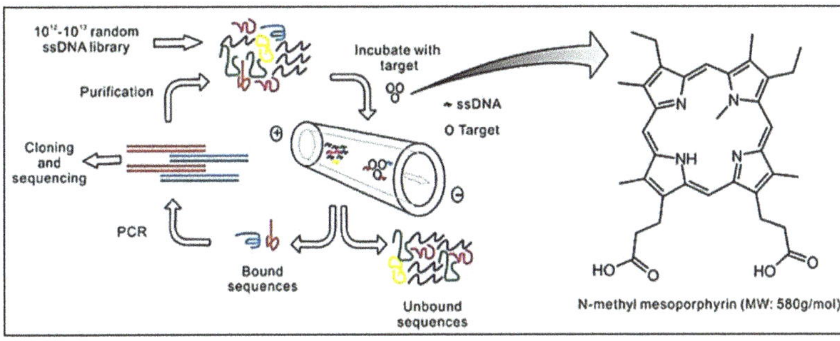

Figure 6.4. Schematic illustration of the capillary electrophoresis-SELEX process. Reproduced with permission from [24]. Copyright (2013) American Chemical Society.

satisfactory enhancement can be accomplished using PCR. Instead, multiple iterative cycles of enrichment can also evolve a high-affinity aptamer in large abundance [33, 48].

Based on CE-SELEX there are two methods i.e. non-equilibrium capillary electrophoresis (NECE) and equilibrium capillary electrophoresis (ECE) of solution mixtures at equilibrium have been introduced for the determination of the different binding parameters (K_d, k_{on}, and k_{off}) of the aptamer–target molecule interaction [47, 49, 50]. The dissociation constants and dissociation equilibrium are related to the peak of free aptamers and the complexation process, respectively. Since there is a short time required for the equilibrium process, the use of a short-length capillary and suction device at the outlet can increase the rate of separation by suppressing the dissociation of the complex during the electrophoresis process. Isolation of the complex with high purity demands extreme control on the equilibrium time of complexation. The low sample injection volume of CE shrinks the chances of getting appropriate aptamers. However, this drawback can be avoided by continuous sample injection using microscale free-flow electrophoresis (μFFG) which expands the aptamer quantity. The dissociation constants between nanomolar to micromolar amounts allows the selection within three rounds. Despite that, low affinity of aptamers towards the target molecule refers to the large dissociation constant and creates difficulty in the selection of the conventional methods. To overcome this issue new methods were introduced, such as NECE and NCE of the equilibrium mixture and non-SELEX [29, 49–51].

The mixture containing free DNA, free proteins, and the protein-DNA complex can be separated by using NECE of the equilibrium mixture by running the buffer mobile phase under high electric fields. The electropherograms obtained from NECE give the dissociation constant (K_d) of the protein-DNA complex. This method allows the exact determination of binding constants, extremely effective screening, and quantitative analysis of complexes. Since free DNA, free proteins, and the protein-DNA complex are migrated with diverse mobilities, K_d values can be easily determined by using ECE of the equilibrium mixture, which is a kinetic method for screening aptamers. During the separation of the complex, it maintains the equilibrium condition in the solution mixture. Moreover, this method gives better results, and depends upon the NECE due to the values of migration time of the complex, concentration-free DNA and K_d can be measured by NECE. Hence, ECE cannot be attained without measuring the above-mentioned parameters [49, 50, 52]. Conventional SELEX involves multiple cycles of selection and PCR amplification, despite that non-SELEX involves repetitive partitioning without amplification and promotes the screening using NECE and final PCR. The use of nitrocellulose filtration before CE allows the removal of free proteins, which diminishes the library size and reduces the screening time [52].

6.3.4 Microfluidic SELEX

A mini platform for performing an automated SELEX on-chip is referred to as a microfluidic system, which is integrated with micropumps, reagent holding chambers, a transportation unit, a microfluidic control model, temperature control modules, microvalves, a PCR chamber, and a waste chamber. These integrations allow multiple cycle selections within a short period. The microfluidic-SELEX method was developed for the bead (mostly magnetic microbead) based separation, CE-based separation, and sol–gel encapsulation (figure 6.5) [53–55]. This integrated

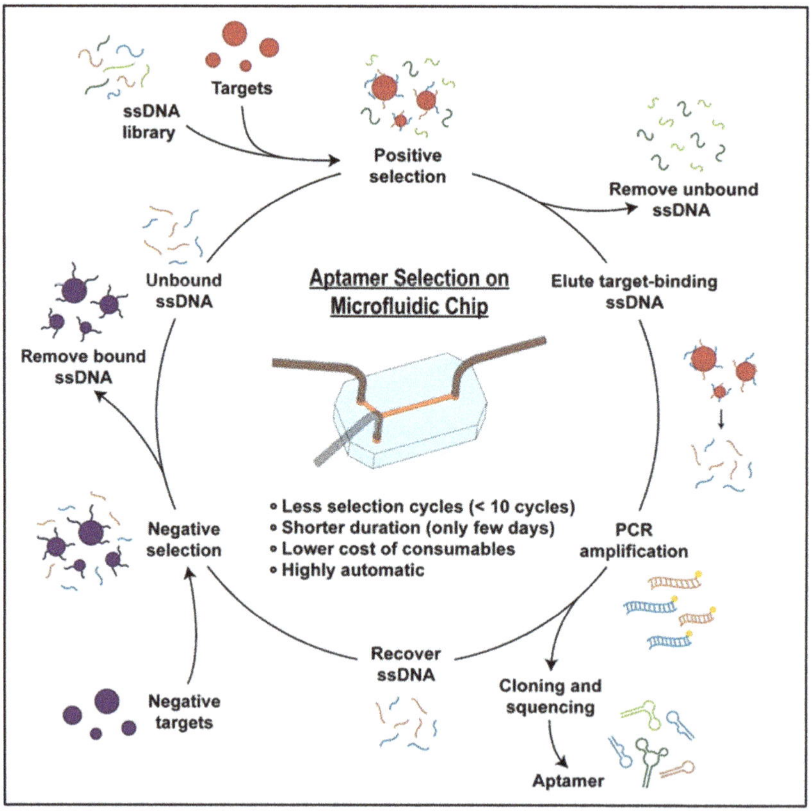

Figure 6.5. Scheme of the microfluidic-based SELEX mechanism for aptamer selection. Reproduced with permission from [54]. Copyright (2021) Frontiers.

on-chip SELEX system is smaller in size, needs smaller amounts of reagents/samples, and allows for performing of the aptamer screening including incubation, extraction, and amplification automatically on an integrated device [56–58]. The chips have a low cost, reproducibility, and disposability, which provides rapid, cost-efficient, reproducible high-affinity ligands and effective selection. Since CE chips enhance the rate of SELEX and separation of aptamers with high affinity within a few cycles due to their greater resolution capability. Consequently, this methodology can be easily implemented to simplify the PCR amplification process in a comprehensive and automated microfluidic platform. In the case of small target molecules, the retention of free nucleic acids and complexes is observed, which causes difficulty in separation; this is just due to this process not being an automated process, which shows the great need for the introduction of microfluidic-based devices in order to make it a fully-automated system [56, 59].

The sol–gel setup is made up of nanoporous silicate glasses that can trap proteins while retaining their activity and biological stability by providing an aqueous environment. This method can hold proteins without any capturing tag and can hold them in their native state. Several target screenings were reported by applying a sol–gel microfluidic chip to immobilization. This system allows adequate binding reactions between aptamers and the immobilized target proteins and thus the isolation of aptamers can be done on the sol–gel microfluidic chip. Microfluidic chip modification along with microheaters can allow thermal elution that shows better elution efficiency compared to elution based on ionic strength. The use of a microheater cannot be done for an on-chip PCR procedure, so an off-chip PCR procedure has been applied for this method. Sol–gel microfluidic devices need syringe pumps for reagent transport and device fabrication is a complex process [60, 61].

Microfluidic technologies for SELEX based on magnetic separation under several conditions, i.e. chip-based separation, magnetically-activated, continuous-flow, are also reported. The fabrication of the ferromagnetic structures in the microchannels is tough, despite the fact that the DNA aptamers for recombinant botulinum neurotoxin type A and streptavidin are isolated using this method. The magnetic bead-based selection can be extended for use with cell targets for fast production of aptamers as cell-surface markers. The un-integrated magnetic bead-based microfluidic devices by microvalves, on-chip PCR modules, or micropumps restrict their real application. The micropump development can be applied as a micromixer by supplying compressed air to the closed microvalve. These developments simplify the control while preventing contamination in the screening process under reduced time and concentration. Aptamers for alpha-fetoprotein (AFP) and C-reactive protein (CRP) are reported based on a multi-function microfluidic chip [55, 59].

6.3.5 *In vivo* SELEX

In vivo, the SELEX (figure 6.6) [62] approach is applied to recognize aptamers that could be *in situ* restricted to the tumor, that exhibit the potential to be exploited for specific delivery as well as the conformation of operative diagnostic agents. Since

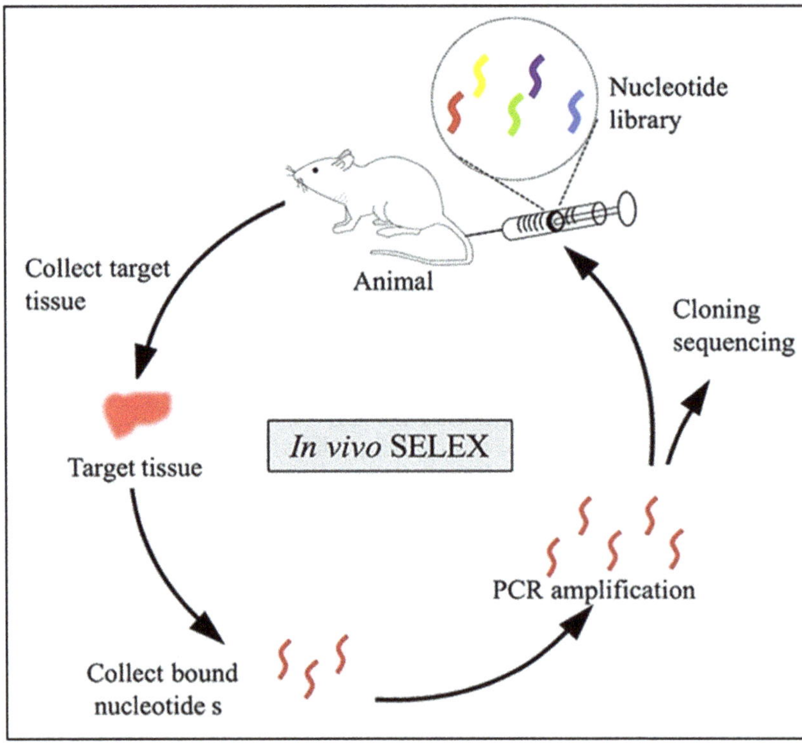

Figure 6.6. Schematic representation of *in vivo* SELEX for aptamer selection against tissue in living anima. Reproduced with permission from [62]. Copyright (2017) Wiley Online Library.

in vivo SELEX is a sophisticated strategy. This method allows for the simultaneous isolation of aptamers, employing negative selection mechanisms to effectively eliminate undesired targets. The *in vitro* cell-based selection approach has a major drawback in that the selected aptamers going to fail under *in vivo* conditions due to poor tissue permeability and change in conformation of proteins under an *in vivo* environment. By maintaining the *in vitro* microenvironment, a cell-based approach for specific binding of prostate tumor cells in nanomolar concentrations was achieved using negative selection followed by selection against the PC-3 cell line by using spheroid cells of human prostate cancer [10, 12, 63]. Despite these strategies, the *in vivo* selection is performed in a diseased living animal cell. The *in vivo* aptamer screening was performed for nuclease-resistant RNA in mice-bearing murine CT26 colon carcinoma liver metastases, which binds an RNA helicase (p68) that regulates colorectal cancer tumors. The selected RNA molecules are separated and amplified under *in vitro* conditions [15, 64]. Surface plasmon resonance can be applied for the determination of binding constants (K_a/K_d) and fluorescence molecular tomography can be used for tumor imaging in deeply implanted organs [65, 66]. Besides that, the individual deference of aptamers limits the amplification via limiting the polymerase activity. Similarly, the cost of SELEX and its safety risks also limit the *in vivo* aptamer screening.

6.4 Summary

Aptamers are powerful tools that exhibit a high interest in the diagnostics and therapeutics of cancer biomarkers over antibody-based diagnostics due to several advantages such as cost-effectiveness, easy and rapid synthesis, high stability, selectivity and high binding affinity. The traditional SELEX method is commonly applied for the synthesis and selection of aptamers. However, a various modified SELEX method such as Cell-SELEX, CE-SELEX, microfluidic-SELEX and *in vivo* SELEX has been utilized to further improve the selection strategy to make highly efficient aptamers. The post-SELEX methods are carefully implemented to address the problems of the SELEX method since it can affect aptamer properties such as binding efficiency and their functioning. Apart from this, aptamer-based diagnostic methods are continuously in progress. However, a big gap is associated with their biomedical application between the initial result and commercialization of the product. Therefore, the new strategiesmust improve the aptamer selection to make high-throughput aptamers in cancer diagnostics applications.

Conflicts of interest

The authors declare no conflict of interest.

Acknowledgments

The authors sincerely thank Director, CSIR-AMPRI for his interest in this work. PR and SY are grateful to CSIR, India for SRF. MAS is thankful to DST-SERB for JRF.

References

[1] Ellington A D and Szostak J W 1990 In vitro selection of RNA molecules that bind specific ligands *Nature* **346** 818–22

[2] Stanciu L A, Wei Q and Barui A K 2021 Recent advances in aptamer-based biosensors for global health applications *Annu. Rev. Biomed. Eng.* **23** 433–59

[3] Vandghanooni S, Sanaat Z, Farahzadi R and Eskandani M 2021 Recent progress in the development of aptasensors for cancer diagnosis: focusing on aptamers against cancer biomarkers *Microchem. J.* **23** 106640

[4] Musumeci D, Platella C, Riccardi C, Moccia F and Montesarchio D 2017 Fluorescence sensing using DNA aptamers in cancer research and clinical diagnostics *Cancers* **9** 174

[5] Sun H and Zu Y 2015 A highlight of recent advances in aptamer technology and its application *Molecules* **20** 11959–80

[6] Ciancio D R, Vargas M R, Thiel W H, Bruno M A and Giangrande P H 2018 Aptamers as diagnostic tools in cancer *Pharmaceuticals* **11** 86

[7] Tello A, Cao R and Gomez H 2016 Conformational changes of enzymes and aptamers immobilized on electrodes *Bioconj. Chem.* **27** 2581–91

[8] Kulbachinskiy A V 2007 Methods for selection of aptamers to protein targets *Biochemistry (Moscow)* **72** 1505–18

[9] Wu X, Shaikh A B, Yu Y, Li Y and Ni S 2017 Potential diagnostic and therapeutic applications of oligonucleotide aptamers in breast cancer *Int. J. Molecular Sci.* **18** 851

[10] Liu M, Yu X, Chen Z, Yang T, Yang D, Liu Q, Du K and Li B 2017 Aptamer selection and applications for breast cancer diagnostics and therapy *J. Nanobiotechnol.* **15** 1–16
[11] Darmostuk M, Rimpelova S, Gbelcova H and Ruml T 2015 Current approaches in SELEX: an update to aptamer selection technology *Biotechnol. Adv.* **33** 1141–61
[12] Catuogno S and Esposito C L 2017 Aptamer cell-based selection: overview and advances *Biomedicines* **5** 49
[13] Qi S, Duan N, Khan I M, Dong X, Zhang Y, Wu S and Wang Z 2022 Strategies to manipulate the performance of aptamers in SELEX, post-SELEX and microenvironment *Biotechnol. Adv.* **55** 107902
[14] Ilgu M and Nilsen-Hamilton M 2016 Aptamers in analytics *Analyst* **141** 1551–68
[15] Yan J, Xiong H, Cai S, Wen N, He Q, Liu Y, Peng D and Liu Z 2019 Advances in aptamer screening technologies *Talanta* **200** 124
[16] Pagratis N C, Bell C, Chang Y F, Jennings S, Fitzwater T, Jellinek D and Dang C 1997 Potent 2′-amino-, and 2′-fluoro-2-deoxyribonucleotide rna inhibitors of keratinocyte growth factor *Nat. Biotechnol.* **15** 68–73
[17] Kato Y, Minakawa N, Komatsu Y, Kamiya H, Ogawa N, Harashima H and Matsuda A 2005 New NTP analogs: The synthesis of 4′-thioUTP and 4′-thioCTP and their utility for SELEX *Nucleic Acids Res.* **33** 2942–51
[18] Georgiadis M M, Singh I, Kellett W F, Hoshika S, Benner S A and Richards N G J 2015 Structural basis for a six nucleotide genetic alphabet *J. Am. Chem. Soc.* **137** 6947–55
[19] Lin Y, Qiu Q, Gill S C and Jayasena S D 1994 Modified RNA sequence pools for *in vitro* selection *Nucleic Acids Res.* **22** 5229–34
[20] Förster C, Zydek M, Rothkegel M, Wu Z, Gallin C, Geßner R, Lisdat F and Fürste J P 2012 Properties of an 'LNA'-modified ricin RNA aptamer *Biochem. Biophys. Res. Commun.* **419** 60–5
[21] Kim D-M, Go M-J, Lee J, Na D and Yoo S-M 2021 Recent advances in micro/nanomaterial-based aptamer selection strategies *Molecules* **26** 5187
[22] Kohlberger M and Gadermaier G 2022 SELEX: critical factors and optimization strategies for successful aptamer selection *Biotechnol. Appl. Biochem.* **69** 1771–92
[23] Wu L, Wang Y, Xu X, Liu Y, Lin B, Zhang M, Zhang J, Wan S, Yang C and Tan W Aptamer-based detection of irculating Tatrgets for precision medicine *Chem. Rev.* **121** 12035–105
[24] Bowser M and Yang J 2013 Capillary electrophoresis-SELEX selection of catalytic DNA aptamers for a small-molecule porphyrin target *Anal. Chem.* **85** 1525–30
[25] Ştefan G, Hosu O, de Wael K, Lobo-Castañón M J and Cristea C 2021 Aptamers in biomedicine: selection strategies and recent advances *Electrochim. Acta* **376** 137994
[26] Arshavsky-Graham S and Heuer C 2022 Aptasensors versus immunosensors—which will prevail? *Engineering in Life Sciences* **22** 319–33
[27] Bruno J G and Kiel J L 2002 Use of magnetic beads in selection and detection of biotoxin aptamers by electrochemiluminescence and enzymatic methods *Biotechniques* **32** 178–83
[28] Kumar T, Bruno J G and Dhiman A 2017 ABCs of DNA aptamer and related assay development *Biotechnol. Adv.* **35** 275–301
[29] Tan W, Donovan M J and Jiang J 2013 Aptamers from cell-based selection for bioanalytical applications *Chem. Rev.* **113** 2842–62
[30] Takahashi M, Sakota E and Nakamura Y 2016 The efficient cell-SELEX strategy, Icell-SELEX, using isogenic cell lines for selection and counter-selection to generate RNA aptamers to cell surface proteins *Biochimie* **131** 77–84

[31] Chen H W, Medley C D, Sefah K, Shangguan D, Tang Z, Meng L, Smith J E and Tan W 2008 Molecular recognition of small-cell lung cancer cells using aptamers *Chem. Med. Chem.* **3** 991–1001

[32] Shangguan D, Li Y, Tang Z, Cao Z C, Chen H W, Mallikaratchy P, Sefah K, Yang C J and Tan W 2006 Aptamers evolved from live cells as effective molecular probes for cancer study *Proc Natl Acad Sci USA* **103** 11838–43

[33] Bing T, Zhang N and Shangguan D 2019 Cell-SELEX, an effective way to the discovery of biomarkers and unexpected molecular events *Adv. Biosyst.* **3** 1900193

[34] Liu L S, Wang F, Ge Y and Lo P K 2020 Recent developments in aptasensors for diagnostic applications *ACS Appl. Mater. Interfaces* **13** 9329–58

[35] Nguyen V-T, Kwon Y S, Kim J H and Gu M B 2014 Multiple GO-SELEX for efficient screening of flexible aptamers *Chem. Commun.* **50** 10513–6

[36] Tan Y *et al* 2014 Single-walled carbon nanotubes (SWCNTs)-assisted cell-systematic evolution of ligands by exponential enrichment (Cell-SELEX) for Improving screening efficiency *Anal. Chem.* **86** 9466–72

[37] Zumrut H E, Ara M N, Fraile M, Maio G and Mallikaratchy P 2016 Ligand-guided selection of target-specific aptamers: a screening technology for identifying specific aptamers against cell-surface proteins *Nucleic Acid Ther.* **26** 190–8

[38] Zumrut H E, Ara M N, Maio G E, Van N A, Batool S and Mallikaratchy P R 2016 Ligand-guided selection of aptamers against T-cell receptor-cluster of differentiation 3 (TCR-CD3) expressed on Jurkat.E6 cells *Anal. Biochem.* **512** 1–7

[39] Souza A G, Marangoni K, Fujimura P T, Alves P T, Silva M J, Bastos V A F, Goulart L R and Goulart V A 2016 3D Cell-SELEX: development of RNA aptamers as molecular probes for PC-3 tumor cell line *Exp. Cell. Res.* **341** 147–56

[40] Mayer G, Ahmed M S L, Dolf A, Endl E, Knolle P A and Famulok M 2010 Fluorescence-activated cell sorting for aptamer SELEX with cell mixtures *Nat. Protoc.* **5** 1993–2004

[41] Chen M, Yu Y, Jiang F, Zhou J, Li Y, Liang C, Dang L, Lu A and Zhang G 2016 Development of cell-SELEX technology and its application in cancer diagnosis and therapy *Int. J. Mol. Sci.* **17** 1–14

[42] Yang X, Li N and Gorenstein D G 2011 Strategies for the discovery of therapeutic aptamers *Expert Opin. Drug Discov.* **6** 75–87

[43] Zhong Y, Zhao J, Li J, Liao X and Chen F 2020 Advances of aptamers screened by Cell-SELEX in selection procedure, cancer diagnostics and therapeutics *Anal. Biochem.* **598** 113620

[44] Zumrut H E and Mallikaratchy P R 2020 Ligand guided selection (LIGS) of artificial nucleic acid ligands against cell surface targets *ACS Appl. Bio Mater.* **3** 2545–52

[45] Mosing R K and Bowser M T 2009 Isolating aptamers using capillary electrophoresis–SELEX (CE–SELEX) *BT—Nucleic Acid and Peptide Aptamers: Methods and Protocols* ed G Mayer (Humana Press) pp 33–43

[46] Hamedani N S and Müller J 2016 Capillary electrophoresis for the selection of DNA aptamers recognizing activated protein C *Methods Mol. Biol.* **1380** 61–75

[47] Luo Z, Zhou H, Jiang H, Ou H, Li X and Zhang L 2015 Development of a fraction collection approach in capillary electrophoresis SELEX for aptamer selection *Analyst* **140** 2664–70

[48] Barman J 2015 Targeting cancer cells using aptamers: cell-SELEX approach and recent advancements *RSC Adv.* **5** 11724–32

[49] Berezovski M, Musheev M, Drabovich A and Krylov S N 2006 Non-SELEX selection of aptamers *J. Am. Chem. Soc.* **128** 1410–1
[50] Berezovski M, Drabovich A, Krylova S M, Musheev M, Okhonin V, Petrov A and Krylov S N 2005 Nonequilibrium capillary electrophoresis of equilibrium mixtures: a universal tool for development of aptamers *J. Am. Chem. Soc.* **127** 3165–71
[51] Sefah K, Shangguan D, Xiong X, Donoghue M B O and Tan W 2010 Development of DNA aptamers using Cell-SELEX *Nat. Protoc.* **5** 1169–85
[52] Dong Y and Diagnosis F 2021 *Aptamers for Medical Applications* (Springer)
[53] Wu Y X and Kwon Y J 2016 Aptamers: the 'evolution' of SELEX *Methods* **106** 21–8
[54] Liu Y, Wang N, Chan C, Lu A, Yu Y and Zhang G 2021 The application of microfluidic technologies in aptamer selection *Frontiers Cell Dev. Biol.* **9** 730035
[55] Wang H, Liu Y, Liu C, Huang J, Yang P and Liu B 2010 Microfluidic chip-based aptasensor for amplified electrochemical detection of human thrombin *Electrochem. Commun.* **12** 258–61
[56] Dembowski S K and Bowser M T 2018 Microfluidic methods for aptamer selection and characterization *Analyst* **143** 21–32
[57] Hybarger G, Bynum J, Williams R F, Valdes J J and Chambers J P 2006 A microfluidic SELEX prototype *Anal. Bioanal. Chem.* **384** 191–8
[58] Lou X, Qian J, Xiao Y, Viel L, Gerdon A E, Lagally E T, Atzberger P, Tarasow T M, Heeger A J and Soh H T 2009 Micromagnetic selection of aptamers in microfluidic channels *Proc. Natl Acad. Sci.* **106** 2989–94
[59] Weng C H, Huang C J and Lee G B 2012 Screening of aptamers on microfluidic systems for clinical applications *Sensors* **12** 9514–29
[60] Park S M, Ahn J Y, Jo M, Lee D K, Lis J T, Craighead H G and Kim S 2009 Selection and elution of aptamers using nanoporous sol–gel arrays with integrated microheaters *Lab Chip* **9** 1206–12
[61] Ahn J Y, Jo M, Dua P, Lee D K and Kim S 2011 A sol–gel-based microfluidics system enhances the efficiency of RNA aptamer selection *Oligonucleotides* **21** 93–100
[62] Goto S, Tsukakoshi K and Ikebukuro K 2017 Development of aptamers against unpurified proteins *Biotech. Bioeng.* **114** 2706–16
[63] Ruscito A and Derosa M C 2016 Small-molecule binding aptamers: selection strategies, characterization, and applications *Frontiers Chem.* **4** 1–14
[64] Mi J, Ray P, Liu J, Kuan C T, Xu J, Hsu D, Sullenger B A, White R R and Clary B M 2016 In vivo selection against human colorectal cancer xenografts identifies an aptamer that targets RNA helicase protein DHX9 *Mol. Ther. Nucleic Acids* **5** e315
[65] di Primo C, Dausse E and Toulmé J J 2011 Surface plasmon resonance investigation of RNA Aptamer–RNA ligand interactions *Methods Mol. Biol.* **764** 279–300
[66] Sparks R P, Jenkins J L and Fratti R 2019 Use of surface plasmon resonance (SPR) to determine binding affinities and kinetic parameters between components important in fusion machinery *Methods Mol. Biol.* **1860** 199–210

Chapter 7

Aptasensors for point-of-care diagnostics of cancer

Deepshikha Shahdeo and Sonu Gandhi

Cancer is a deadly disease around the world. Diagnosis at the initial stages can help the patient to access the finest treatment against this threat. However, traditional methods of diagnosis are not very effective, and most cancers are discovered at the late stage. Therefore, it is critical to develop a quick, portable, and sensitive method to detect the cancer at early stages. Among several detection techniques, biosensors have shown a promising result in terms of rapid detection of different biomarkers for cancerous cells. Aptamer-based biosensors (aptasensors) have lately offered several advantages over other antibody-based assays, such as easy synthesis, thermal stability, and lower cost of fabrication. The combination of aptamer with the sensing element resulted in the birth of the term 'aptasensor'. Many research groups have successfully used aptamers as capture probes in the development of platforms for cancer detection. In this chapter, we have briefly explained about the most recent approaches of aptasensors for cancer diagnosis. To conclude, we also shed some light on the limitation, advantages, and future perspective of the same.

7.1 Introduction

Cancer is one of the most deadly diseases and fourth most widely diagnosed worldwide (Cisterna *et al* 2016). Despite notable progress in the field of treatment, it is still a major cause of morbidity and mortality (Kuipers *et al* 2015). Nearly 10 million deaths were recorded in 2020 (Pineros *et al* 2021). Sedentary lifestyle, being overweight, high alcohol and meat consumption, smoking and increasing age are considered as some of the risk factors that can lead to cancer (Rampado *et al* 2019). Currently, surgery, radiotherapy, and chemotherapy are some of the conventional techniques used for the detection and treatment of cancer. However, chemotherapy is the main treatment but it comes with its own side effects and toxicity (Shahdeo and Gandhi 2022). It is non-specifically distributed in the body, and inefficiently

doi:10.1088/978-0-7503-5012-9ch7

inhibits the tumor growth. This challenge limits the level of funding and interest of big pharmaceutical companies. Therefore, researchers are trying to develop comparatively advanced techniques for the early detection of cancer. Nanocarriers are emerging as an advanced tool for the imaging, targeting, and treatment of cancer (Gandhi *et al* 2016, Tomitaka *et al* 2015). Along with the treatment, early and rapid detection of cancer biomarkers is also very crucial to save hundreds of lives. Researchers are also focusing on the development of some advanced and portable sensors for sensitive and initial-stage diagnosis of cancer. Nowadays, aptamers are emerging as a promising tool to overcome challenges.

Aptamers are single-stranded, short oligonucleotide (DNA/RNA) sequences that can assemble into a three-dimensional (3D) unique assembly that selectively binds to the specialized analyte, which can range from small molecules to whole cells (Bai *et al* 2015, Pandey *et al* 2018). Currently, antibodies are widely used as a recognition element in several biosensors, however, it comes with its own drawback. Antibody-based sensors are difficult to deploy in the field due to their precise temperature requirement and storage issues. Unlike antibodies, aptamers are highly stable at a wide range of temperatures and are as selective and sensitive as antibodies (Sekhon *et al* 2021). Due to their low cost of production and great stability, aptamers can be generated for different targets, such as small molecules, proteins, whole cells, and intact viral and bacterial cells (Zahra *et al* 2021). After all these years, aptamers are gaining in popularity, however, only a handful of aptamers are commercially available for therapeutics and diagnostics. In 2004, Macugen, a well-known therapeutic aptamer, was launched by Pfizer for the treatment of neovascular age-related macular degeneration (AMD). In addition to that, Zimura, Fovista, and Pegnivacogin are some of the other therapeutic aptamers used for the treatment of macular degeneration, which are in the advanced clinical trial stage (Ng *et al* 2006). Aptamers can also be employed to recognize cancer biomarkers and this can lead to major advancement in cancer detection and therapy (Porciani *et al* 2018). In the past few decades, various aptamers were screened and validated against numerous biomolecules such as tumor cells, pesticides (Liu *et al* 2019), antibiotics (Hosseinzadeh and Mazloum-Ardakani 2020), multiple toxins (Zhao *et al* 2018b), viral and bacterial proteins and different disease related biomarkers (Hassan and DeRosa 2020). Many aptasensors have been developed that perhaps use a range of transmission mechanisms to detect cancer and cancer biomarkers, including electrochemistry, fluorescence, and chemiluminescence.

7.2 Method of selection of aptamers

Aptamers are usually selected from the combinatorial library screening method called SELEX (Systemic Evolution of Ligands by Exponential Enrichment; Thiviyanathan and Gorenstein 2012). Aptamers are selected by screening the library of nucleic acids and it is an *in vitro* method of selection. Gold, Tuerk, Szostak and Ellington (Tuerk and Gold 1990) have reported the SELEX method, which involves iterative cycles of screening and amplification of the desired sequence via PCR at each round of screening. Recently, the aptamer selection technique has been modified, where the nucleic acid library is synthesized on the non-cleavable beads,

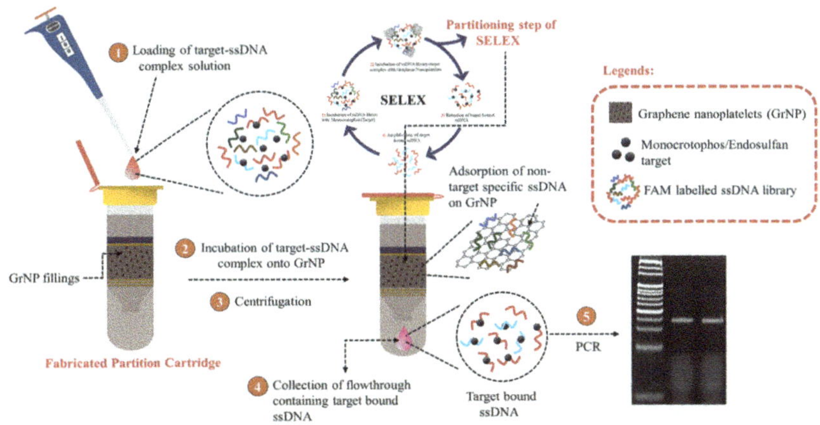

Figure 7.1. Selection of aptamers via SELEX. ssDNA library was incubated with the analyte and later passed through a column called a graphene-modified partition cartridge, where non-specific ssDNA binds to graphene, while target-bound ssDNA collected as flowthrough. Reproduced with permission from (Narlawar and Gandhi 2021). Copyright (2021) Elsevier.

and high affinity binders are determined (He *et al* 2012). Microfluidic chips are also available for the selection of aptamers, which drastically reduces the time of screening. Narlawar *et al* developed a partition cartridge for the convenient separation of selected aptamers after SELEX as shown in figure 7.1. A mixture of target-bound and non-specific ssDNA was screened with the assistance of graphene. Initially, the ssDNA library was incubated with the analyte/target and later, analyte-bound and non-specific ssDNA were loaded onto the graphene-modified partition cartridge. Non-specific unbound ssDNA was allowed to get adsorbed onto the graphene and the bound ssDNA fraction was collected as flowthrough and confirmed by PCR (Narlawar and Gandhi 2021).

The above-mentioned steps were repeated numerous times to increase the amount of strong binder. To reduce the enrichment of non-specific ssDNA, several modifications such as changes in washing and binding conditions were changed in the SELEX procedure. To produce potential aptamer sequences, five to twenty rounds of selection are usually undertaken (Animesh and Singh 2020).

7.3 Aptasensor fabrication for cancer diagnostics

Biosensors are analytical devices that covert the chemical and biological signals into a readable electrical signal. It consists of a biorecognition element (antibody, aptamer, DNA, biomarker; Tripathi *et al* 2018), which binds to the target analyte, a transducer, which translates the interaction between analyte and biorecognition element into a quantifiable signal, an amplifier, which performs amplification of the samples, and a processor to detect and analyze the result. Biosensors are categorized as electrochemical, colorimetric, optical, piezoelectric, or thermal sensors based on the transducing elements (Banga *et al* 2019, Fei *et al* 2015, Piliarik *et al* 2009, Roberts and Gandhi 2020, Shahdeo and Gandhi 2022, Shahdeo *et al* 2020).

Integration of biorecognition elements onto the transducer is a challenging process. Aptamers are highly flexible and can be readily modified with different groups such as biotin, avidin, thiol (Kawaguchi *et al* 2007, Moitra *et al* 2020), FAM (Duan *et al* 2012), FITC, amino, carboxyl, etc, to provide a support system and enhance electrical signal (Connor *et al* 2005, Kim *et al* 2007, Gupta *et al* 2016). Currently, electrochemical sensors are prominently used for the development of aptasensors. In case of cancer detection, aptamers can specifically bind to the analyte, even in the presence of protein contaminants present in the biological fluid used for diagnosis. Aptasensors have the potential to detect even ultralow levels of analyte. Aptasensor-based detection strategies are either label-free, or label-based. Surface plasmon resonance (Cui and Zhou 2020, Densmore *et al* 2008, Najitha Banu *et al* 2014), Raman spectroscopy, and impedance spectroscopy are some of the examples of label-free aptasensors. Meanwhile, flourine-doped electrode (FTO)-based (Roberts *et al* 2019, Roberts *et al* 2021, 2022, Talan *et al* 2018), field-effect transistors (FET) (Cui and Zhou 2020, Islam *et al* 2019, Kawamura and Miyata 2016, Roberts *et al* 2020), fluorescence, chemiluminescence, and nanoparticle-based (Chouhan *et al* 2021, Mahari and Gandhi 2022, Zhu *et al* 2013a) methods are some of the label-based sensors.

7.3.1 Electrochemical sensors

Researchers have focused a lot on the fabrication of electrochemical aptasensors for the detection of several cancer biomarkers. Electrochemical-based aptasensors are sensors that use specific aptamers against different analytes as an affinity biorecognition element. Usually in electrochemical sensors, aptamers are coated onto the surface of electrodes and allowed to bind with the analyte molecule present in the solution. Biochemical interaction between the analyte and aptamers is transduced into the electrical signal, which is further measured by the processor. Methylene blue (MB) and bis-anthraquinone-modified propanediol are some of the examples of redox labels. In the positive sample, interaction of aptamers with the analyte results in a change in the redox molecules, which leads to change in the electrochemical signal. Electrochemical sensors are the advanced sensors that work on the principle of change in current or voltage. They can either be potentiometric or amperometric, according to their perspective of measurement. Potentiometric sensors are based on the detection of change in the potential generated by the surface ion in the solution, on the other hand amperometric sensors operate on observing the change in current due to oxidation and reduction of electroactive redox species at constant potential. Different cancer biomarkers such as prostate-specific antigen (PSA), carcinoembryonic antigen (CEA), human epidermal growth factor Receptor 2 (HER2), cancer antigen 125 (CA125), alpha fetoprotein (AFP) and interleukin 6 can be detected by generating the aptamers against the destined biomarker and immobilizing it as a biorecognition element on the sensor.

Souada *et al* have designed a label-free aptasensor for diagnosis of PSA as shown in figure 7.2. Specific aptamers for PSA were generated and immobilized on the quinone-based polymers, which acted as redox-electroactive species. After addition of the positive sample, aptamer conformation switched after binding to analyte, which

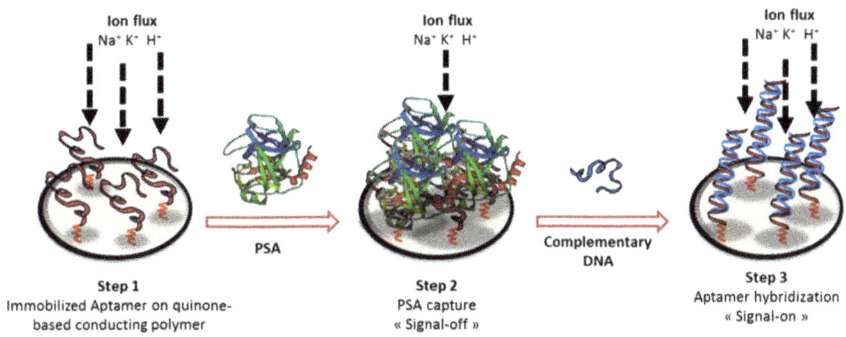

Figure 7.2. Different steps of mechanism of action of aptasensor for detection of PSA (biomarker for prostate cancer); Step 1 depicts the grafting of aptamers on the surface of quinone modified polymer; Step 2 represents the addition of PSA, resulting in change in conformation of aptamer and switch of signal; Step 3 represents the addition of complementary DNA resulted in aptamer hybridization and switch on. Reproduced with permission from (Souada *et al* 2015). Copyright (2015) Elsevier.

resulted in the change in the ion flux at the polymer-electrode interface. This change in the redox current intensity was measured (Souada *et al* 2015). Qureshi *et al* (2015b) have fabricated an aptasensor for detection of HER2, which is a biomarker for breast cancer. Anti-HER2 ssDNA aptamers were generated and functionalized on the surface of an electrode. The response of the interaction was measured by the non-Faradaic impedance spectroscopy (nFIS) method. This method was based on the change of charge distribution after the interaction of the biomarker and ssDNA. This aptasensor was found to be very sensitive and can detect HER2 in the range of 0.2–2 ng ml^{-1}.

Platelet-derived growth factor (PDGF) is another cancer biomarker that has been extensively studied by researchers. Rebecca *et al* developed a sensor based on an aptamer that detects PDGF, directly from the blood. Methylene blue-modified aptamers were used as a biorecognition element. Alternating current voltammetry was employed to monitor the analyte-aptamer binding. In the serum sample, the sensor has showed a sensitivity of 1.25 ng ml^{-1} (Lai *et al* 2007). Secondary aptamers labeled with HRP were used to develop an aptasensor via aptamer sandwich assay for the detection of Michigan cancer foundation-7 (MCF-7) (Zhu *et al* 2013b), which is a breast cancer cell line. A glassy carbon electrode (GCE) was used as the base electrode, where multiwall carbon nanotubes (MWCNTs) and poly(glutamic acid) was used as a biocompatible composite for enhancing the sensitivity of the sensor. Aptamers specific to mucin-1 (MUC1) were allowed to get immobilized on the surface of nanocomposite and another secondary aptamer (a silver nanoparticle-labeled aptamer) was further applied to enhance the selectivity and amplification of signal during detection of MCF-7. Under the optimal condition, the limit of detection was found to be 25 cells, in the dilution range of 1.0 × 102 to 1.0 × 107 cells ml^{-1} (Yazdanparast *et al* 2018).

In the recent years, researchers are combining aptamers and antibodies for enhancing the sensitivity of electrochemical sensors. Qureshi *et al* developed an apta-immunosensor for detection of vascular endothelial growth factor-165 (VEGF) in human serum. Herein, researchers have fabricated a two-probe capturing assay.

Aptamers for VEGF were immobilized on the surface of the sensor, which captures the VEGF protein present in the serum. Further anti-VEGF antibodies conjugated with magnetic beads were allowed to bind to the aptamer-antigen complex. nFIS was used to measure the change in capacitance at different AC electrical frequencies. According to the result, it was estimated that coupling of the aptamer and antigen can increase the sensitivity 2 to 4-fold (figure 7.3) (Qureshi *et al* 2015a). In another

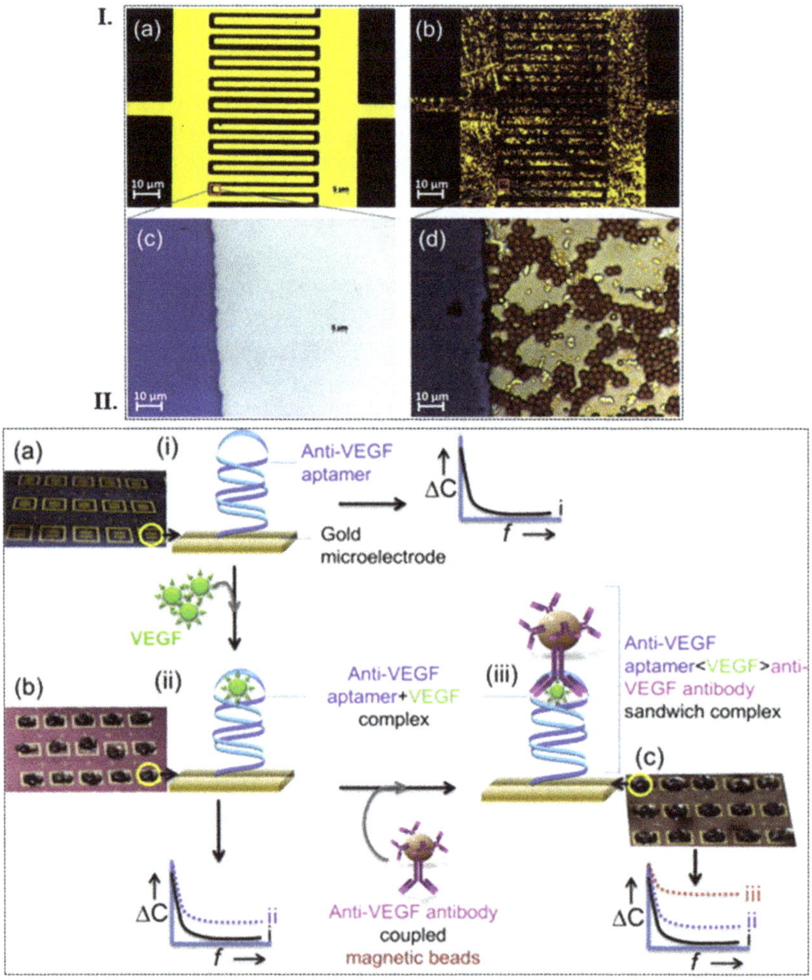

Figure 7.3. Development of apta-immunosensor for detection of VEGF in human serum; (I) Microscopic image representing the surface of electrode (a) surface of control electrode; (b) after the coupling of aptamer-antigen–antibody; (c) zoomed image of control electrode surface; (d) zoomed image of electrode with Apta-antibody complex. Reproduced with permission from (Qureshi *et al* 2015a). Copyright (2015) Elsevier. (II) Visual representation of apta-immunosensor illustrating capacitance variations with AC electrical frequency. Three stages are outlined: (a) aptamer-functionalized sensor surfaces, (b) incubation with 0.1x serum spiked with VEGF protein, and (c) sandwiching with MB-Abs on the aptamer-VEGF protein complex. Real capacitor array images at each stage ((i)–(iii)) are provided.

case, antibodies acted as a capture probe and aptamers were used as an indicator/enhancer probe. Zhu *et al* developed an immunosensor, where HER2, which overexpresses in breast cancer cells, were detected, employing antibody and gold nanoparticle (AuNP)-functionalized aptamers. Aptamers were physio-adsorbed on the surface of AuNPs (Zhu *et al* 2013b, Kasoju *et al* 2020a, Kasoju *et al* 2020b) followed by addition of hydrazine. This nanocomposite was further self-assembled with assembled 2,5-bis(2-thienyl)–1H-pyrrole-1-(p-benzoic acid) (DPB), which has a tendency to reduce the silver ion in the presence of the analyte. Reduction of silver ions resulted in staining of the cells, which can be visualized under an optical microscope and further be quantified by stripping voltammetry (Zhu *et al* 2013c). Urokinase plasminogen activator (uPA), a 54 kDa serine protease that is significant for the cancer invasion and metastasis (Noh *et al* 2013, Shahdeo *et al* 2021a, 2021b), is considered as a universal prognostic biomarker of cancer. Overexpression of uPA can lead to ovarian cancer and it is a valuable biomarker for the diagnosis of cancer (Zhao *et al* 2015a, 2015b, Roberts *et al* 2019, Malecka *et al* 2021).

Osteopontin (OPN) is a sialoprotein and one of the prominent proteins present in the extracellular matrix of tooth and bones (Lund *et al* 2009). It is involved in a variety of physiological processes, including bone remodeling, inflammation, immunological control, and vascularization. OPN is a crucial mediator of inflammation and a key factor in carcinogenesis, having a variety of functions. Cao *et al* developed a cucurbit[7]uril (CB[7])-functionalized pyrolytic graphite electrode. The interaction between OPN and the aptamer resulted in the digestion of methylene blue-labeled DNA. This digested biomolecule was captured by the (CB[7]) and subsequently generated a voltametric response with respect to the concentration of OPN (Cao *et al* 2014). In another experiment, a simple aptasensor was developed using ferri-ferrocyanide as a redox indicator. Herein, the Au-electrode was coated with 3,3-dithiodipropionic acid to attach the biotinylated aptamer. Further, a thin layer of streptavidin was attached to the surface via carbodiimide chemistry (Meirinho *et al* 2015). Later, the voltametric response was measured after addition of the analyte. With an increase in the concentration of analyte, the current intensity decreased. This aptasensor showed the detection limit of 3.7 nM OPN.

7.3.2 Optical biosensors

Optical biosensors are the most versatile type of biosensors, utilizing a wide range of spectroscopy techniques, including UV–vis absorption (Atta *et al* 2015, Bala *et al* 2017, Ermini *et al* 2014, Pei *et al* 2018), phosphorescence, luminescence, and fluorescence (Alizadeh *et al* 2021, Damborska *et al* 2017, Sametband *et al* 2007). In an optical biosensor, binding of analyte with biorecognition element can be detected optically. These aptasensors are light based and can measure the change in wavelength of light passed through the molecule. The enzyme-linked immunosorbent assay (ELISA) is the most well-known commercial optical method for antigen detection (Kawamura and Miyata 2016, Kong *et al* 2010, Majdinasab *et al* 2020). Different ELISA kits are available on the market, which are widely used for clinical diagnostic purposes. Surface plasmon resonance (SPR) is the other technique used for observing the interaction between a ligand and a receptor. Optical methods have their own advantages and disadvantages. They are usually simple to operate and give quick results. However, they do not have high sensitivity as compared to their other counterparts (De Souza Castilho *et al* 2011). In this decade, optical sensors have gained enough interest in the screening of cancer biomarkers. Fluorescence-based aptasensors are considered the most trustworthy and reliable optical aptasensor in cancer diagnostics. The molecular beacon strategy is another technique which is emerging as a boon in diagnostics field. Molecular beacons are nucleic acid hybridization probes that are designed to form the hairpin loop structures with a dye and a quencher at the 3′ and 5′ ends. The fluorophore and quencher are adjacent in the absence of the target, which results in no fluorescence signal, however in the presence of the analyte, this hairpin loop opens up, resulting in creating a distance between both the arms. This distance between the dye and quencher allows the dye to fluoresce. Fluorescent dyes like cy3, cy5, FITC, and FAM, quantum dots, and nanoparticles are the most often-used fluorophores. Xiao *et al* introduced Forster resonance energy transfer (FRET)-based sensors and cyclic enzymatic signal amplification (CTCESA). Graphene oxide can bind with ssDNA via hydrophobic and π-stacking interactions and can act as an excellent quencher due to its electronic properties. Aptamers are designed as hairpin aptamer probes (HAPs) and this HAP can specifically bind to the target analyte. In the absence of target, fluorescence was quenched via the GO-based FRET method. However, in the presence of the target, a conformation change occurred that led to an increase in the fluorescence (Xiao *et al* 2017). Similarly, another group has developed an aptasensor to detect the presence of adenosine in urine samples. In the sensor, quantum dots (QDs) acted as the donor, while polypyrrole adhered to QDs with a detection limit of 9.3 nM (Hashemian *et al* 2016). CA125 is a cancer biomarker used in clinical diagnosis and is presently one of the best serum-based tumor-markers to date. Hamd-Ghadareh *et al* developed a biosensor for diagnosis of CA125 via an antibody-ssDNA hybrid complex. It is an optical-type immunosensor, where CA125 antibodies were immobilized on the surface of AuNPs, and PAMAM-dendrimer was added further to increase the sensitivity as shown in figure 7.4. CA125 can be used to quench the fluorescence of CDs in the presence of thiol-terminated PAMAM-AuNPs. The obtained result revealed that the built biosensor is highly sensitive, cost effective, renewable, and easy to handle, with a lot of potential as a platform for CA125 detection in blood samples, ovarian cancer cell detection, and cancer cell imaging (Hamd-Ghadareh *et al* 2017). Carcinoembryonic antigen (CEA) is other cancer biomarker which plays an important role for screening and detection of tumors. Zhao *et al* developed a 'turn on' fluorescent sensor for rapid detection of CEA (Zhao *et al* 2018b). Pei *et al* have proposed a competitive aptasensor for multiplexed cancer biomarker detection (Pei *et al* 2020). In another experiment cell surface antigen (CD63) was detected on the surface of exosomes. Yu *et al* coupled the CD63 aptamer on magnetic beads and used a Cy3-labeled antisense ssDNA sequence to mask the aptamer's binding site. When human lung adenocarcinoma cells (A549) produce exosomes, they compete with the Cy3-labeled sequence on the binding site, causing the short sequence to be shed into the supernatant. The fluorescence intensity of the supernatant was then determined. As few as 1.01 exosomes ml^{-1} might be detected using this method (Yu *et al* 2019).

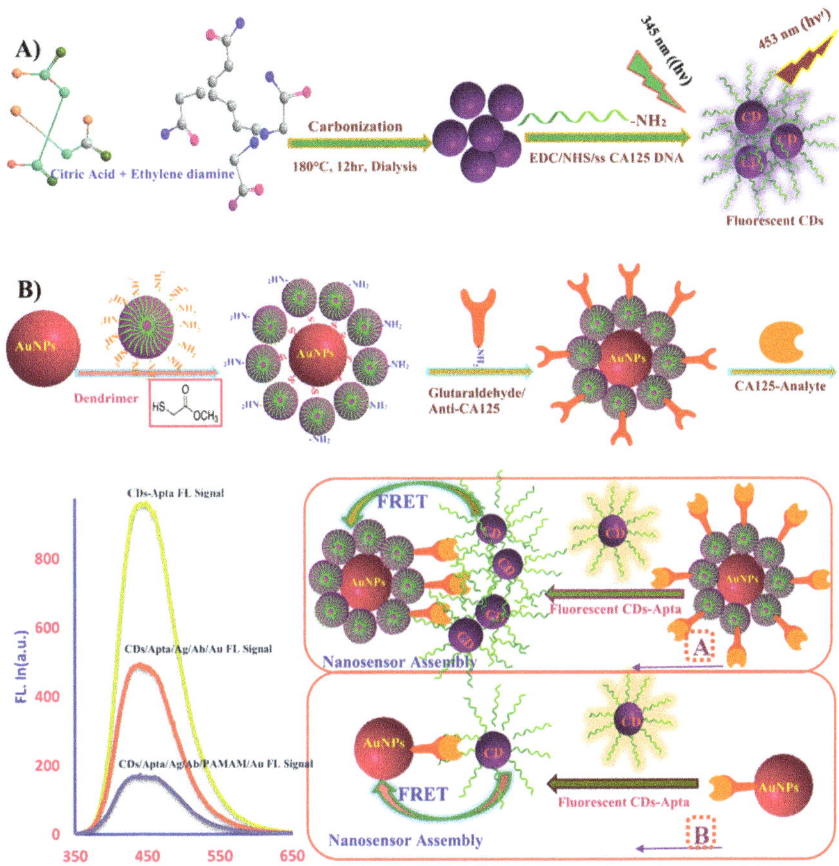

Figure 7.4. The FRET-based detection system's methodology. Firstly, fluorescent CDs were attached to DNA; subsequently, in the presence of CA125 analyte, the CDs-Apta fluorescence response was suppressed by AuNPs-PAMAM-Ab through FRET. Reproduced with permission from (Hamd-Ghadareh *et al* 2017). Copyright (2017) Elsevier.

Optical aptasensors are based on chemiluminescence. Luminescence is a phenomenon in which light is released from a molecule that is not induced by heat, and it can be divided into two types on the basis of their trigger sources (energy): electrochemiluminescence (ECL) and chemiluminescence (CL). Aptasensors constructed based on these techniques are commonly used for detection of biomarkers overexpressed in cancerous cells. Several aptasensors have been developed using the chemiluminescence resonance energy transfer concept (CRET) (Cha *et al* 2014, Yamasuji *et al* 2011). For example, employing glow chemiluminescence of guanine nucleotides, a team of scientists developed a chemiluminescent aptasensor to detect the PSA biomarker in human blood samples. Several CL aptasensors have already been introduced for early cancer detection. Due to the sheer excellent results, it is considered the most sensitive optical method. Jie *et al* developed electrochemiluminescence signal probe using QDs for the early diagnosis of cancer biomarkers in clinical samples (Jie and Jie 2016).

Surface plasmon resonance (SPR) has a potential to track the molecular interaction in real time. It is one of the optical sensing techniques widely used for checking the interaction between analyte and recognition element (Chang 2021). In SPR-based biosensors, aptamers or biomolecules are coated on the surface of a nanomaterial that has SPR properties, such as AuNPs or silver nanoparticles (Shahdeo *et al* 2022a). When the target comes in contact with the aptamer, it results in a change in the refractive index, which is dependent on the resonance (incident) starting angle and weight of the biomolecule (Homola 2003, Homola *et al* 1999, Kawamura and Miyata 2016). SPR works in collaboration with different nanomaterials such as nanoparticles, nanorods, iron oxide nanoparticles (Chouhan *et al* 2021, Shahdeo *et al* 2022b), nano-urchins, and nanosheets, for the signal amplification in a low concentrated sample (Mishra *et al* 2019). In one study, researchers have employed the aptamer-coated gold nanorods for detection of MCF-7. MCF-7 cells were recognized by the mucin-1 aptamer coated with the nanomaterial. Signals after the interaction was detected in the Localized surface plasmon resonance (LSPR) spectra (Li *et al* 2016). Liu *et al* developed a SPR sensor for detection of microRNA (miRNA) and cancer cells. A thiolated hairpin loop-mediated oligo-sequence was immobilized on the surface of AuNPs along with a complementary sequence of miRNA. In the presence of miRNA, the stem loop of the oligo-sequence unfolds, and AuNPs associated with DNA hybridize forming a DNA super-sandwich to which AgNPs absorb, which improves SPR response and further results in the miRNA detection (Liu *et al* 2017). Guo *et al* conducted electrochemical and SPR experiments to investigate detection kinetics. They proposed an aptasensor based on the AgNCs@Apt@UiO-66 nanocomposite, which revealed substantial results to detect CEA. Their SPR aptasensor is reported to have better performance, regenerability, selectivity, repeatability, sensitivity, and stability (Guo *et al* 2017). Another example of an electro-SPR aptasensor was conducted by Duan *et al.* They developed a novel nanostructured biosensing platform using a two-dimensional (2D) nanocomposite comprising graphitic carbon nitride (g-C3N4) nanosheets and MoS_2 quantum dots (MoS_2 QDs), which was then decorated with chitosan-stabilized Au nanoparticles (CS-AuNPs). When compared to the individual components, including MoS_2 QDs, g-C3N4, and CS-AuNPs, the MoS_2QDs@g-C3N4@CS-AuNP-based aptasensor demonstrates excellent bio-binding affinity for the prostate-specific antigen (PSA)-targeted aptamer strands. When it comes to detecting PSA, the electrochemical aptasensor showed a limit of detection (LOD) of 0.71 pg ml^{-1} (Duan *et al* 2018) as shown in figure 7.5. Loyez *et al* developed multiple narrowband resonances (near-infrared wavelength range), to detect the circulating tumor cells. To detect metastatic breast cells, the sensor surface was immobilized with specific aptamers against mammaglobin-A as receptors. This is an ultraquick aptasensor that takes only a few minutes to detect the breast cancer cells (Loyez *et al* 2020).

Aptasensors based on surface-enhanced Raman scattering (SERS) have been explored as a possible avenue for description in the area of nanoscience, especially in cancer-related applications (Nandi *et al* 2020, Yadav *et al* 2021, Zahra *et al* 2021). Raman spectroscopy is an optical technique, which is used to determine the functional group as well as chemical composition of a compound, including serum

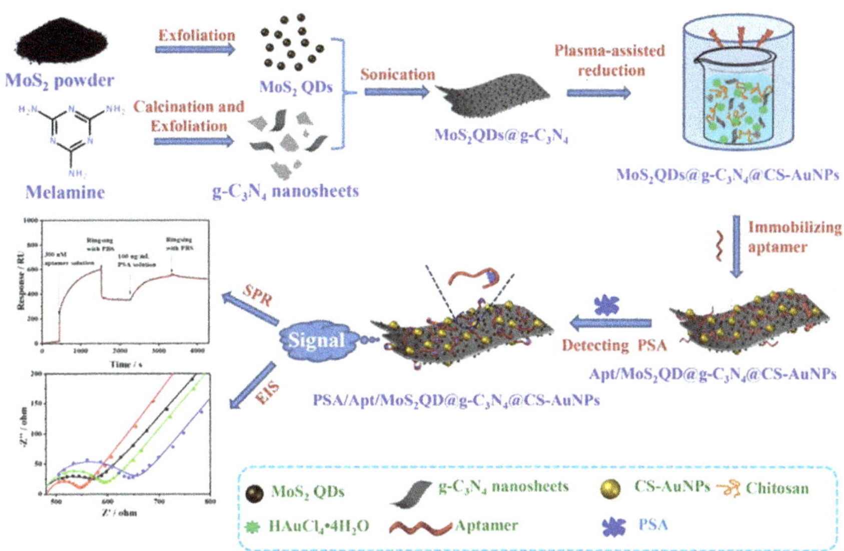

Figure 7.5. The fabrication of MoS_2QD@g-C3N4 and MoS_2QD@g-C3N4@CS-AuNPs nanocomposite; Attachment of aptamer on the surface of MoS_2QD@g-C3N4@CS-AuNPs; to detect the PSA concentration, and; collection of signals employing SPR and electrochemical. Reproduced with permission from Duan *et al* (2018). Copyright (2018) Elsevier.

samples, based on the incident photons of a light source. The combination of Raman spectroscopy-based technology with aptamers has the capacity to recognize the selection of target molecules more accurately, and also improved the sensitivity. Two significant benefits of SERS imaging are the ability to measure a sample with great spatial resolution (within visible range) and the ability to perform multiple discrete tests from a single sample at the same time (Blanco-Formoso and Alvarez-Puebla 2020). In a single experiment, many target molecules can be identified using SERS, which is an efficient vibration-based spectroscopic technique.

A SERS-based aptasensor for detection of EpCAM protein was developed by Bhamidipati *et al.* The sensor was fabricated by modifying the substrate with EpCAM aptamer along with gold nanostars. Different dilutions of analyte were added and their SERS response was measured. Sun *et al* developed a similar aptasensor to identify cytochrome c (Cyt c) for diagnosis of non-small cell lung cancer (NSCLC). Hydrophobic filter paper was decorated with the gold urchins functionalized with Cyt c aptamer. Interaction between Cyt c and the aptamer resulted in a change in the conformation, which created a SERS signal. The LOD was found to be 1.148 pg ml^{-1} (Sun *et al* 2020). Ning *et al* synthesized a SERS-aptamer based sensor for the detection of multiple biomarkers simultaneously. Nanotags (Gold–silver–silver nanotrepangs) and magnetic beads were used for detection purposes.

Colorimetric aptasensors are widely used for detection due to their ease of fabrication, ease of use, high convenience to analyze, and offer point-of-care detection. It is based on the identification of a color change. Xu *et al* developed a colorimetric assay for cancer cell diagnosis. In this work, messenger DNA (mDNA) was aligned with magnetic bead coated specific aptamers designed for the cancer cell. In the presence of positive sample, aptamer would bind to the analyte, result in the release of mDNA, which was cleaved into single-stranded fragments. These fragments were adsorbed on the surface of AuNPs and prevent the particle aggregation. With an increase in the concentration of analyte, stability of the AuNPs increased and the LOD was found to be 4 cells in buffer, as shown in figure 7.6 (Xu *et al* 2020). A highly sensitive sensor was developed to detect the exosomes isolated from pancreatic and breast cancer cells (Wu *et al* 2015, Xu *et al* 2020). Shayesteh *et al* created an aptamer containing poly-adenine and gold nanoparticles, for the development of a probe-free colorimetric aptasensor for prostate-specific antigen (PSA) detection in urine samples. Change in the color and shift in the UV–vis spectra confirmed the binding of PSA with the aptamer (Kim *et al* 2020).

Xia *et al* created a rapid and probe-free aptasensor for visual detection of exosomes. Single-walled carbon nanotubes were conjugated with DNA (Wang *et al* 2017). Similarly, Wang *et al* used graphitic carbon nitride nanosheets conjugated

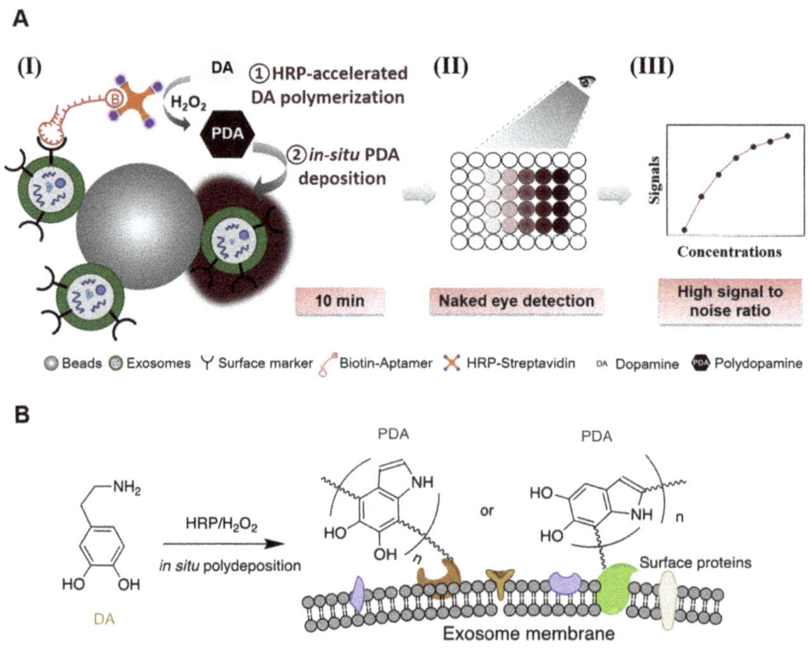

Figure 7.6. Different steps of fabrication of colorimetric sensor for detection of exosomes. (A) (I) Exosomes were attached to beads and captured by the biotin-labeled specific aptamers and later incubated with HRP-labeled streptavidin. Interaction resulted in conversion of colorless substrate into brown-black colored product (II) With increase in the concentration of exosomes, color intensity increased which can be seen by the naked eye. (III) Signal is recorded at 400 nm. (B) The *in situ* poly-deposition process of PDA onto the surface of exosomes. Reproduced with permission from (Xu *et al* 2020). Copyright (2020) Elsevier.

with a CD63 aptamer for ultrasensitive detection of exosomes to diagnose breast cancer. In the absence of the analyte, the aptamer remained bound with the nanosheet, however, in the presence of the analyte, it detached and bound to CD63. It resulted in a change in color from dark blue to light blue.

7.4 Future perspective

Advances in science and technology have resulted in a significant improvement in cancer detection at an early stage. The development of new biomarkers and the discovery of new biomarkers not only have improved sensitive diagnostic modules but also demonstrated a dramatic improvement in the condition of cancer patients and a rise in their chances of surviving. Aptamers are highly selective, sensitive and specific in their approach for target binding. Invention of aptamer-based biosensing has a substantial impact on the clinical field. It has the potential to overcome the shortcomings of other biorecognition elements such as antibodies. It has created a great impact with respect to the reshaping the biosensing technology. Furthermore, aptamers are chemically prepared in the laboratory, which again reduces the usage of animal facilities and eliminates the batch-to-batch variability. Aptamers are considered to be highly stable, reproducible, cost effective and flexible with respect to their counterparts. Several aptasensors have been developed for different analytes such as heavy metal, antibiotic contamination, viral and bacterial protein detection and for cancer diagnostics. Although several aptamer-based sensors are available, these techniques are still at their initial stage at clinical trials. Application of aptasensors is currently restricted at the laboratory level.

7.5 Conclusion

Herein, several aptasensors based on electrochemical and optical platforms for cancer diagnostics were discussed. Moreover, the involvement of different biomarkers such as PSA, CA125, MCF-7, mucin-1, growth factors and exosomes were elaborated in detail. Researchers have focused on the development of chemically synthesized biorecognition elements, which can overcome the shortcomings of current diagnostic techniques. Optical and electrochemical sensors discussed here exhibit a remarkable sensitivity and specificity, however, some of the technology and challenges related to the feasibility of these aptasensors still needs to be addressed. In addition to that, aptamers generated for cancer diagnostics need further investigation prior to clinical application. Overall, it is evident that the emergence of aptasensors is paving a new path for new possibilities in science and it is still on the way to a bright future.

Author contributions

Conceptualization—SG; investigation—SG and DS; writing—original draft preparation—DS and SG; writing—review and editing, SG; supervision—DS and SG.

Conflicts of interest

The authors declare no conflict of interest.

Acknowledgments

We are grateful for the research endowment under the Intensification of Research in High Priority Area (IRHPA) program (Grant No. IPA/2020/000069), Core Research Grant (Grant No. CRG/2020/003014), Women Excellence Award (Grant No. WEA/2020/000036) from Science and Engineering Research Board (SERB), New Delhi, and Extramural Research (Grant No. BT/PR34216/AAQ/1/765/2019) Department of Biotechnology, New Delhi.

References

Alizadeh N, Hashemi J and Shahdost-Fard F 2021 Spectrofluorimetric study of the complexation of ochratoxin A and Cu^{2+}: towards the hybrid fluorimetric sensor and visual detection of ochratoxin A in wheat flour samples from farm to fork *Food Chem.* **350** 129204

Animesh S and Singh Y D 2020 A comprehensive study on aptasensors for cancer diagnosis *Curr. Pharm. Biotechnol.* **22** 1069–84

Atta N F, Galal A and El-Ads E H 2015 Graphene—a platform for sensor and biosensor applications *Biosensors: Micro and Nanoscale Applications* (InTech)

Bai W *et al* 2015 Gold nanoparticle-based colorimetric aptasensor for rapid detection of six organophosphorous pesticides *Environ. Toxicol. Chem.* **34** 2244–9

Bala R *et al* 2017 Detection of organophosphorus pesticide—Malathion in environmental samples using peptide and aptamer based nanoprobes *Chem. Eng. J.* **311** 111–6

Banga I *et al* 2019 Biosensors and their application for the detection of avian influenza virus *Nanotechnology in Modern Animal Biotechnology* (Elsevier) pp 1–16

Blanco-Formoso M and Alvarez-Puebla R A 2020 Cancer diagnosis through SERS and other related techniques *Int. J. Mol. Sci.* **21** 2253

Cao Y *et al* 2014 Aptamer-based homogeneous protein detection using cucurbit[7]uril functionalized electrode *Anal. Chim. Acta* **812** 45–9

Cha T *et al* 2014 Rapid aptasensor capable of simply diagnosing prostate cancer *Biosens. Bioelectron.* **62** 31–7

Chang C C 2021 Recent advancements in aptamer-based surface plasmon resonance biosensing strategies *Biosensors* **11** 233

Chouhan R S *et al* 2021 Magnetic nanoparticles—a multifunctional potential agent for diagnosis and therapy *Cancers* **13** 2213

Cisterna B A *et al* 2016 Targeted nanoparticles for colorectal cancer *Nanomedicine* **11** 2443–56

Connor E E *et al* 2005 Gold nanoparticles are taken up by human cells but do not cause acute cytotoxicity *Small* **1** 325–7

Cui F and Zhou H S 2020 Diagnostic methods and potential portable biosensors for coronavirus disease 2019 *Biosens. Bioelectron.* **165** 112349

Damborska D *et al* 2017 Nano material-based biosensors for detection of prostate specific antigen *Microchim. Acta* **184** 3049–67

Densmore A *et al* 2008 Spiral-path high-sensitivity silicon photonic wire molecular sensor with temperature-independent response *Opt. Lett.* **33** 596

De Souza Castilho M *et al* 2011 Magneto immunoassays for plasmodium falciparum histidine-rich protein 2 related to malaria based on magnetic nanoparticles *Anal. Chem.* **83** 5570–7

Duan F *et al* 2018 Bifunctional aptasensor based on novel two-dimensional nanocomposite of MoS_2 quantum dots and g-C3N4 nanosheets decorated with chitosan-stabilized Au nanoparticles for selectively detecting prostate specific antigen *Anal. Chim. Acta* **1036** 121–32

Duan N *et al* 2012 Gold nanoparticle-based fluorescence resonance energy transfer aptasensor for ochratoxin a detection *Anal. Lett.* **45** 714–23

Ermini M L *et al* 2014 Bioanalytical approaches for the detection of single nucleotide polymorphisms by surface plasmon resonance biosensors *Biosens. Bioelectron.* **61** 28–37

Fei Y *et al* 2015 Characterization of receptor binding profiles of influenza a viruses using an ellipsometry-based label-free glycan microarray assay platform *Biomolecules* **5** 1480–98

Gandhi S, Arami H and Krishnan K M 2016 Detection of cancer-specific proteases using magnetic relaxation of peptide-conjugated nanoparticles in biological environment *Nano Lett.* **16** 3668–74

Guo C *et al* 2017 Aptamer-templated silver nanoclusters embedded in zirconium metal-organic framework for bifunctional electrochemical and spr aptasensors toward carcinoembryonic antigen *ACS Appl. Mater. Interfaces* **9** 41188–99

Gupta A *et al* 2016 Ultrastable and biofunctionalizable gold nanoparticles *ACS Appl. Mater. Interfaces* **8** 14096–101

Hamd-Ghadareh S *et al* 2017 An amplified comparative fluorescence resonance energy transfer immunosensing of CA125 tumor marker and ovarian cancer cells using green and economic carbon dots for bio-applications in labeling, imaging and sensing *Biosens. Bioelectron.* **96** 308–16

Hashemian Z *et al* 2016 Aptasensor based on fluorescence resonance energy transfer for the analysis of adenosine in urine samples of lung cancer patients *Biosens. Bioelectron.* **79** 334–40

Hassan E M and DeRosa M C 2020 Recent advances in cancer early detection and diagnosis: role of nucleic acid based aptasensors *TrAC Trends Anal. Chem.* **124** 115806

He W *et al* 2012 X-aptamers: a bead-based selection method for random incorporation of druglike moieties onto next-generation aptamers for enhanced binding *Biochemistry* **51** 8321–3

Homola J 2003 Present and future of surface plasmon resonance biosensors *Anal. Bioanal. Chem.* **377** 528–39

Homola J, Yee S S and Gauglitz G 1999 Surface plasmon resonance sensors: review *Sensors Actuators* B **54** 3–15

Hosseinzadeh L and Mazloum-Ardakani M 2020 Advances in aptasensor technology *Adv. Clin. Chem.* **99** 237–79

Islam S *et al* 2019 A smart nanosensor for the detection of human immunodeficiency virus and associated cardiovascular and arthritis diseases using functionalized raphene-based transistors *Biosens. Bioelectron.* **126** 792–9

Jie G and Jie G 2016 Sensitive electrochemiluminescence detection of cancer cells based on a CdSe/ZnS quantum dot nanocluster by multibranched hybridization chain reaction on gold nanoparticles *RSC Adv.* **6** 24780–5

Kasoju A, Shahdeo D, Khan A A, Shrikrishna N S, Mahari S, Alanazi A M, Bhat M A, Giri J and Ghandi S 2020a Fabrication of microfluidic device for Aflatoxin M1 detection in milk samples with specific aptamers *Sci. Rep.* **10** 4627

Kasoju A, Shrikrishna N S, Shahdeo D, Khan A A, Alanazi A M and Gandhi S 2020b Microfluidic paper device for rapid detection of aflatoxin B1 using an aptamer based colorimetric assay *RSC Adv.* **10** 11843–50

Kawaguchi T *et al* 2007 Fabrication of a novel immunosensor using functionalized self-assembled monolayer for trace level detection of TNT by surface plasmon resonance *Talanta* **72** 554–60

Kawamura A and Miyata T 2016 Biosensors *Biomaterials Nanoarchitectonics* (Elsevier) pp 157–76

Kim M, Kim K and Lee J H 2020 A cost-effective and rapid aptasensor with chemiluminescence detection for the early diagnosis of prostate cancer *Microchem. J.* **155** 104763

Kim S J *et al* 2007 Novel miniature SPR immunosensor equipped with all-in-one multi-microchannel sensor chip for detecting low-molecular-weight analytes *Biosens. Bioelectron.* **23** 701–7

Kong Y *et al* 2010 Development of a monoclonal antibody-based enzyme immunoassay for the pyrethroid insecticide deltamethrin *J. Agric. Food Chem.* **58** 8189–95

Kuipers E J *et al* 2015 Colorectal cancer *Nat. Rev. Dis. Primers.* **1** 15065

Lai R Y, Plaxco K W and Heeger A J 2007 Aptamer-based electrochemical detection of picomolar platelet-derived growth factor directly in blood serum *Anal. Chem.* **79** 229–33

Li Y *et al* 2016 A simple aptamer-functionalized gold nanorods based biosensor for the sensitive detection of MCF-7 breast cancer cells *Chem. Commun.* **52** 3959–61

Liu M *et al* 2019 Aptasensors for pesticide detection *Biosens. Bioelectron.* **130** 174–84

Liu R *et al* 2017 Surface plasmon resonance biosensor for sensitive detection of microRNA and cancer cell using multiple signal amplification strategy *Biosens. Bioelectron.* **87** 433–8

Loyez M *et al* 2020 Rapid detection of circulating breast cancer cells using a multiresonant optical fiber aptasensor with plasmonic amplification *ACS Sens.* **5** 454–63

Lund S A, Giachelli C M and Scatena M 2009 The role of osteopontin in inflammatory processes *J. Cell Commun. Signal.* **3** 311

Mahari S and Gandhi S 2022 Electrochemical immunosensor for detection of avian Salmonellosis based on electroactive reduced graphene oxide (rGO) modified electrode *Bioelectrochemistry* **144** 108036

Majdinasab M, Ben Aissa S and Marty J L 2020 Advances in colorimetric strategies for mycotoxins detection: toward rapid industrial monitoring *Toxins* **13** 13

Malecka K, Mikuła E and Ferapontova E E 2021 Design strategies for electrochemical aptasensors for cancer diagnostic devices *Sensors* **21** 736

Meirinho S G *et al* 2015 Development of an electrochemical RNA-aptasensor to detect human osteopontin *Biosens. Bioelectron.* **71** 332–41

Mishra P, Munjal T and Gandhi S 2019 Nanoparticles for detection, imaging, and diagnostic applications in animals *Nanoscience for Sustainable Agriculture* (Springer) pp 437–77

Moitra P *et al* 2020 Selective naked-eye detection of SARS-CoV-2 mediated by N gene targeted antisense oligonucleotide capped plasmonic nanoparticles *ACS Nano* **14** 7617–27

Najitha Banu A, Balasubramanian C and Moorthi P V 2014 Biosynthesis of silver nanoparticles using *Bacillus thuringiensis* against dengue vector, *Aedes aegypti* (Diptera: Culicidae) *Parasitol. Res.* **113** 311–6

Nandi S *et al* 2020 Biosensor platforms for rapid HIV detection *Adv. Clin. Chem.* **98** 1–34

Narlawar S S and Gandhi S 2021 Fabrication of graphene nanoplatelets embedded ‘partition cartridge’ for efficient separation of target-bound ssDNA during SELEX *Mater. Today Adv.* **12** 100174

Ng E W M *et al* 2006 Pegaptanib, a targeted anti-VEGF aptamer for ocular vascular disease *Nat. Rev. Drug. Discov.* **5** 123–32

Noh H, Hong S and Huang S 2013 Role of urokinase receptor in tumor progression and development *Theranostics* **3** 487–95

Pandey A K *et al* 2018 Prediction of shorter oligonucleotide sequences recognizing aflatoxin M1 *Biotechnol. Appl. Biochem.* **65** 397–406

Pei K *et al* 2018 Colorimetric ELISA for ochratoxin A detection based on the urease-induced metallization of gold nanoflowers *Sensors Actuators* B **262** 102–9

Pei X *et al* 2020 Competitive aptasensor for the ultrasensitive multiplexed detection of cancer biomarkers by fluorescent nanoparticle counting *Analyst* **145** 3612–9

Piliarik M, Vaisocherová H and Homola J 2009 Surface plasmon resonance biosensing. *Methods Mol. Biol.* **503** 65–88

Pineros M *et al* 2021 Scaling up the surveillance of childhood cancer: a global roadmap *JNCI: J. Natl. Cancer Inst.* **113** 9–15

Porciani D *et al* 2018 Modular cell-internalizing aptamer nanostructure enables targeted delivery of large functional RNAs in cancer cell lines *Nat. Commun.* **9** 1–13

Qureshi A, Gurbuz Y and Niazi J H 2015a Capacitive aptamer-antibody based sandwich assay for the detection of VEGF cancer biomarker in serum *Sensors Actuators* B **209** 645–51

Qureshi A, Gurbuz Y and Niazi J H 2015b Label-free capacitance based aptasensor platform for the detection of HER2/ErbB2 cancer biomarker in serum *Sensors Actuators* B **220** 1145–51

Rampado R *et al* 2019 Nanovectors design for theranostic applications in colorectal cancer *J. Oncol.* **2019** 2740923

Roberts A *et al* 2020 Graphene functionalized field-effect transistors for ultrasensitive detection of Japanese encephalitis and Avian influenza virus *Sci. Rep.* **10** 1–12

Roberts A *et al* 2021 Label-free detection of SARS-CoV-2 Spike S1 antigen triggered by electroactive gold nanoparticles on antibody coated fluorine-doped tin oxide (FTO) electrode *Anal. Chim. Acta* **1188** 339207

Roberts A *et al* 2022 Electroactive reduced graphene oxide for highly sensitive detection of secretory non-structural 1 protein: a potential diagnostic biomarker for Japanese encephalitis virus *Biosens. Bioelectron.* **198** 113837

Roberts A and Gandhi S 2020 Japanese encephalitis virus: a review on emerging diagnostic techniques *Front. Biosci. (Landmark)*

Roberts A, Tripathi P P and Gandhi S 2019 Graphene nanosheets as an electric mediator for ultrafast sensing of urokinase plasminogen activator receptor-A biomarker of cancer *Biosens. Bioelectron.* **141** 111398

Sametband M *et al* 2007 Application of nanoparticles for the enhancement of latent fingerprints *Chem. Commun.* **2007** 1142

Sekhon S S *et al* 2021 2D graphene oxide–aptamer conjugate materials for cancer diagnosis *npj 2D Mater. Appl.* **5** 1–19

Shahdeo D *et al* 2020 Graphene based sensors *Compr. Anal. Chemstry* **91** 175

Shahdeo D *et al* 2021 Self-assembled chitosan polymer intercalating peptide functionalized gold nanoparticles as nanoprobe for efficient imaging of urokinase plasminogen activator receptor in cancer diagnostics *Carbohydrate Polym.* **266** 118138

Shahdeo D and Khan A A *et al* 2022a Molecular diagnostic of ochratoxin a with specific aptamers in corn and groundnut via fabrication of a microfluidic device *Front Nutr* **9** 851787

Shahdeo D and Roberts A *et al* 2022b Polymeric biocompatible iron oxide nanoparticles labeled with peptides for imaging in ovarian cancer *Biosci. Rep.* **42** 20212622

Shahdeo D, Chandra A B and Gandhi S 2021 Urokinase plasminogen activator receptor-mediated targeting of a stable nanocomplex coupled with specific peptides for imaging of cancer *Anal. Chem.* **93** 11868–77

Shahdeo D and Gandhi S 2022 Next generation biosensors as a cancer diagnostic tool *Biosensor Based Advanced Cancer Diagnostics* (Academic)

Souada M *et al* 2015 Label-free electrochemical detection of prostate-specific antigen based on nucleic acid aptamer *Biosens. Bioelectron.* **68** 49–54

Sun Y *et al* 2020 Highly sensitive detection of cytochrome c in the NSCLC serum using a hydrophobic paper based–gold nanourchin substrate *Biomed. Opt. Express* **11** 7062

Talan A *et al* 2018 Ultrasensitive electrochemical immuno-sensing platform based on gold nanoparticles triggering chlorpyrifos detection in fruits and vegetables *Biosens. Bioelectron.* **105** 14–21

Thiviyanathan V and Gorenstein D G 2012 Aptamers and the next generation of diagnostic reagents *Proteomics. Clin. Appl.* **6** 563

Tomitaka A *et al* 2015 Lactoferrin conjugated iron oxide nanoparticles for targeting brain glioma cells in magnetic particle imaging *Nanoscale* **7** 16890–8

Tripathi P P *et al* 2018 Cell penetrating peptides in preclinical and clinical cancer diagnosis and therapy. *Oncotarget* **9** 37252–67

Tuerk C and Gold L 1990 Systematic evolution of ligands by exponential enrichment: RNA ligands to bacteriophage T4 DNA polymerase *Science* **249** 505–10

Wang Y M *et al* 2017 Enhancement of the intrinsic peroxidase-like activity of graphitic carbon nitride nanosheets by ssDNAs and its application for detection of exosomes *Anal. Chem.* **89** 12327–33

Wu W *et al* 2015 Recent progress on magnetic iron oxide nanoparticles: synthesis, surface functional strategies and biomedical applications. *Sci. Technol. Adv. Mater.* **16** 023501

Xiao K *et al* 2017 A label-free and high-efficient GO-based aptasensor for cancer cells based on cyclic enzymatic signal amplification *Biosens. Bioelectron.* **91** 76–81

Xu L *et al* 2020 Development of a simple, sensitive and selective colorimetric aptasensor for the detection of cancer-derived exosomes *Biosens. Bioelectron.* **169** 112576

Yadav S *et al* 2021 SERS based lateral flow immunoassay for point-of-care detection of SARS-CoV-2 in Clinical Samples *ACS Appl. Bio Mater.* **4** 2974–95

Yamasuji M *et al* 2011 Chemiluminescence detection of telomere DNA in human cells on a membrane by using fluorescein-5-isothiocyanate-labeled primers *Anal. Biochem.* **413** 50–4

Yazdanparast S *et al* 2018 Dual-aptamer based electrochemical sandwich biosensor for MCF-7 human breast cancer cells using silver nanoparticle labels and a poly(glutamic acid)/MWNT nanocomposite *Mikrochim. Acta* **185** 405

Yu X *et al* 2019 An aptamer-based new method for competitive fluorescence detection of exosomes *Nanoscale* **11** 15589–95

Zahra Q, Khan Q A and Luo Z 2021 Advances in optical aptasensors for early detection and diagnosis of various cancer types *Front. Oncol.* **11** 19

Zhao B *et al* 2015a Mapping the topographic epitope landscape on the urokinase plasminogen activator receptor (uPAR) by surface plasmon resonance and X-ray crystallography *Data Brief* **5** 107–13

Zhao B *et al* 2015b Stabilizing a flexible interdomain hinge region harboring the SMB binding site drives upar into its closed conformation *J. Mol. Biol.* **427** 1389–403

Zhao L *et al* 2018a A fluorescent biosensor based on molybdenum disulfide nanosheets and protein aptamer for sensitive detection of carcinoembryonic antigen *Sensors Actuators* B **273** 185–90

Zhao L *et al* 2018b Aptamers and aptasensors for highly specific recognition and sensitive detection of marine biotoxins: recent advances and perspectives *Toxins* **10** 427

Zhu Q *et al* 2013a Amperometric immunosensor for simultaneous detection of three analytes in one interface using dual functionalized graphene sheets integrated with redox-probes as tracer matrixes *Biosens. Bioelectron.* **43** 440–5

Zhu X *et al* 2013b Sensitive detection of human breast cancer cells based on aptamer-cell-aptamer sandwich architecture *Anal. Chim. Acta* **764** 59–63

Zhu Y, Chandra P and Shim Y B 2013c Ultrasensitive and selective electrochemical diagnosis of breast cancer based on a hydrazine-Au nanoparticle-aptamer bioconjugate *Anal. Chem.* **85** 1058–64

Chapter 8

Optical aptasensors for the early diagnosis of cancer biomarkers

Debanjan Ghosh, Sakshi Hardaha, Aadil Ashraf and Soumyadeep Mukherjee

Early diagnosis of cancer is the new SOS to curb the menace and timely treatment of patients across the globe. Novel and effective measures to detect cancer and its markers are brimming up in the medical diagnostic sector every now and then. Optical aptamers based on biosensor technology are the next-generation high-throughput technology in development. Solid preciseness, cost-effective fabrication, high sensitivity, long-term usage, absolute accuracy, and patient acceptance are the major factors that are addressed in addition to identifying the appropriate biomarker candidate involved. This chapter comprehends the utility and mechanism of action of optical aptamers, their latest developments, and advances over conventional methods in diagnosing various benign and metastatic cancer biomarkers.

8.1 Introduction

Cancer is a type of disease caused by normal cells losing the usual control over their division, differentiation, and apoptosis and becoming tumor cells. So, a tumor results from an abnormal proliferation of cells without differentiation and apoptosis. Cancer is now the world's second most significant cause of mortality, trailing only behind cardiovascular diseases. Breast, stomach, colorectal, liver and lung cancer are the most frequent cancers, generating a high mortality rate yearly [1]. As a result, early cancer detection has been the key to preventing organ damage and improving cancer patient survival. Currently, various cancer diagnostic techniques are available, including mammography, cervical cytology, colonoscopy, molecular detection, immunohistochemistry, and cancer imaging. They have their own limitations and may give false-positive results [2]. In immunohistochemistry, staining results may vary considerably. Molecular detection techniques are quite expensive and require a lot of tumor tissue to detect the presence of cancer. Thus, the quantitative measurement of cancer-specific biomarkers plays a critical role in implementing

doi:10.1088/978-0-7503-5012-9ch8

preventive strategies and monitoring prognosis and recurrence outcomes. Many enzyme immunoassays are currently in use to detect cancer biomarkers. Although these assays are precise in their antigen–antibody interaction, they are not extensively relied upon because of antibodies' high production cost and relatively low stability. Therefore, aptamers can be considered an alternative to antibodies for early diagnosis of cancer biomarkers [3].

Aptamers can be defined as short DNA or RNA molecules (oligonucleotides, ONs) or their related analogs that have the ability to bind to a numerous range of targets with high selectivity and specificity. The aptamers include metal ions, organic dyes, nucleotides, amino acids, peptides, proteins, enzymes, whole cells, and even entire organisms, such as viruses or bacteria, due to their unique three-dimensional folding [4]. They are typically recognized using a technique known as Systematic Evolution of Ligands by Exponential Enrichment (SELEX). It is an *in vitro* stepwise process that allows the selection of high-affinity ligands for the chosen chemical or biological targets from libraries of 1015–1016 different oligonucleotide sequences [5]. The non-binding aptamers are generally discarded. They utilize various interactions, which include electrostatic and hydrophobic interactions, van der Waals forces, π–π stacking, and structural complementarity, to interact with their targets [4]. Aptamers have several advantages. Aptamers have several advantages firstly they can recognize a variety of biological substrates using high affinity and specificity. Secondly, aptamers have excellent thermal stability and can tolerate repeated denaturation and renaturation. Third, aptamers are simple to synthesize and functionalize. Aptamers are ideal recognition elements for biosensors because of their desirable properties.

Various biosensors have been developed owing to various properties of signal transduction, such as fluorescence resonance energy transfer (FRET), surface plasmon resonance (SPR), chemiluminescence, and other calorimetric methods. Fluorescent sensors have garnered much more attention than other biosensors due to their high sensitivity, simple operation, quick reaction, non-destructive and minor damage to cells and ability to provide real-time information.

Fluorescent aptasensors offer promising potential for analyte detection by integrating aptamers as the element for recognition and fluorescence analytical methods, which helps in the transduction of signals [3].

This chapter will summarize recent advances in optical aptasensors (fluorescence, chemiluminescence, surface plasmon resonance, and calorimetric) for targeting tumor-related biomarkers such as vascular endothelial growth factor (VEGF), prostate-specific antigen (PSA), carcinoembryonic antigen (CEA), thrombin and mucin 1 (MUC1). Cancer biomarkers have essential and diverse features that make them unique and highly detectable by optical biosensors. These features include their concentration in the blood, precise location in the body and association–dissociation kinetics with its cognate aptamer. The use of optical aptasensors in the detection of various cancer biomarkers will be discussed in the upcoming section. The various optical aptasensors include fluorescence, chemiluminescence, calorimetric and SPR-based aptasensors. We also highlight the merits and demerits of aptasensors and the upcoming challenges associated with them.

8.2 Fluorescence-based aptasensors

The most commonly used optical biosensors for cancer detection are fluorescent aptasensors. They have gained popularity due to their reproducibility, simplicity, sensitivity, efficiency, and cheap rates [6]. There are specifically two types of aptamer-based fluorescent biosensors: label-free aptamers and fluorescently labeled aptamers. These aptamers generally use the technique of fluorescence resonance energy transfer (FRET) to produce 'ON' and 'OFF' signals. The ON signal represents an increase (i.e. 'signal-on') whereas the OFF signal represents a reduction (i.e. 'signal-off'). The concentration of the target can be quantitatively measured by noting the signal change (increase or decrease) which represents the binding of the aptamer with its target [7].

This chapter offers an overview of fluorescent-based optical aptasensors that commonly use fluorescent techniques to detect significant cancer biomarkers, essentially proteins/receptors in both soluble and cancer cell membrane-bound forms. This chapter summarizes the most recent fluorescent aptasensors available, which can target cancer-related biomarkers such as VEGF, CEA, PSA, Elastase, thrombin and mucin.

8.2.1 VEGF

As a signaling protein, vascular endothelial growth factor (VEGF) functions in regulating vascular development as well as permeabilization (angiogenesis) [8]. The most common and potent pro-angiogenic variant of VEGF, VEGF165, is generally overexpressed in various cancer types and thus has been recognized as a significant serum biomarker for cancer.

Li *et al* invented a technique that was based on structural switching of DNA assembly and isothermal amplification, which could easily target VEGF165 in serum samples as shown in figure 8.1 [9]. This method made use of six separate DNA

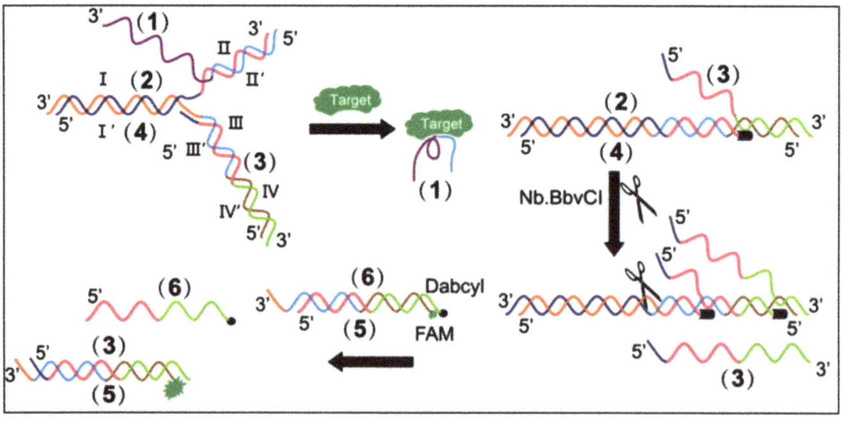

Figure 8.1. This diagram depicts the VEGF detection methodology developed by Li *et al*. This method switches DNA assembly structure and amplifies it isothermally after cleavage by nicking endonuclease. Reproduced with permission from [9]. Copyright (2016) Elsevier.

sequences: the VEGF aptamer (1), primer (2), protector (3), a template (4), fluorescent-labeled strand (5), and a quencher labeled strand (6). (1), (2), (3), and (4) strands hybridize in the absence of VEGF, generating a complex assembly that resists strand displacement and an extension activity. The presence of the target releases the aptamer sequence (1) from the assembly. This in turn exposes the II' domain of (2), which can interact with the III' domain of (4), displacing the III domain of (3). The polymerization reaction is triggered by the creation of the (2)/(4) complex, which is catalyzed by a polymerase using the deoxynucleotide triphosphates. The next displacement cycle, nicking, and polymerization events are initiated when a nicking endonuclease cleaves the duplex (2)/(4) at its unique recognition site during polymerization. The DNA (3) that is generated at the end of each cycle displaces the dabcyl-labeled-(6) strand from the duplex (5)/(6). The FAM dye fluorescence is regained after removing (5) from (6). Thus, fluorescence is detected. This method can detect up to 3.5 pg ml^{-1} of VEGF165 in serum samples.

The strong quenching ability of GO with the assistance of a nicking endonuclease to amplify signal was used by Li *et al* to create a platform for the detection of VEGF (figure 8.2) [10]. A stable complex of two aptamer subunits Apt1 and Apt2 is not formed in the absence of VEGF, and the addition of GO results in fluorescence quenching. When VEGF is present a duplex DNA region comprising the VEGF/aptamer is formed. The duplex DNA can be recognized by the nicking endonuclease and it cleaves Apt1 into two short pieces of DNA. The short FAM-labeled DNA fragment binds weakly to GO and the fluorescence intensity gradually increases after multiple cycles of enzyme cleavage. This method was susceptible, and VEGF can be detected up to limits of 1 pM.

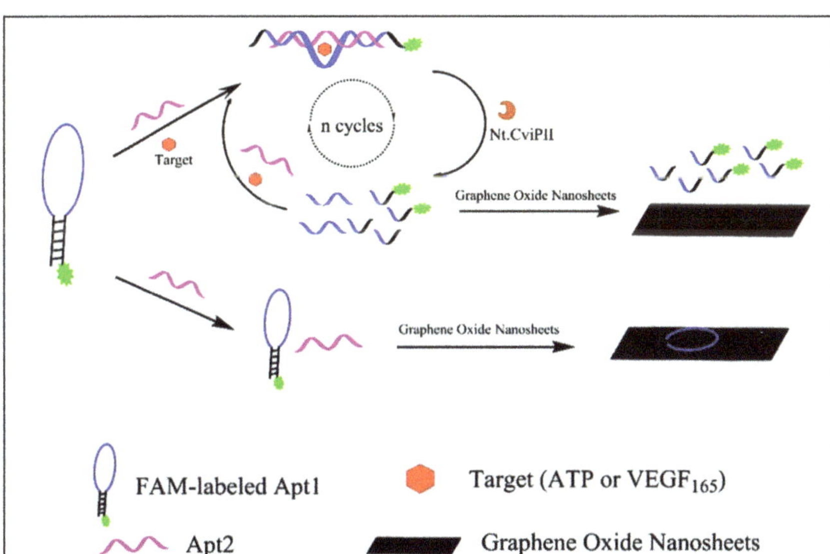

Figure 8.2. Schematic representation of the GO-based fluorescent aptasensor for VEGF detection. Reproduced with permission from [10]. Copyright (2015) Royal Society of Chemistry.

8.2.2 CEA

Carcinoembryonic antigen (CEA), a human glycoprotein, is a broad-spectrum cancer marker that is used to diagnose various clinical disorders, including ovarian cancer, pancreatic cancer, gastric cancer, and, most notably, colorectal cancer [11]. Healthy people have less CEA levels in the blood than cancer patients which makes CEA a potent cancer biomarker. As a result, reliable quantification of CEA in the blood is critical for early cancer diagnosis and therapy evaluation. Specific sensors for CEA detection have gained considerable interest in recent years. This chapter discusses some of the particular sensors for CEA detection.

A fluorescent aptasensor was developed by Zhao *et al* for easy, rapid, and sensitive CEA detection [12]. As shown in figure 8.3, the fluorescence of the fluorophore-labeled CEA aptamer was quenched as it got adsorbed via hydrophobic and π-stacking interactions on the surface of MoS_2 nanosheets. In the presence of CEA, the CEA-specific aptamer changed its structure by interacting with CEA, resulting in fluorescence recovery. This assay demonstrated reproducibility and excellent selectivity. This technique could detect CEA to levels as low as 34 pg ml^{-1}.

8.2.3 PSA

The most compelling and trusted biomarker for detecting prostate cancer is prostate-specific antigen (PSA), which is a single-chain glycoprotein (33–34 kDa). It has been found that average PSA serum concentrations in men are less than 4 ng ml^{-1} and it rises when prostate cancer develops [3]. As a result, early clinical diagnoses of

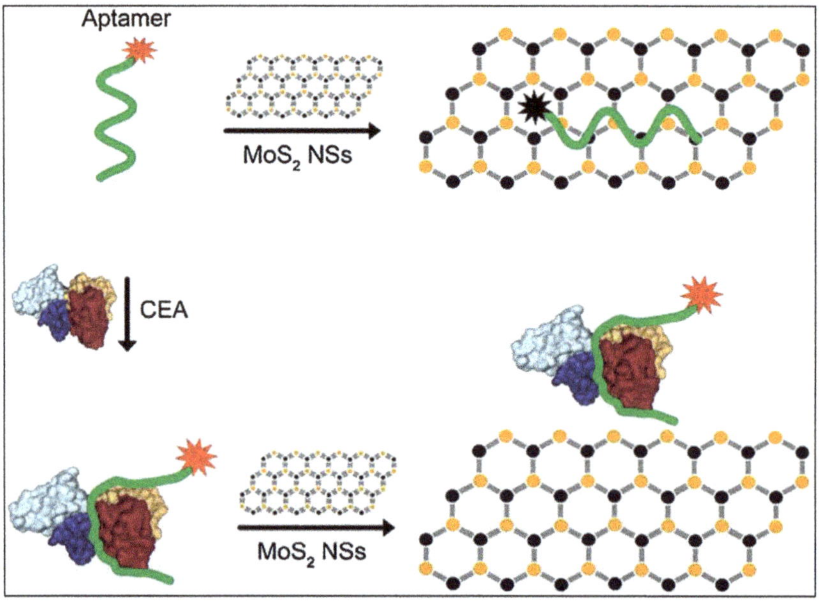

Figure 8.3. Schematic representation of the MoS_2 nanosheet-based fluorescent biosensor for CEA detection. Reproduced with permission from [12]. Copyright (2018) Elsevier.

prostate cancer can be made by measuring the concentration of PSA in serum and tumor tissues. Thus, it would be easier to treat patients suffering from prostate cancer.

To detect PSA in serum, a fluorescent anisotropy (FA) test was developed by Zhao and colleagues [13]. This test uses a dye-labeled aptamer that can be adsorbed onto the Cu-based metal–organic gel (Cu-MOG). The adsorption onto the Cu-MOG gel in the absence of PSA increases the FA value considerably. The presence of PSA lowers the FA value as well as the fluorescence due to the separation of aptamers from the MOG surface. This method can detect PSA in serum to levels of 0.33 ng ml^{-1}.

Recently, a label-free DNA-AgNC/aptamer hybridization probe was developed by Fang *et al* to detect PSA in serum (figure 8.4) [14]. The fluorescence of DNA-AgNCs can be increased when the PSA aptamer base pairs with it. At the same time, the fluorescence of DNA-AgNC is reduced when PSA competitively binds to its aptamer. The aptamer cannot raise the fluorescence of DNA-AgNC in the presence of PSA. This sensor can quantitatively determine PSA in spiked human serum.

8.2.4 Elastase

Neutrophils are the innate immune system's initial line of defense. They are essential in chronic and acute inflammation and act by defending against non-self and infectious agents. Human neutrophil elastase (HNE), which is a serine proteinase, is the primary enzyme secreted by neutrophil granulocytes. Tumor proliferation and metastasis are promoted by HNE, making it one of the primary reasons for cancer progression. Furthermore, the levels of HNE rise during carcinogenesis, making HNE a promising biomarker for cancer detection [7].

Charlton *et al* [15] made use of a randomized DNA-valine phosphonate library to identify an aptamer against HNE produced from active neutrophils. After appropriate fluorescent labeling, the same research group employed this aptamer for

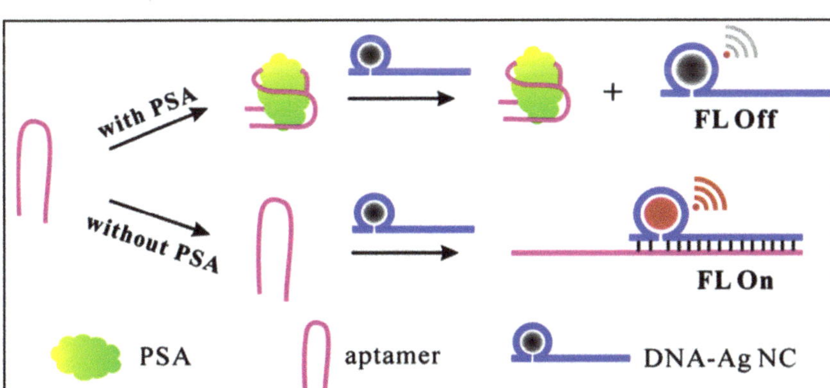

Figure 8.4. Schematic of the PSA detection based on inhibiting the fluorescence enhancement of DNA-AgNC induced by PSA aptamer. Reproduced with permission from [14]. Copyright (2019) Elsevier.

in vivo and *in vitro* diagnostic studies. Fortunately, the fluorescent intensity of the aptamer was proved by the researchers for both *in vivo* and *in vitro* studies.

A fluorescent aptasensor was recently developed by He *et al* that relied on the competitive binding for the detection of HNE [16]. Three oligonucleotides are employed in this assay. The first one is the HNE aptamer. The molecular beacon and a short DNA sequence are the second and third oligonucleotides, respectively. Fluorescein and dabcyl are coupled to the 5′ and 3′ ends of the molecular beacon, respectively. The short DNA sequence is partly complementary to the aptamer sequence and partly to the loop of the molecular beacon (figure 8.5). In the absence of HNE, the aptamer is incubated with a short DNA sequence. It is then allowed to react with the molecular beacon after incubation. As a result of the interaction between the aptameric sequence and the short DNA, the molecular beacon cannot interact with the short DNA sequence. Hence, fluorescence is turned off. In the presence of HNE, the aptamer cannot interact with the short DNA as it binds to HNE. This allows the short DNA sequence to hybridize with the molecular beacon and produce a bright fluorescence signal due to the separation of fluorescent from the quencher. HNE could be detected to levels of 47 pM using this approach.

8.2.5 Thrombin

Thrombin is a critical protein known for its physiological role in hemostasis, thrombosis, and other blood coagulation events [7]; Alzheimer's and cancer are related to changed thrombin concentration levels in the blood.

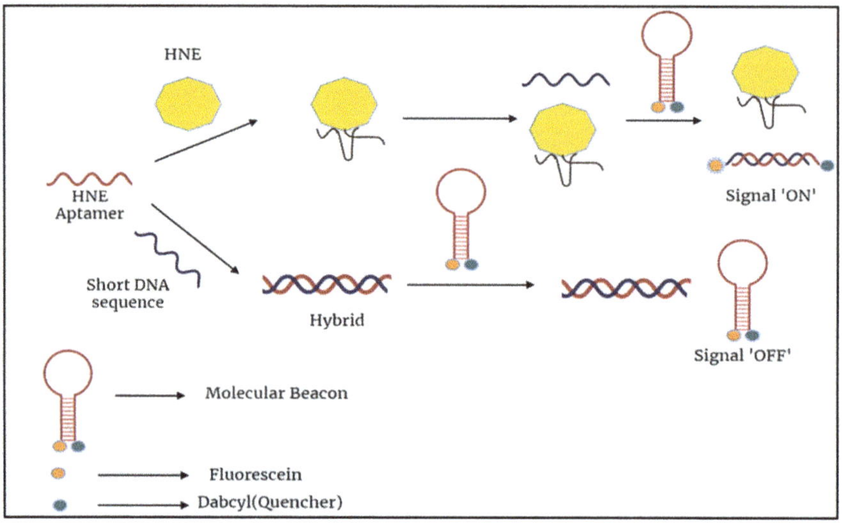

Figure 8.5. Schematic representation of elastase detection strategy based on the competitive binding involving the elastase aptamer, a molecular beacon, and a short DNA sequence.

Thrombin detection is based on fluorescence sensing systems developed by Deng and coworkers who primarily made use of thrombin binding antigen (TBA) to detect the presence of thrombin [17].

Recently, Du *et al* used fluorescence resonance energy transfer (FRET) to develop a novel label-free thrombin detection assay [18]. The cationic conjugated polymer (CCP) acts as the energy donor to an Ir(III) complex, which acts as the acceptor (figure 8.6). π–π stacking and electrostatic interactions act to hold the energy donor and the acceptor in the system, resulting in fluorescence amplification by FRET. TBA29 disrupts the planned order between CCP and the Ir(III) complex, and the FRET between CCP and the Ir(III) complex is insignificant (quenching effect). The folding of the aptamer in the presence of thrombin restores fluorescence, which allows the quantitative detection of thrombin ('signal-on' mode). The test detects thrombin at concentrations as low as 0.05 pM and could easily discriminate against other proteins.

The use of gold nanoparticles (AuNPs) or nanostructures as fluorescence quenchers is done by various research groups. TBA15 is used as a probe in association with these fluorescence quenchers. In presence of thrombin, the fluorescence is turned on when the fluorophore gets separated from the Au surfaces. The fluorescent TBA15 derivatives are attached to AuNPs via specific adsorption (figure 8.7(A)). TBA may also form duplexes via complementary sequences covalently linked to the NPs (figures 8.7(B) and (C)) [19]. TBA may also be attached to chitosan-coated Au nanostructures via electrostatic attractions [20]. Quenching effects are obtained with these structures. Fluorescence is recovered when the aptamer binds to thrombin forming a G-quadruplex structure. Fluorescence is turned on when the structure dissociates from the gold surface.

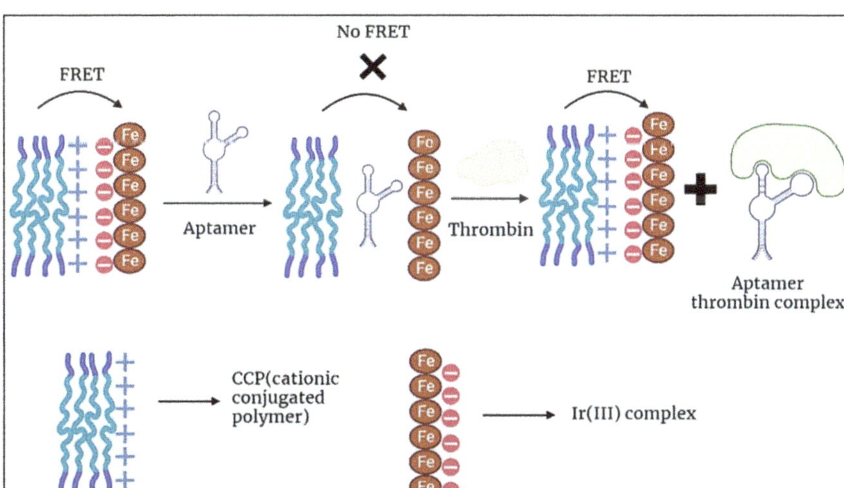

Figure 8.6. The fluorescence resonance energy transfer between CCP and Ir (III) complex is disrupted by the aptamer TBA29. Fluorescence is turned on when thrombin interacts with aptamer TBA29 and the interaction between CCP and Ir (III) is restored.

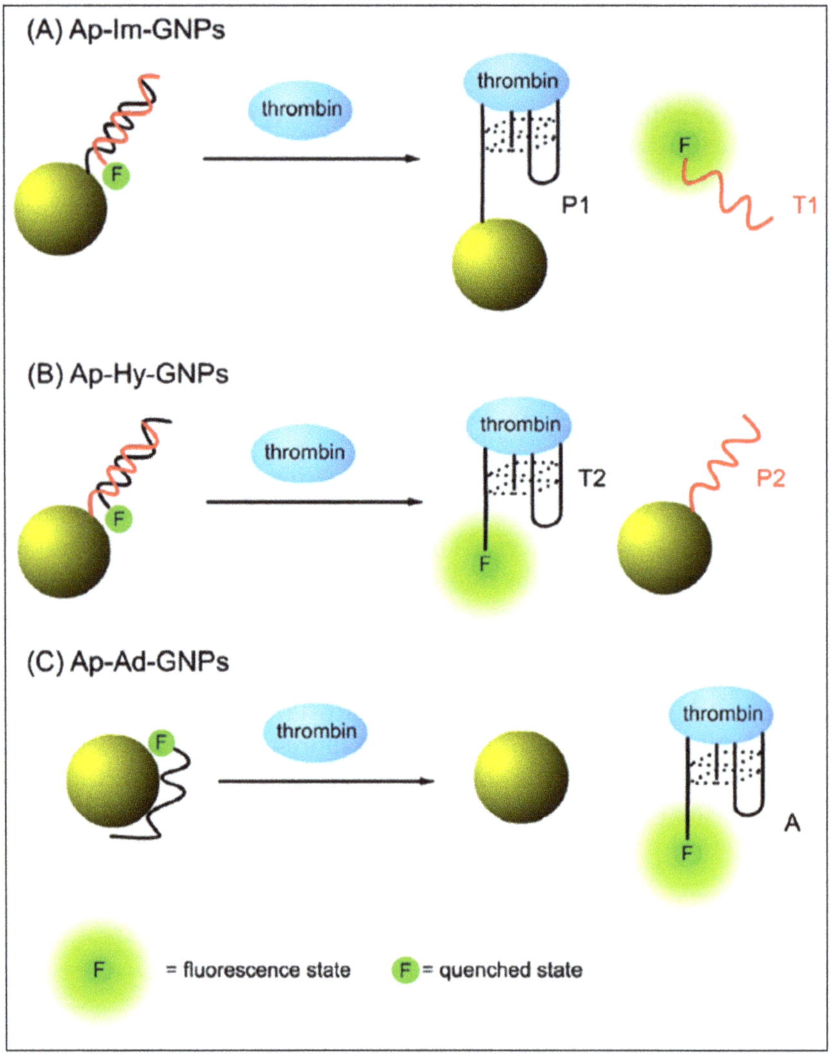

Figure 8.7. (A) Schematic illustration of the detection of thrombin with Ap–Im–GNPs, (B) Ap–Hy–GNPs, and (C) Ap–Ad–GNPs. Reproduced with permission from [19]. Copyright (2008) Elsevier.

8.2.6 Mucin

Mucins are a protein family with a considerable molecular weight that is extensively O-glycosylated. Cell surface-associated mucins and secreted (gel-forming) mucins are the two sub-families of mucin [21]. The transmembrane mucin, Mucin 1 (MUC1) is heavily glycosylated, containing an extracellular domain that extends up to 200–500 nm from the cell surface. MUC1 is abundant in malignant tumors such as breast, ovarian, prostate, lung, and pancreatic cancers [22, 23]. 90% of breast malignancies are registered with MUC1 overexpression. It has been also observed that MUC1 is relocalized to the entire cell surface in almost all epithelial carcinomas. As a result of its direct access to membrane cells, MUC1 is a signal for poor prognosis in various malignancies and an attractive target for imaging.

Ma *et al* created a hybridization chain reaction (HCR)-based technique for detecting MUC1 peptides [24]. The oligonucleotide sequences employed in the assay are the MUC1 aptameric sequence, hairpin duplex, and two hairpin probes, H1 (hairpin probe 1) and H2 (hairpin probe 2). A stable hairpin duplex is formed from the complementary sequence, which extends from the MUC1 aptamer. The ends of the hairpin probes are labeled with FAM dyes. The hairpin structure of the aptamer is opened when it interacts with mucin. This triggers a chain reaction involving both the hairpin probes. The addition of graphene oxide results in the reduction of fluorescence by adsorbing free H1 and H2. This assay can detect mucin up to 3.33 pM and the optimum reaction time for HCR is 1 h.

He *et al* [25] used graphene oxide in their process as well. The Cy5-conjugated MUC1 fluorescent aptamer was quenched by GO in this method. The fluorescence is recovered when the aptamer detaches from the GO surface and interacts with the mucin protein, forming a compound. Mucin is detected using this approach in actual serum samples also. The detection limit of this assay is 28 nM.

8.3 Chemiluminescence-based aptasensors

Due to its cost-effective and straightforward approach, another kind of aptasensor gaining popularity nowadays is the chemiluminescence-based aptasensor [26]. Electromagnetic radiation in the form of ultraviolet, visible, or infrared radiation is released when an excited chemical species undergoes decay and returns to its ground state in terms of electric charge. This phenomenon is known as chemiluminescence (CL) [27]. The fact that it does not depend on any external light source makes this type of aptasensor more efficient by reducing any background signal produced due to an external light source [28]. The luminescence released depends only on chemical reactions to overcome the problem of reduced photon signals and enhance the signals. Nowadays, various metal nanoparticles, enzymes, or transition metals are used for luminescence [29]. Aptasensors used for diagnostic purposes in cancer is broadly classified into two categories depending on the source that triggers the phenomenon of luminescence. They are typically classified as chemiluminescence (CL) and electrochemiluminescence (ECL) [30].

8.3.1 VEGF

The property of luminol to produce chemiluminescent signals on oxidation has been widely used to develop aptasensors for diagnosing and early detection of cancers. When the horseradish peroxidase (HRP) enzyme is present, luminol gets oxidized by hydrogen peroxide (H_2O_2), producing high-intensity signals [31]. This approach has been used to develop a CL assay to identify the vascular endothelial growth factor (VEGF), a potential oncogenic biomarker found in blood circulation. The proteins of the VEGF family are involved in organogenesis in the embryonic state. It also helps in angiogenesis and leads to the creation of new blood vessels. Angiogenesis assists in the spreading of cancer by metastasis [32, 33]. This assay involves the formation of a sandwich-type immunocomplex. VEGF-specific aptasensors are coated on silicon oxide surfaces. The captured VEGF, circulating in the blood by aptamers, get recognized by the HRP antibody. Chemiluminescent signals are produced when HRP catalyzes the oxidation of luminol by H_2O_2. These signals are detected by a single-photon avalanche diode (SPAD). The SPAD-based aptasensor is able to locate the target molecules even if it is present in picomoles. It remains stable for 42 days and can be reused for finding the target molecules for up to seven cycles [34].

8.3.2 PDGF

A homolog of the platelet-derived growth factor (PDGF), PDGF-BB, has a critical role in the advancement of the tumor. This protein has been used as a biomarker to develop a CL-based aptasensor as shown in figure 8.8. Anti-human PDGF-BB raised in rabbits gets attached to the surface by means of an N-oxysuccinimide ester (referred to as NOS group) bond. The PDGF-BB gets attached to the antibody in the experimental setup, which the biotin-attached aptamer recognizes. This leads to the formation of a ternary complex. Streptavidin gold nanoparticles attach to the ternary complex. The catalytic attachment of gold metal onto the AuNPs' surface was facilitated when AuNPs on the surface reacted with $HAuCl_4$ and NH_2OH. After oxidative gold metal dissolution, a substantial number of Au^{3+} ions were released from the hydroxylamine expanded AuNPs, as assessed by a sensitive and straightforward luminol CL reaction. This particular aptasensor allows for detecting target proteins as low as 60 pM and even in serum samples that have been diluted. This assay involving a sandwich of components has provided high precision, amplified signals and accurate detection of target proteins [35].

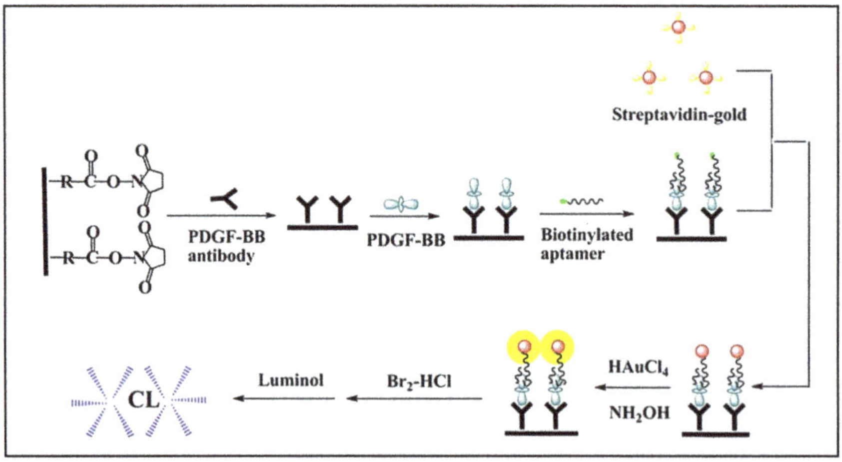

Figure 8.8. Mechanism of CL assay used for detection of PDGF-BB by utilizing biotinylated aptamer and hydroxylamine enlarged AuNPs as the recognition element and label. Reproduced with permission from [35]. Copyright (2013) Elsevier.

8.3.3 CEA

An all-in-one dual-aptasensor (figure 8.9) with 1,1′-oxalyldiimidazole (ODI) chemiluminescence detection was created using two DNA aptamers (CEA aptamer and hemin aptamer) which are connected together by means of five adenine residues. Carcinoembryonic antigen (CEA) has been reported as a tumour biomarker in cancers like breast cancer. Hemin, on binding with the DNA aptamer, has HRP-mimicking G-quadruplex DNAzyme. There is a competition between CEA and hemin for binding with the dual-DNA aptamer over a 30-minute incubation period at room temperature in a detection cell. The quantity of resorufin yielded when Amplex Red reacted with H_2O_2 was dependent on the amount of HRP-mimicking G-quadruplex DNAzyme formed after hemin was bound to the dual-DNA aptamer when introduced to the detection cell after incubation. When ODI and H_2O_2 were added to the detecting cell, a bright red light was noticed. Using ODI-CL instead of luminol Cl, this method has higher sensitivity and higher emission rates. This 'all-in-one' dual aptasensor can efficiently detect low concentrations of target molecules as low as 0.58 ng ml^{-1} [36].

8.3.4 HCL-60 cancer cells

A novel approach for detecting HL-60 cancer cells was developed using the ECL approach. Two novel items—g-C_3N_4 nanosheets (graphite-like carbon nitride) and Ag-PAMAM (Ag-polyamidoamine luminol nanocomposites) were used. The spectra of emission of g-C_3N_4 due to redox reactions match with the absorption spectrum of Ag-PAMAM-luminol NCs. This would be accompanied by redox ECL of luminol occurring at the same time. The Ag-PAMAM-luminol nanocomposites (NCs) were made first. Composite pDNA-Ag-PAMAM was generated when Ag-PAMM were allowed to hybridize using probe DNA (pDNA) and

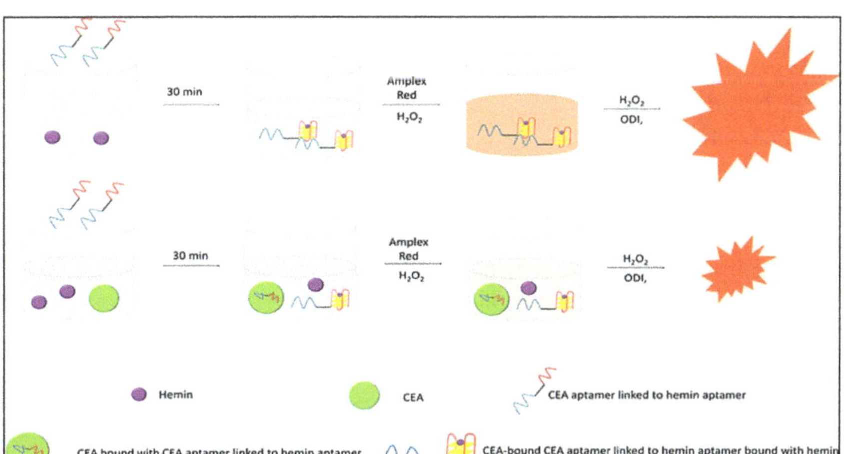

Figure 8.9. Schematic representation of how an all-in-one dual-aptasensor is used to quantify the CEA. Reproduced with permission from [36]. Copyright (2017) Elsevier.

bio-bar-code DNA (bbcDNA) on magnetic microbeads with the aptamer after functionalization. The addition of different amounts of HL-60 cells led to the production of pDNA-Ag-PAMAM after the aptamer reacted with the glycoprotein present on the cell surface. Immobilized g-C_3N_4 was functionalized with capture DNA on the electrode surface. The Ag-PAMAM-luminol NCs were then introduced to the electrode so that hybridization occurs with complementary DNA and it gets static on the electrode. The concentration of pDNA-Ag-PAMAM bioconjugate on the electrode escalated as cell concentrations escalated. When the common co-reactant H_2O_2 was available, the ECL signal of g-C_3N_4 NSs reduced, but the ECL intensity of luminol was significantly magnified. This change in the ratio of signals led to detecting the quantity of HL-60 cancer cells. It can efficiently locate 150 cells in 1 ml of the solution [37].

8.3.5 Prostate-specific antigen (PSA)

Peope suffering from prostate cancer have high levels of circulating prostate-specific antigen (PSA) in their blood. This PSA has been recognized as a potential biomarker of prostate cancer by the US FDA. Earlier diagnostic methods involved a sandwich-enzyme immunoassay. This method had several disadvantages, which include high costs, lengthy procedures, and enzymes that are unstable and lose efficiency when kept at room temperature. To avoid these circumstances an aptamer-based diagnostic tool was developed. A PSA aptamer (P: 5′-TTTTTAATTAAAGCTCGCC ATCAAATAGCTTT-3′) was linked to a hemin aptamer (H: 5′-TAAAGGGTAGGG CGG GTTGGGTAAAT-3′) with the help of five adenine residues to form a dual aptamer, which was further conjugated with biotin residue. After immobilizing the aptamer on a paramagnetic bead, they were incubated with human serum for twenty minutes at room temperature to allow competitive binding of PSA or hemin. A magnetic separator was used to separate the aptamers after the incubation was over. The dual aptamers were mixed with Amplex Red and H_2O_2 in Tris–HCl (pH 8) inside a microcentrifuge tube. Amplex Red reacted with H_2O_2 in the presence of a DNAzyme. This DNAzyme imitates the function of the horseradish peroxidase enzyme. As a result of the reaction between the dual aptamer and hemin, resorufin is formed. The higher the levels of DNAzyme, the higher the concentration of resorufin is formed. 1,1′-oxalyldiimidazole (ODI) chemiluminescence reagents such as ODI and H_2O_2 were added to resorufin. This led to the emission of bright red light. If the concentration of PSA is more compared to tyhe DNAzyme, competition occurs at the binding site. This is followed by a decrease in the brightness of the red light due to the binding of PSA to the dual aptamer instead of the DNAzyme. With the help of this approach, even scarce levels of PSA can be detected with high accuracy. 0.1 ng of PSA per ml is the limit of detection (LOD = 3 s/slope) for this aptasensor method (figure 8.10) [38].

Another DNA aptasensor to detect PSA has been designed with a high concentration of guanine residues in the sequence of the aptamer. This aptamer is linked with a 6-carboxyfluorescein (6-FAM) residue. This cheap aptasensor has been designed on the phenomenon of chemiluminescent resonance energy transfer (CRET) in guanine chemiluminescence detection. The amount or intensity of light

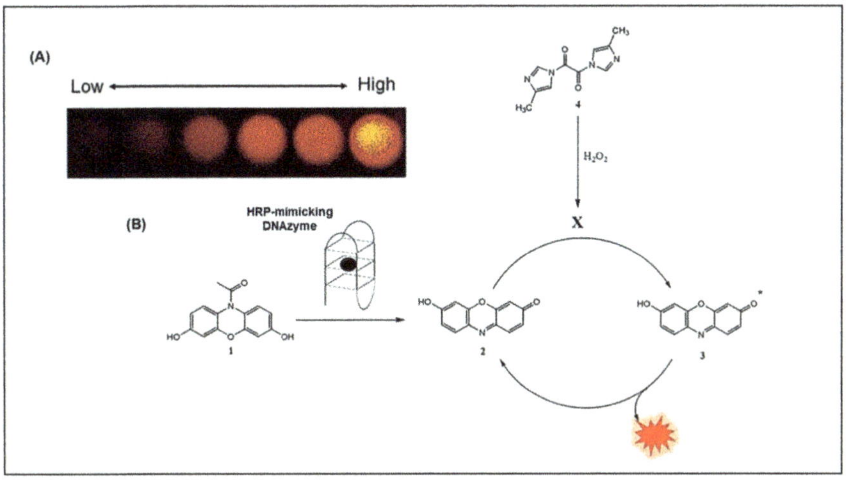

Figure 8.10. (A) Formation of resorufin when Amplex Red reacts with H_2O_2 in the presence of HRP-mimicking DNAzyme and its brightness. (B) Mechanism of the reaction between ODI-CL in the presence of HRP-mimicking DNAzyme, 1: Amplex Red, 2. Resorufin under the ground state, 3. Resorufin under the excited state, 4. ODI, X: high-energy intermediate. Reproduced with permission from [38]. Copyright (2020) Elsevier.

emitted by the guanine aptamer gets highly reduced when the G-rich DNA aptamer-conjugated 6-FAM gets bound with PSA. This technique is efficient for detecting small amounts of PSA in human serum when incubated for only thirty minutes. This aptasensor can detect over a large range of PSA concentrations, ranging from 1.9 ng ml^{-1} to 125ng ml^{-1}. The lowest amount of PSA that can be detected is 1.0 ng ml^{-1}. This approach is quite promising because the correlation coefficient of detection levels for this technique and the typical immunoassays denotes a strong linear relationship between them [39].

8.4 Colorimetric aptasensors

Colorimetric aptasensors detect biomarkers based on color change when they bind to the target, which can be seen with the unaided eye or simple instruments [30, 40]. Thus, it offers a simple, low-cost, user-friendly, and accessible diagnostic approach that may be used at the bedside [30, 41]. Colorimetric detection uses enzymes, enzyme mimics, and nanomaterials as sources [30]. Studies have frequently used enzymes, including HRP and alkaline phosphatase (ALP), to detect cancer biomarkers [30]. ALP-conjugated anti-antibody bound to an aptamer was employed in the detection of MUC1 protein that serves as a biomarker of breast, bladder, and other epithelial tumors. The resulting aptamer-antibody hybrid sandwich ELISA could sense even one microgram per milliliter of the protein based on the intensity of colored p-nitrophenol (pNP) generated [41].

HRP was used in a colorimetric aptasensor for the detection of exosomes produced from cancerous pancreatic and breast cells. In the presence of H_2O_2, it catalyzes the polymerization of colorless dopamine to black-brown polydopamine.

The proportion of target associated with the HRP-binding aptamer directly corresponds with the color intensity, allowing for highly sensitive quantitative exosome detection [42]. Enzyme mimics came into use to address the problem of enzyme instability. Furthermore, these provide sustained catalytic activity at a cheaper cost. In order to detect carcinoembryonic antigen (CEA), Zou *et al* created an aptamer-based colorimetric test using a G-quadruplex-hemin DNAzyme that, like peroxidase, turned 3,3,5,5-tetramethylbenzidine (TMB) to an oxidized yellow-colored compound. The aptasensors could spot the target antigen at even 0.06 ng ml^{-1} concentrations in the human serum [43].

Nanomaterials offer the advantages of a large surface area compared to volume, numerous functionally active moieties flanking the surface, simple synthesis, intriguing catalytic activity, interesting optical features, unique electrical characteristics, and thermal conductivity [30, 40]. A higher surface area allows more interacting molecules to adsorb, minimizing aggregation and thus providing better signals for biomarker detection [40]. In addition to these, metallic nanoparticles (MNPs) have a significant extinction coefficient and show the property of the localized surface plasmon resonance (LSPR) effect. These features lend MNPs strong optical characteristics that vary with distance. When the differently modified MNPs are near together, their absorption spectra and, thus, the scattering profile shift, changing the sample's color and region of absorption [44]. Aggregation and redispersion of MNPs are followed by color changes [30, 44]. In a study, when gold nanoparticles (NPs) were hybridized with aptamers, the NPs aggregated, resulting in a purple solution. In the presence of nucleolin protein, however, the aptamer hybridizes to the protein, dispersing NPs and resulting in the red-colored solution. This assay could detect rare metastasizing cancer cells expressing nucleolin protein [45]. Shayesteh *et al* designed a colorimetric assay involving no labels that could detect prostate-specific antigen (PSA) present in the sample at a concentration of even 20 pg ml^{-1} based on a color shift from red to blue. They used modified aptamers and gold NPs for detection using the same principle of aggregation and dispersion [46]. However, this approach involving aggregation of NPs has a limitation: when the target sequence is provided, some non-binding target sites of aptamers bordering the target site do not entirely disassociate from NPs. This hinders the aggregation of NPs, leading to poor sensor performance. This problem was partially overcome by removing a few flanking sequences. This method, however, is time-demanding and requires prior and precise knowledge of the aptamer sequence [47]. NPs can also be used as enzyme mimics. Platinum-gold (PtAu) NPs were used as peroxidase mimics to detect the presence of MUC1 and VEGF, the biomarkers for cancerous cells present in the breast. With the help of oxidation of TMB to a yellow-colored product, the NPs could clearly identify ten cancerous cells per milliliter of the sample with the naked eye [48].

Not only NPs, but also other nanomaterials like nanotubes and nanosheets have been utilized in aptasensors. Single-walled carbon nanotubes were used as a peroxidase mimic that, when bound to aptamers, showed a blue shift from a colorless solution, but when bound to circulating exosomes derived from cancerous breast cells, the color intensity dropped. These aptamers could detect a minimum of

5.2×10^5 particles μl^{-1} of the sample [49]. In another study, nanosheets made from graphitic carbon nitride were used as peroxidase mimics to sense the exosomes, derivatives of cancerous breast cells [50].

Besides this, several colorimetric detection sources can be coupled to create a more sensitive biomarker detection method. By combining a trivalent DNAzyme with peroxidase-like activity and MNPs, Ying *et al* constructed a colorimetric aptasensor. With this approach, even 5.08 nM and 5.60 nM of MUC1 could be found in buffer and serum samples, respectively [51].

Apart from all these applications, colorimetric aptasensors possess certain limitations, such as the time-consuming construction process, the limited range of optimized pH solutions, and the effect of color of the sample on results that make them challenging to use in multi-target detection [40, 44]. However, by integrating colorimetric aptasensors with other detection techniques or modes, certain limitations of colorimetric aptasensors can be solved. Fang *et al* came up with an aptasensor for CEA detection (figure 8.11) that could overcome the limitation of time and sensitivity. They employed HRP burrowed in hollow AuNPs (HGNPs) and the aptamer's ability to switch its structure upon binding to the target as the basis for colorimetric detection using the naked eye, UV-visible spectroscopy, and differential pulse voltammetry. The aptasensor detected a minimum of 0.78 ng ml^{-1} CEA in about 45 min [52]. To detect MUC1 biomarkers, Wang and his coworkers prepared a special aptasensor combining colorimetric and surface-enhanced Raman

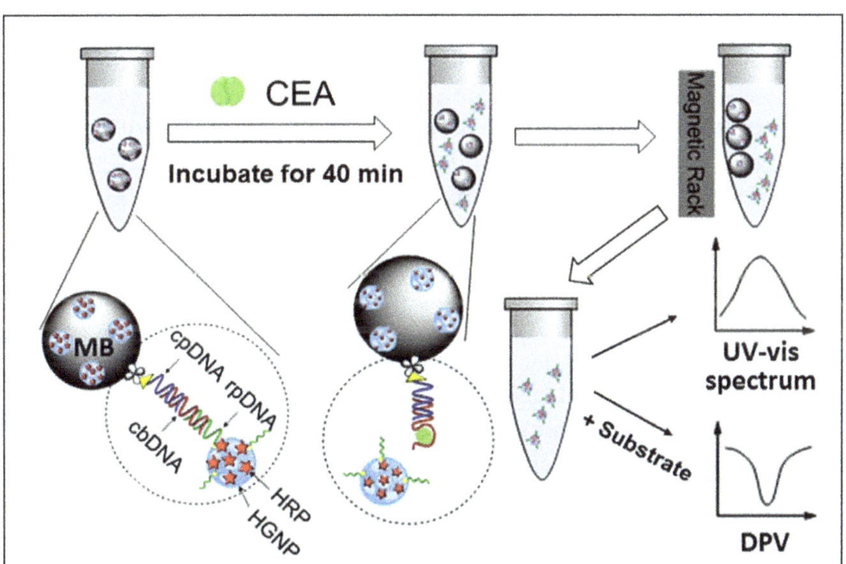

Figure 8.11. Schematic representation of colorimetric aptasensor designed by Fang *et al* for the CEA detection. The aptasensor comprises a combination DNA (cbDNA) linking the magnetic beads bound capture DNA (cDNA) to the reporter DNA on HRP-loaded HGNP. The addition of CEA causes structural changes in cbDNA, releasing HRP-loaded HGNP that leads to color development and target detection. Reproduced with permission from [52]. Copyright (2020) Elsevier.

scattering (SERS) detection modes. SERS provides sensitivity to the assay, while colorimetry enables fast detection overcoming the weak and nearly undetectable signals generated by SERS alone. Using aptamer functionalized magnetic nanobeads for colorimetry and probing gold-silver (Au-Ag) NPs using MUC1 specific sequence and reporters for SERS, a detection limit of 0.1 units per milliliter was reached [53].

8.5 SPR-based aptasensors

Optical methods are beneficial as they possess a faster response, are user-friendly, highly sensitive, and are a non-invasive high-throughput form of diagnosis. Aptamers are employed as a bio-recognition element in optical aptasensors, and other optical techniques utilized as a signal transducing component. When engaging with various analytes, optical aptasensors exhibit variations in luminescence and light absorption that can be used to categorize them. These aptasensors frequently exhibit low reagent demands, are inexpensive, simple to label, and operate quickly. SPR-based optical aptasensors are among the effective methods used to diagnose early cancer detection. Early cancer identification is a contentious issue in the field of study since early detection can help patients live longer and have a better prognosis. For early cancer diagnosis, highly sensitive and durable technologies are required [54]. The key benefits of employing SPR-based aptasensors for clinical diagnostics are specific selectivity and precision, as well as inexpensive manufacturing costs.

Introduced in the early '90s by Pharmacia Biosensors AB, a Swedish firm established via Pharmacia AB, launched the first commercial SPR-based instrumentation on the market which evolved as amongst the sophisticated technologies addressing varied parameters of macromolecular binding *in situ* as well as in high-throughput real-time screening. SPR is based upon the principle of refractive index monitoring used towards the metal/dielectric media interface. Through a high refractive index (RI) prism with a thin coating of Au (preferably) or Ag, incident light (p-polarized) of a certain wavelength and at a specific angle is coupled to the propagating surface plasmons (50 nm). Resonance conditions are altered by modifications to the sensor surface, which causes intensity variations in reflected light at a specific angle. A charge-coupled device (CCD) camera records the light reflected, enabling the simultaneous real-time display of several interactions on the biosensor as well as the related sensorgram. The percent change in reflectance versus time is plotted on the kinetic sensorgram providing the quintessential data within a limited period hand has high reliability.

The molecular interaction affinity, kinetics, and specificity can be elucidated extensively in enzyme-substrate [55], protein-DNA [56, 57], protein–protein [58, 59], lipid-membrane protein [60, 61], polysaccharide-protein [62], cellular and viral proteins [63], the amalgamation of varied biomolecules together in the form of exosomes [64, 65], epitope mapping [66], etc. Sensing SPR signals can be paired with a variety of transducer designs, including the Kretschmann configuration [67], nanoparticle-based LSPR [67], long-range SPR [68], fiber-optic configuration [69], and phase sensing [70] that accomplish stable and reliable background signal suppression, targeted binding prevention, and signal amplification. In addition to their chemical inertness properties like high electrical conductivity for reducing conduction losses, biocompatibility, improved alteration in the optical properties at the nanomaterial surface, and efficient transduction of varied signals in a biochemical pathway, noble metal nanoparticles (NPs) have emerged as the leading probe resources for SPR-based cancer detection biomarkers [71].

Advances in SPR-based aptamers by Loyez *et al* on developing an all-fiber SPR aptasensor that detects metastatic breast cancer cells in five minutes using several narrowband resonances (near-infrared wavelength range). The aptasensor's performance is improved twofold when functionalized AuNPs are added [69]. Diseased states of cancer, and autoimmune abnormalities, have the soluble form of ICAM-1 in their serum. Aptamers for the soluble form of ICAM-1 were chosen and incorporated into a magnetic separation system with SPR sensor chips to create an SPR aptasensor by Dursan *et al* [70]. Gur *et al* successfully detected the CA 125 biomarker for the earlier diagnosis of ovarian cancer using an incredibly sensitive and label-devoid SPR sensor based on polymeric NPs that are molecularly imprinted [72, 73]. The large surface area of the CA 125-imprinted p(HEMA-MATrp) NPs and the MATrp monomer interplay with the template conferred a greater number of accessible and comparable cavities to the template, allowing sensitive and targeted detection of CA 125 even in a complex media. This was accomplished by using the p(HEMA-MATrp) NPs on an SPR gold chip surface. An efficient and affordable detection method for locating the CA 125 tumor marker has been devised by producing artificial recognition components complementary to the template rather than antibodies. To explore detection kinetics, Guo *et al* conducted electrochemical and SPR experiments. They created an aptasensor based on the AgNCs@Apt@UiO66 nanocomposite, and the findings for CEA detection were substantial. Their SPR aptasensor is thought to function well in terms of regeneration, selectivity, repeatability, sensitivity, and stability. Wang *et al* created a very efficient and responsive SPR aptasensor for exosomal detection methods based on dual AuNP-assisted signal amplification. Exciting applications for the approach have been discovered in clinical and scientific research [73, 74].

New plasmonic biosensing techniques that accomplish reliable and stable signal amplification, background signal silencing, and quasi-binding prevention are required due to the combination of extremely low concentrations of cancer-related biomolecules, particularly in the early stages of the disease, and the molecular complexity of biofluids. In order to improve cancer biomarker detection in clinical diagnosis, researchers are now looking into novel approaches for amplifying the transducer signals for target recognition at lower tiers. The most common signal amplifying technique utilized in clinical practice to date, for example, is the employment of antibodies or modified nanoparticles for secondary detection [68].

Biomarker detection supplemented with high specificity and sensitivity in the early stages of a disease directly in *in vivo*, avoiding the requirement for any labeling mechanism to yield the detectable signal, is a critical issue to be solved in SPR-based biosensing (label-free). Advanced plasmonic biosensing techniques are required due to the amalgamation of extremely low concentrations of cancer-related biomolecules, particularly in the early stages of the disease, and the molecular variability of biofluids, that has a significant impact on the reliability of signal detection.

To overcome the lingering obstacles to the adoption of SPR sensing in medical care, research efforts are currently concentrated on improving the sensitivity and reliability of current SPR techniques. The examination of various biological receptor types for robust and sensitive detection, the investigation of the complete complex medium, and the clinical variability of biofluids are all significant issues that need to be addressed. The development of multifunctional nanomaterials that can concurrently identify and curb cancer cells for tumor biomarker monitoring should be the main goal of future research. To increase their practical utility, monitoring systems must be architectured properly in a way to detect cancer biomarkers in the plasma, sera, and tissue fluids. Many other issues must be addressed to complete the SPR-based biosensing idea, particularly in terms of downsizing, reproducibility, portability, and increased detection sensitivity.

8.6 Conclusion

This chapter highlights current breakthroughs in aptamer-based amplification sensing methodologies for the early detection of cancer biomarkers using various optical techniques. Early cancer identification plays a crucial role in increasing treatment options for patients' more prolonged survival. Therefore, researchers are thinking about the advances in various types of optical aptasensors to detect cancer cells and biomarkers. So, we have reviewed some of the recent optical aptasensors which can detect cancer biomarkers. A series of fluorescent aptasensors for cancer-associated biomarkers are successfully created nowadays, taking advantage of aptamers' high affinity and specificity to their targets and the numerous benefits of fluorescence determination compared to other optical techniques. These aptamers are highly selective and sensitive, but many other optical-based aptasensors don't work correctly in clinical settings. Hence, the researchers overcome this challenge as they look for the most advanced aptamers that can work properly and provide a means for clinical significance and better prognosis.

Currently, the aptamers are selected through a time consuming and a tedious process called the SELEX process, which has a low success rate and hinders some of the applications of biosensors. Scientists are chipping in new technologies like magnetic separation and affination chromatography with SELEX to improve success rates.

Firstly, the development of aptamers is a cumbersome process. Secondly, additional aptamers are needed that can target multiple cancer biomarkers. Thirdly, many aptamers are presently under clinical trial in the laboratory, and they need to be exported to the market to make them useful. Most importantly, aptamers are oligonucleotides that are susceptible to degradation by nucleases, which can indirectly affect the performance of the biosensor and can lead to false signals, reducing the efficacy of the aptasensor. Therefore, researchers can easily exploit this research field in the future to make the most out of it. The applications of optical aptasensors will spread by leaps and bounds shortly. The application will not be limited to targeting *in vitro* cancer biomarkers. Still, it can also target *in vivo* markers, and cancer bioimaging could also be possible soon. We could also see aptamers targeting multiple biomarkers with high efficiency and excellent performance in the near future. Altogether, to develop aptasensors and make them useful in our daily lives, we need to screen more aptamers that can achieve our desired goal. Overall, many adjustments and refinements are required in order to make aptamers turn into a clinical reality. Nevertheless, aptasensors can become one of the most potent early cancer detection tools. Aptasensor technology has the potential to pave its path for a brighter future.

Conflict of interest

The authors state that they have no known competing financial interests or personal ties that could appear to have influenced the work described in this study.

Author contributions

All the authors have contributed equally to the work.

Funding agency

This work is not funded by any organization or institute.

Acknowledgments

This work is supported by CSIR-AMPRI. We are thankful to Dr Arpana Parihar for providing guidance and support for the work.

References

[1] Nair M, Sandhu S S and Sharma A K 2018 Cancer molecular markers: a guide to cancer detection and management *Semin. Cancer Biol.* **52** 39–55

[2] Liu M *et al* 2017 Aptamer selection and applications for breast cancer diagnostics and therapy *J. Nanobiotechnol.* **15** 81

[3] Zhao X, Dai X, Zhao S, Cui X, Gong T, Song Z, Meng H, Zhang X and Yu B 2021 Aptamer-based fluorescent sensors for the detection of cancer biomarkers *Spectrochim. Acta* A **247** 119038

[4] Mayer G 2009 The chemical biology of aptamers *Angew. Chem. Int. Ed.* **48** 2672–89

[5] Darmostuk M, Rimpelova S, Gbelcova H and Ruml T 2015 Current approaches in SELEX: an update to aptamer selection technology *Biotechnol. Adv.* **33** 1141–61

[6] Zahra Q, Khan Q A and Luo Z 2021 Advances in optical aptasensors for early detection and diagnosis of various cancer types *Front Oncol.* **11** 632165

[7] Musumeci D, Platella C, Riccardi C, Moccia F and Montesarchio D 2017 Fluorescence sensing using DNA aptamers in cancer research and clinical diagnostics *Cancers* **9** 174

[8] Ferrara N and Davis-Smyth T 1997 The biology of vascular endothelial growth factor *Endocr. Rev.* **18** 4–25

[9] Li J, Sun K, Chen Z, Shi J, Zhou D and Xie G 2017 A fluorescence biosensor for VEGF detection based on DNA assembly structure switching and isothermal amplification *Biosens. Bioelectron.* **89** 964–9

[10] Li X, Ding X and Fan J 2015 Nicking endonuclease-assisted signal amplification of a split molecular aptamer beacon for biomolecule detection using graphene oxide as a sensing platform *Analyst* **140** 7918–25

[11] Goldenberg D M, Neville A M, Carter A C, Go V L W, Holyoke E D, Isselbacher K J, Schein P S and Schwartz M 1981 CEA (carcinoembryonic antigen): its role as a marker in the management of cancer *J Cancer Res. Clin. Oncol.* **101** 239–42

[12] Zhao L, Cheng M, Liu G, Lu H, Gao Y, Yan X, Liu F, Sun P and Lu G 2018 A fluorescent biosensor based on molybdenum disulfide nanosheets and protein aptamer for sensitive detection of carcinoembryonic antigen *Sensors Actuators* B **273** 185–90

[13] Zhao T T, Peng Z W, Yuan D, Zhen S J, Huang C Z and Li Y F 2018 Metal-organic gel enhanced fluorescence anisotropy for sensitive detection of prostate specific antigen *Spectrochim. Acta* A **192** 328–32

[14] Fang B Y, An J, Liu B and Zhao Y D 2019 Hybridization induced fluorescence enhanced DNA-Ag nanocluster/aptamer probe for detection of prostate-specific antigen *Colloids Surf. B.* **175** 358–64

[15] Charlton J, Kirschenheuter G P and Smith D 1997 Highly potent irreversible inhibitors of neutrophil elastase generated by selection from a randomized DNA—valine phosphonate library *Biochemistry* **36** 3018–26

[16] He J L, Wu Z S, Zhang S B, Shen G L and Yu R Q 2010 Fluorescence aptasensor based on competitive-binding for human neutrophil elastase detection *Talanta* **80** 1264–8

[17] Deng B, Lin Y, Wang C, Li F, Wang Z, Zhang H, Li X-F and Le X C 2014 Aptamer binding assays for proteins: the thrombin example—a review *Anal. Chim. Acta* **837** 1–15

[18] Du C, Hu Y, Zhang Q, Guo Z, Ge G, Wang S, Zhai C and Zhu M 2018 Competition-derived FRET-switching cationic conjugated polymer-Ir(III) complex probe for thrombin detection *Biosens. Bioelectron.* **100** 132–8

[19] Wang W, Chen C, Qian M and Zhao X S 2008 Aptamer biosensor for protein detection using gold nanoparticles *Anal. Biochem.* **373** 213–9

[20] Nambi Krishnan J, Park S H and Kim S 2017 Aptamer-based single-step assay by the fluorescence enhancement on electroless plated nano Au substrate *Sensors* **17** 2044

[21] Kufe D W 2009 Mucins in cancer: function, prognosis and therapy *Nat. Rev. Cancer* **9** 874–85

[22] Wreesmann V B *et al* 2004 Genome-wide profiling of papillary thyroid cancer identifies MUC1 as an independent prognostic marker *Cancer Res.* **64** 3780–9

[23] Khodarev N N, Pitroda S P, Beckett M A, MacDermed D M, Huang L, Kufe D W and Weichselbaum R R 2009 MUC1-induced transcriptional programs associated with tumorigenesis predict outcome in breast and lung cancer *Cancer Res.* **69** 2833–7

[24] Ma C, Liu H, Tian T, Song X, Yu J and Yan M 2016 A simple and rapid detection assay for peptides based on the specific recognition of aptamer and signal amplification of hybridization chain reaction *Biosens. Bioelectron.* **83** 15–8

[25] He Y, Lin Y, Tang H and Pang D 2012 A graphene oxide-based fluorescent aptasensor for the turn-on detection of epithelial tumor marker mucin 1 *Nanoscale* **4** 2054

[26] Wang H, Wang D M, Gao M X, Wang J and Huang C Z 2014 Potassium-induced G-quadruplex DNAzyme as a chemiluminescent sensing platform for highly selective detection of K^+ *Anal. Methods* **6** 7415–9
[27] Bowie A R, Sanders M G and Worsfold P J 1996 Analytical applications of liquid phase chemiluminescence reactions—a review *J. Biolumin. Chemilumin.* **11** 61–90
[28] Huang Y, Zhao S, Chen Z F, Shi M, Chen J and Liang H 2012 An amplified chemiluminescence aptasensor based on bi-resonance energy transfer on gold nanoparticles and exonuclease III-catalyzed target recycling *Chem. Commun.* **48** 11877
[29] Eivazzadeh-Keihan R, Pashazadeh P, Hejazi M, de la Guardia M and Mokhtarzadeh A 2017 Recent advances in nanomaterial-mediated Bio and immune sensors for detection of aflatoxin in food products *TrAC Trends Anal. Chem.* **87** 112–28
[30] Kou X, Zhang X, Shao X, Jiang C and Ning L 2020 Recent advances in optical aptasensor technology for amplification strategies in cancer diagnostics *Anal. Bioanal. Chem.* **412** 6691–705
[31] Barni F, Lewis S W, Berti A, Miskelly G M and Lago G 2007 Forensic application of the luminol reaction as a presumptive test for latent blood detection *Talanta* **72** 896–913
[32] Finley S D, Engel-Stefanini M O, Imoukhuede P and Popel A S 2011 Pharmacokinetics and pharmacodynamics of VEGF-neutralizing antibodies *BMC Syst. Biol.* **5** 193
[33] Kut C, mac Gabhann F and Popel A S 2007 Where is VEGF in the body? A meta-analysis of VEGF distribution in cancer *Br. J. Cancer* **97** 978–85
[34] Pasquardini L *et al* 2015 SPAD aptasensor for the detection of circulating protein biomarkers *Biosens. Bioelectron.* **68** 500–7
[35] Wang P, Song Y, Zhao Y and Fan A 2013 Hydroxylamine amplified gold nanoparticle-based aptameric system for the highly selective and sensitive detection of platelet-derived growth factor *Talanta* **103** 392–7
[36] Khang H, Cho K, Chong S and Lee J H 2017 All-in-one dual-aptasensor capable of rapidly quantifying carcinoembryonic antigen *Biosens. Bioelectron.* **90** 46–52
[37] Wang Y Z, Hao N, Feng Q M, Shi H W, Xu J J and Chen H Y 2016 A ratiometric electrochemiluminescence detection for cancer cells using g-C 3 N 4 nanosheets and Ag–PAMAM–luminol nanocomposites *Biosens. Bioelectron.* **77** 76–82
[38] Kim M, Kim K and Lee J H 2020 A cost-effective and rapid aptasensor with chemiluminescence detection for the early diagnosis of prostate cancer *Microchem. J.* **155** 104763
[39] Cha T, Cho S, Kim Y T and Lee J H 2014 Rapid aptasensor capable of simply diagnosing prostate cancer *Biosens. Bioelectron.* **62** 31–7
[40] Shaban S M and Kim D H 2021 Recent advances in aptamer sensors *Sensors* **21** 979
[41] Ferreira C S M, Papamichael K, Guilbault G, Schwarzacher T, Gariepy J and Missailidis S 2008 DNA aptamers against the MUC1 tumour marker: design of aptamer–antibody sandwich ELISA for the early diagnosis of epithelial tumours *Anal. Bioanal. Chem.* **390** 1039–50
[42] Xu L, Chopdat R, Li D and Al-Jamal K T 2020 Development of a simple, sensitive and selective colorimetric aptasensor for the detection of cancer-derived exosomes *Biosens. Bioelectron.* **169** 112576
[43] Zou M and Wang S 2017 An Aptamer-based self-catalytic colorimetric assay for carcinoembryonic antigen *Bull. Korean Chem. Soc.* **38** 1143–8
[44] Mo T *et al* 2022 Aptamer-based biosensors and application in tumor theranostics *Cancer Sci.* **113** 7–16

[45] Borghei Y S, Hosseini M, Dadmehr M, Hosseinkhani S, Ganjali M R and Sheikhnejad R 2016 Visual detection of cancer cells by colorimetric aptasensor based on aggregation of gold nanoparticles induced by DNA hybridization *Anal. Chim. Acta* **904** 92–7
[46] Shayesteh O H and Ghavami R 2020 A novel label-free colorimetric aptasensor for sensitive determination of PSA biomarker using gold nanoparticles and a cationic polymer in human serum *Spectrochim. Acta* A **226** 117644
[47] Alsager O A, Alotaibi K M, Alswieleh A M and Alyamani B J 2018 Colorimetric aptasensor of vitamin D3: a novel approach to eliminate residual adhesion between aptamers and gold nanoparticles *Sci. Rep.* **8** 12947
[48] Wang K, Fan D, Liu Y and Wang E 2015 Highly sensitive and specific colorimetric detection of cancer cells via dual-aptamer target binding strategy *Biosens. Bioelectron.* **73** 1–6
[49] Xia Y *et al* 2017 A visible and colorimetric aptasensor based on DNA-capped single-walled carbon nanotubes for detection of exosomes *Biosens. Bioelectron.* **92** 8–15
[50] Wang Y M, Liu J W, Adkins G B, Shen W, Trinh M P, Duan L Y, Jang J-H and Zhong W 2017 Enhancement of the intrinsic peroxidase-like activity of graphitic carbon nitride nanosheets by ssDNAs and its application for detection of exosomes *Anal. Chem.* **89** 12327–33
[51] Liu S, Xu N, Tan C, Fang W, Tan Y and Jiang Y 2018 A sensitive colorimetric aptasensor based on trivalent peroxidase-mimic DNAzyme and magnetic nanoparticles *Anal. Chim. Acta* **1018** 86–93
[52] Wang Q L, Cui H F, Li C L, Song X, Lv Q Y and Li Z Y 2020 A multimode aptasensor based on hollow gold nanoparticles and structure switching of aptamer: fast and sensitive detection of carcinoembryonic antigen *Sensors Actuators Rep.* **2** 100021
[53] Li N *et al* 2020 A SERS-colorimetric dual-mode aptasensor for the detection of cancer biomarker MUC1 *Anal. Bioanal. Chem.* **412** 5707–18
[54] Hong P, Li W and Li J 2012 Applications of aptasensors in clinical diagnostics *Sensors* **12** 1181–93
[55] Geitmann M and Danielson U H 2004 Studies of substrate-induced conformational changes in human cytomegalovirus protease using optical biosensor technology *Anal. Biochem.* **332** 203–14
[56] Akgönüllü S, Koyun S, Yavuz H, Erdem A and Denizli A 2022 Preparation of surface plasmon resonance aptasensor for human activated Protein C sensing *Methods Mol. Biol.* **2393** 37–56
[57] Teh H F, Peh W Y X, Su X and Thomsen J S 2007 Characterization of Protein–DNA interactions using surface plasmon resonance spectroscopy with various assay schemes *Biochemistry* **46** 2127–35
[58] Kim M, Park K, Jeong E J, Shin Y B and Chung B H 2006 Surface plasmon resonance imaging analysis of protein–protein interactions using on-chip-expressed capture protein *Anal. Biochem.* **351** 298–304
[59] Vance S A and Sandros M G 2015 Zeptomole detection of C-reactive protein in serum by a nanoparticle amplified surface plasmon resonance imaging aptasensor *Sci. Rep.* **4** 5129
[60] Taylor J D, Linman M J, Wilkop T and Cheng Q 2009 Regenerable tethered bilayer lipid membrane arrays for multiplexed label-free analysis of lipid–protein interactions on Poly (dimethylsiloxane) microchips using SPR imaging *Anal. Chem.* **81** 1146–53

[61] Maynard J A, Lindquist N C, Sutherland J N, Lesuffleur A, Warrington A E, Rodriguez M and Oh S-H 2009 Surface plasmon resonance for high-throughput ligand screening of membrane-bound proteins *Biotechnol. J.* **4** 1542–58

[62] Mariani S and Minunni M 2014 Surface plasmon resonance applications in clinical analysis *Anal. Bioanal. Chem.* **406** 2303–23

[63] Nguyen H, Park J, Kang S and Kim M 2015 Surface plasmon resonance: a versatile technique for biosensor applications *Sensors* **15** 10481–510

[64] Chen W *et al* 2021 Surface plasmon resonance biosensor for exosome detection based on reformative tyramine signal amplification activated by molecular aptamer beacon *J. Nanobiotechnol.* **19** 450

[65] Grasso L, Wyss R, Weidenauer L, Thampi A, Demurtas D, Prudent M, Lion N and Vogel H 2015 Molecular screening of cancer-derived exosomes by surface plasmon resonance spectroscopy *Anal. Bioanal. Chem.* **407** 5425–32

[66] Sibille P and Strosberg A D 1997 A FIV epitope defined by a phage peptide library screened with a monoclonal anti-FIV antibody *Immunol. Lett.* **59** 133–7

[67] Wang S, Dong Y and Liang X 2018 Development of a SPR aptasensor containing oriented aptamer for direct capture and detection of tetracycline in multiple honey samples *Biosens. Bioelectron.* **109** 1–7

[68] Bellassai N, D'Agata R, Jungbluth V and Spoto G 2019 Surface plasmon resonance for biomarker detection: advances in non-invasive cancer diagnosis *Front. Chem.* **7** 570

[69] Loyez M, Hassan E M, Lobry M, Liu F, Caucheteur C, Wattiez R, DeRosa M C, Willmore W G and Albert J 2020 Rapid detection of circulating breast cancer cells using a multiresonant optical fiber aptasensor with plasmonic amplification *ACS Sens.* **5** 454–63

[70] Dursun A D, Dogan S, Kavruk M, Busra Tasbasi B, Sudagidan M, Deniz Yilmaz M, Yilmaz B, Ozalp V C and Tune B G 2022 Surface plasmon resonance aptasensor for soluble ICAM-1 protein in blood samples *Analyst* **147** 1663–8

[71] Karami P, Khoshsafar H, Johari-Ahar M, Arduini F, Afkhami A and Bagheri H 2019 Colorimetric immunosensor for determination of prostate specific antigen using surface plasmon resonance band of colloidal triangular shape gold nanoparticles *Spectrochim. Acta* A **222** 117218

[72] Gür S D, Bakhshpour M and Denizli A 2022 Nanoscale SPR sensor for the ultrasensitive detection of the ovarian cancer marker carbohydrate antigen 125 *New J. Chem.* **46** 7263–70

[73] Wang Q, Zou L, Yang X, Liu X, Nie W, Zheng Y, Cheng Q and Wang K 2019 Direct quantification of cancerous exosomes via surface plasmon resonance with dual gold nano-particle-assisted signal amplification *Biosens. Bioelectron.* **135** 129–36

[74] Guo C, Su F, Song Y, Hu B, Wang M, He L, Peng D and Zhang Z 2017 Aptamer-templated silver nanoclusters embedded in zirconium metal–organic framework for bifunctional electrochemical and SPR aptasensors toward carcinoembryonic antigen *ACS Appl. Mater. Interfaces* **9** 41188–99

Chapter 9

Lab-on-a-chip systems for aptamer-based cancer biomarker screening

Ali Firoozbakhtian, Morteza Hosseini, Javad Gilnezhad and Mohammad Reza Ganjali

It is anticipated that lab-on-chip (LOC) devices would spur innovation and advancement in the realms of diagnostics and treatments. To fully realize the potential of these devices, however, there are also difficulties related to the creation and widespread use of LOC devices, such as complexity, standardization, integration, materials, and cost. The present chapter discusses cancer biomarkers and the fabrication of LOC devices for the detection of cancer.

9.1 Introduction

Cancer is ranked the second leading cause of death and is regarded as one of the most frequent worldwide. There were an estimated more than 19 million cancer cases in 2020 [1] and reports claim that it was responsible for more than 10 million deaths in that year. According to the World Health Organization (WHO), one in eight men and one in eleven women die from this disease and around 40% of those diagnosed survive [2]. The disease can transpire in various forms, i.e. lung cancer, breast cancer, bone cancer, bladder cancer, colon cancer, etc. Thus, early-stage diagnosis of the disease is of high importance while there is still chance of improvement of the patient's welfare. The current methods diagnosing cancer are the likes of enzyme-linked immunosorbent assays (ELISA) [3, 4], serving as the gold standard, radioimmunoassays, immunohistochemistry, and fluorescent spectrometry [5]. The early diagnosis of the disease relies on the detection of either the biomarkers or the single cancerous cells that circulate through the body (CTCs). The former sometimes is subject to be found in the body at very low concentrations even in the absence of cancer; however, its concentration would rise dramatically in the onset of cancer, thus cancer biomarker detection should be performed in combination with other diagnoses to confirm the onset of cancer. The latter, as the name

doi:10.1088/978-0-7503-5012-9ch9

suggests, is the detection of circulating tumor cells confirming the occurrence of cancer. The detection of disease biomarkers is of great importance in the fields of biomedical applications, clinical diagnosis, and medical research [6, 7] and gains more interest and importance when dealing with cancer [8]. The detection of these biomarkers helps with the diagnosis and treatment procedure of the disease [9].

9.2 Biomarkers

The National Cancer Institute (NCI) has defined the term "biomarker" as a biological molecule located in body fluids or tissues that is a sign of normal or abnormal processes or of a condition or disease, e.g. cancer. With the help of biomarkers, one can differentiate between a normal person and a diseased person, and afterwards investigate the stage of the disease and the treatment follow-up. One of the major benefits in the analysis of biomarkers is the possibility of the employment of non-invasive methods. Despite the challenges in the way of biomarker analysis, a great number of biosensors have been introduced for their detection. Here, we will discuss some of the biomarkers used.

9.2.1 Abnormal prothrombin (APT)

The des-γ-carboxy prothrombin is a biomarker associated with liver cancer. Reports say that the protein is detected within 90% of the patients diagnosed with hepatocellular carcinoma [10]. It should be noted that a concentration of 0.1 AU ml^{-1} is present in healthy individuals. Despite the protein being associated with liver cancer, it cannot be solely relied on, since the assays are prone to false-negative and -positive results. To address this issue, two other proteins related to the disease, AFP and AFP-L3, should also be analyzed. The biomarker can be used to detect the early stages of cancer through the fabrication of ultra-sensitive biosensors at home.

9.2.2 Carcinoma embryonic antigen (CEA)

Carcinoembryonic antigen (CEA) is a 180 kDa protein expressed by mucosal cells and found at very low concentrations in the body [11]. The biomarker is associated mainly with colorectal cancer; however, its elevated levels can be seen in pancreas, breast, lung, and ovarian cancers as well [12]. The protein concentration may rise in both cancerous and benign conditions. The normal concentration of the protein ranges between 0 and 2.5 ng ml^{-1}. Should the concentrations reach 10 ng ml^{-1} and above, this shows an extensive level of the disease and anything beyond 20 ng ml^{-1} indicates the spreading of cancer. CEA analysis is performed mainly to study the treatment process. If the levels stay unchanged or don't change much, then one can consider the treatment unsuccessful.

9.2.3 Prostate-specific antigen (PSA)

Prostate-specific antigen (PSA), which also goes by the name of kallikrein-3 or P-30 antigen, is a KLK3 gene-encoded 33 kDa glycoprotein enzyme in humans. The enzyme is produced by both normal and cancerous epithelial cells and is secreted to the seminal fluid [13]. The biomarker is found at very low concentrations in healthy individuals but the concentrations increase at the onset of cancer. The high levels of the biomarker can be the result of both a cancerous condition and a non-cancerous benign prostatic hyperplasia (BPH). The normal range for PSA concentrations is dependent on the age of the person and increases slightly as the individual ages. For instance, a normal range is considered 0–2.5 ng ml^{-1} in one's 40s but is considered normal from 0 to 4.5 ng ml^{-1} in their 60 s. However, it is considered suspicious from 4 to 10 ng ml^{-1} and repeatedevaluation of its levels is suggested [14]. In addition, another marker that can be monitored at the same time for a more accurate and earlier detection of the disease is citrate [15, 16]. Thus, the development of ultra-sensitive biosensors for its POC testing makes early detection of prostate cancer possible.

9.2.4 Cancer antigen 15-3 (CA 15-3)

Cancer antigen 15-3 (also known as MUC1) is a protein produced in the onsets of breast and ovarian cancers. The protein is found at low concentrations in healthy individuals (less than or equal to 30 U ml^{-1}); however, its concentration is subject to an increase at the occurrence of cancer, particularly in the metastasis stage. Although the antigen is associated with breast cancer, it cannot always be relied upon since the levels of the protein do not rise in some classes of breast cancer. The analysis of the biomarker indicates the efficiency of the cancer treatment and its recurrence after the treatment. It should be highlighted that the levels of CA 15-3 also do increase during pregnancy. Thus sensitive, rapid, and cost-effective means of its detection would be useful in the early detection of breast cancer.

9.2.5 Alpha-fetoprotein (AFP)

Alpha-fetoprotein (AFP) is a 70 kDa protein encoded by the AFP gene in humans. The protein is considered a biomarker in the detection of gastrointestinal, liver, ovarian, and testicle cancer and also in non-cancerous liver-related diseases including cirrhosis and hepatitis [17, 18]. The biomarker is not a cancer-specific marker as it is also synthesized in the liver of a developing fetus, which can transfer to the body of the mother [19]. The concentrations of AFP should go down after birth to 20 ng ml^{-1} [17]. Hepatocellular carcinoma (HCC) is considered to have occurred at 400 ng ml^{-1} or higher concentrations of AFP [20]. The protein is used in the detection of symptomless hepatocellular carcinoma as well.

9.2.6 Human epidermal growth factor receptor 2 (HER2)

HER2 is a 185 kDa protein in the breast cells. Normally the protein receptors are responsible for the healthy growth and life cycle of the breast cells [21]. However, in approximately 20% of breast cancers, the genes make numerous copies of themselves where the receptors on the surface of the breast cells become overexpressed. The overexpression of the receptor leads to the formation of different complexes with ligands that control cellular functions (e.g. proliferation, survival, and apoptosis). The normal concentration of the protein in healthy women ranges between 2 and

15 μg l^{-1} [22]. The levels of the protein are highly associated with breast cancer; therefore, fabrication of biosensors sensitive enough to determinist presence could help a lot with the early detection of breast cancer.

9.2.7 Tumor necrosis factor alpha (TNF-α)

Tumor necrosis factor alpha (TNF-α) is a 17 kDa cytokine produced by immune cells, keratinocytes, and cancer cells. Reports show that cancer-initiator chemicals lead to increased secretion of the protein, which would have direct effects on programmed cell death and tumor growth [23]. The cytokine would also have indirect effects on the crippling of DNA repair mechanisms leading to increased DNA mutations. Secreted by the adipose cells, TAM, or the tumor cells, the protein leads to an increase in the expression of aromatase, which would consequently lead to the enhanced proliferation of the luminal breast cancer cells. Hence, the identification of trace amounts of TNF-α helps with the early detection of cancer [24, 25].

9.2.8 Cancer antigen 125 (CA 125)

Cancer antigen 125 is a 200 kDa protein located on the majority of ovarian cancer cells secreted into the blood [26]. Moreover, the protein can be found on other both normal and cancerous cells (e.g. mesothelioma, breast cancer, colorectal cancer, uterine cancer, lung cancer, and stomach cancer) as well. The protein is found at concentrations under 35 U ml^{-1} in healthy individuals or at the first stages of breast cancer, and is increased as the patient's conditions worsen [27]. Its concentrations increase in the blood over the occurrence of cancer or in other conditions, e.g. menstruation, pregnancy, uterine fibroids, and endometriosis. CA 125 analysis is performed in situations when there is a suspicion of cancer, investigating the efficiency of the treatment, and looking for the recurrence of the disease. The decrease in the levels of CA 125 in the blood means that the cancer is being treated appropriately, whereas the unchanged levels of it mean that the treatment has been unsuccessful. The high levels of the protein after the completion of the treatment means that cancer has recurred. Thus, sensitive detection of CA 125 helps with the early detection, efficiency of the treatment, and early diagnosis of the recurrence of cancer.

9.2.9 Mucin 1

Mucin 1 (MUC1) is a 250–1000 kDa membrane-bound heterodimeric glycoprotein secreted to protect and lubricate the surfaces of the epithelial cells. Mucin domains are associated with the regulation of immune response and tumorigenesis. Mucins protect the cells by preventing them from being touched by infectious pathogens. The overexpression, changes in its glycosylation, and misplacement of the protein in the cell have been associated with cancers of the lung, breast, colon, and pancreas [28]. High levels of MUC1 have been linked with a high risk of cancer return and increased metastasis of lymph nodes in breast cancer [29].

9.2.10 Interleukins (ILs)

Interleukins (ILs) are a class of cytokines expressed by various body cells including white blood cells, fibroblasts, and some types of tumor cells. Chronic inflammation is one of the driving forces leading to cancers of the skin, lung, colorectal, and hepatocellular carcinoma [30]. Some classes of ILs are directly involved in the signaling of non-immune cells. At the occurrence of an oncogenic event this signaling in tumor cells can become a mechanism of tumor growth consequently leading to the spread and progression of cancer. IL-1 has been associated with carcinogenesis that is induced by inflammation [31, 32]. IL-8 and IL-6 could also be used as cancer biomarkers. The increase in the levels of them would result in enhanced proliferation, survival, and spreading of cancer throughout the body. The ultra-sensitive detection of these markers would help in the early-stage detection of cancers of the bladder and colon.

9.2.11 C-Reactive protein (CRP)

C-reactive protein (CRP) is a 5-subunit acute phase protein. Each subunit consists of 206 amino acids resulting in a 120 kDa protein. The protein is expressed in response to other interleukins (i.e. IL-1, IL-6, IL-17) and TNF-α from hepatocytes [33]. The protein is found at low concentrations in healthy individuals (<5 mg l^{-1}); however, the concentration rises in cases of inflammation, CVD diseases, bacterial infections, and a variety of cancers (e.g. pancreatic, colorectal, ovarian, etc) [34, 35]. Hence, sensitive detection of the biomarker would help with the clinical decision-making process of the patients.

9.2.12 Platelet-derived growth factor (PDGF)

Platelet-derived growth factors (PDGFs) are a group of proteins secreted by the platelets in the blood. The dimeric glycoprotein consists of two subunits (A and B) and can be formed either with the same subunits or one from each. The protein regulates the growth and division of the mesenchymal cells. They play a vital role in the blood vessels' genesis [36]. In the field of biomarkers for the detection of cancers, the protein with the two B subunits (PDGF-BB) can be measured relative to tumor angiogenesis [37]. The glycoprotein is found at very low concentrations in normal conditions; however, its concentrations rise in the onset of cancers including sarcoma and glioma tumors. Thus, sensitive detection of PDGF-BB can help with a more accurate cancer diagnosis and investigating the efficiency of the treatment [29].

9.2.13 Vascular endothelial growth factor (VEGF)

Vascular endothelial growth factor (VEGF), otherwise known as vascular permeability factor (VPF), is classified as a signaling protein leading to the successful angiogenesis for the expansion of vessels. The protein is a subfamily of PDGFs. The overexpression of VEGF is caused by the rapid growth of tumor cells, which consequently leads to the migration of the cancer cells to other parts of the body.

In the majority of cancer cases the levels of VEGF are higher than normal. The higher levels in the body sometimes accounts for reduced chances of survival. The normal levels of VEGF in healthy individuals range between 1 and 177 pg ml^{-1} whereas in the onset of cancer, the concentrations increase from 18 to 328 pg ml^{-1} [38]. The protein is considered a biomarker for the early detection and investigation of the treatment process. The lowered levels of VEGF can indicate that the treatment has been successful. Since tumors need angiogenesis for their growth and survival, VEGF can also be used as an anticancer target for suppressing the vessels' growth. Hence, sensitive detection of the biomarker's levels is of great importance in dealing with cancer.

9.2.14 Cancer antigen 19-9 (CA19-9)

Carbohydrate antigen sialyl Lewis a (CA 19-9) is a 1000 kDa protein located on the surface of some cancer cells. The protein is associated with the cancers of the digestive tract system and specific types of pancreatic cancers. The normal levels of the protein in healthy individuals are below 37 U ml^{-1}. The CA 19-9 test is mainly performed to find out the efficiency of the treatment and also recurrence of the cancer after the finishing of treatment procedure. High levels of the protein cannot be directly related to the occurrence of cancer in the body as its levels may also rise in both normal and non-cancerous conditions. The protein is found in healthy individuals in the pancreas, lungs, and liver and also may not even be present at all in those suffering from cancer since it is a Lewis antigen [39]. Despite lacking specificity, it is the only FDA-approved biomarker in the detection of pancreatic cancer; thus, ultra-sensitive detection of this marker could help with early detection of cancer and the treatment follow-ups.

9.2.15 Human epididymis secretory protein 4 (HE4)

Encoded by the WFDC2 gene, human epididymis protein-4 (HE4) also known as WAP four-disulfide core domain protein 2, is a protein found to be extremely overexpressed in the cases of cancers of the ovary compared to normal conditions [40]. Studies have shown that the protein assists with the growth, proliferation, and metastasis of ovarian cancer. Thus, its sensitive detection could be of use in the early detection of ovarian cancer.

9.2.16 Squamous cell carcinoma antigen (SCC-Ag)

Squamous cell carcinoma antigen (SCC-Ag) is a biomarker used in the screening of cancers related to the uterine cervix. The 48-kDa-glycolprotein is a serin protease inhibitor is found in both normal and cancerous squamous cells [41]. The normal concentration of the protein in healthy women is measured at 1.9 mg l^{-1} whereas augmented levels between 2 and 2.5 mg l^{-1} could indicate a cut-off point. The levels of the biomarker increase in both cancerous and non-cancerous conditions (e.g. head and neck, lung, vulva and vagina squamous cell carcinomas and liver and kidney-related diseases). Thus, the glycoprotein is not a specific biomarker for cervical cancer [42]. However, there is a positive correlation between the levels of the protein and stage of the cancer. Hence one can detect the protein and analyze its concentration to investigate the efficiency of the treatment process. Should the levels of SCC rise after the finishing of the treatment, chances are that the cancer has returned.

9.2.17 Multidrug resistance-associated protein 1 (MRP-1)

Multidrug resistance-associated protein 1 (MRP-1) is one of the ABC transporter proteins found in the plasma membrane of both normal and cancerous cells (e.g. kidney, liver, brain, testis, etc). The protein is responsible for the limited efficiency of some treatments in some cases of cancers, where the needed therapeutics are sent out of the cell due to the function of this protein. The glycoprotein's levels increase at the onset of cancer and its monitoring could help with a better understanding of how the treatment procedure is going.

9.2.18 Basigin (CD147)

Basigin/CD 147 is a highly glycosylated transmembrane protein that is overexpressed by a variety of cancer cells. The protein plays a rather significant role in the proliferation, growth, and migration of cancer cells and also induces the expression of VEGF and MRPs. Basigin increases the expression of matrix metalloproteinases and would consequently result in the invasion of the tumor cell. Screening of the protein's concentration could help with the early detection of cancer and the follow-up procedures.

9.3 Aptamers

The short, single-stranded DNA/RNA with the ability of specifical binding to target molecules are called aptamers. Aptamers can be used to detect almost any type of chemical and biological target, including proteins, ions, small molecules, and cells. Aptamers are selected from oligonucleotide sequencing libraries by a process called SELEX, which represents the systematic evolution of ligands using exponential enrichment [43]. The process starts with the incubation of 10^{14}–10^{15} random DNA or RNA sequences to target molecules (figure 9.1). After incubation, excess unbound oligonucleotides are removed and bound oligonucleotides are eluted from the molecule of interest. Employing an amplification step (through PCR), first the oligonucleotides are amplified and then purified from the rest of the PCR products and the process would go on for another selection round. The process goes on for 5–15 rounds when no further noticeable enrichment of the nucleic acids is seen. With the goals of increasing the efficiency and rapidity of the procedures, other SELEX-based techniques have been proposed, including capillary electrophoresis SELEX (CE-SELEX), Flu-Mag SELEX, Capture SELEX, and MonoLEX [44, 45]. Magnetic-assisted rapid aptamer selection (MARAS) is another SELEX-based method that can generate aptamers that are highly affinitive, eliminating the need for repeating cycles [46]. The smaller size of aptamers compared with antibodies would ultimately lead to better signaling of aptamer-based assays. Aptamer-based sensors are known to have longer stabilities compared with antibody-based ones due

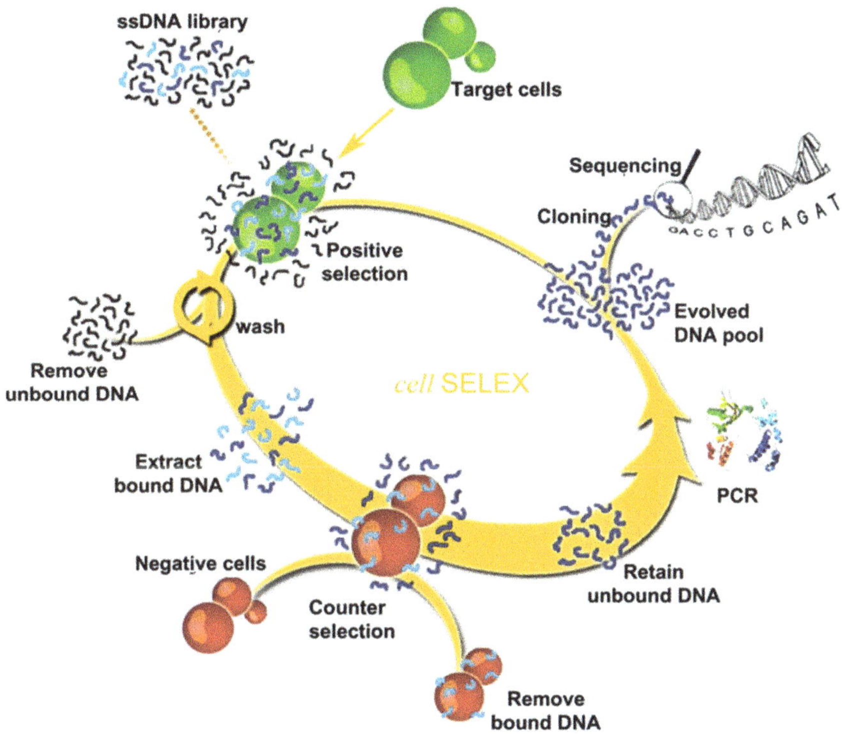

Figure 9.1. Illustration of cell SELEX process. Reprinted with permission from reference [41].

to the higher stability of aptamers [47–50]. One of the most important things one should keep in mind is the maintenance of the health of the cancer cells during the enrichment process. Should the cells die during the process, the enrichment process can be delayed or worse, lead to the enrichment of non-specific binder sequences [51]. Most aptamers are enriched for membrane proteins since they usually bind to them. Various aptamers have been produced that specifically target cancer cells, which can be used in the early detection of the disease.

There are generally two modes of detection with respect to the signal-sensing format. The first one is called signal-on, where the intensity of the signal is subject to an increase with the increasing target concentration. One of the common ways to perform a signal-on sensing format is to employ sandwich assays, where the target of interest is sandwiched between two capture probes that are specific for it. Usually, one of the probes is modified with a reporter molecule whose concentration changes linearly with respect to the concentration of the target. So, the concentration of the target is determined indirectly through the determination of the concentration of the reporter [52, 53]. The signal-on process can also be used directly to measure the concentration of the target. For instance, employing electrochemical impedance spectroscopy (EIS), one can sensitively quantify the presence of targets (in this case cancer cells, or cancer biomarkers) through an increase in the EIS value with the increasing concentration of the target [54–58]. For a better sensitivity of the assay, nanomaterials have been used providing a better electron transfer media or improved biocompatibility for the capturing of the targets. The other method is called the signal-off sensing format, where upon the introduction of the target to the environment, the signal intensity decreases. Signal-off assays are prone to false negative results due to the unwanted adsorption of components on the electrode surface. Voltammetric techniques are one of the most used while working with signal-off assays. Differential pulse voltammetry (DPV) is mostly employed among other voltammetry techniques since the signals are better interpreted [59, 60]. Other voltammetry techniques like cyclic voltammetry (CV), linear sweep voltammetry (LSV), and anodic stripping voltammetry (ASV) have also been employed in the signal-off detection of cancer biomarkers [61–63]. Electrogenerated chemiluminescence (ECL) is also an electrochemical technique widely used in bioanalysis [64, 65]. ECL can offer signal-on as well as signal-off sensing format assays and with its ease and practicality of use has gained much attention over the years. Several diagnostic companies are known to employ ECL in their bioanalysis (e.g. Roche diagnostics) suggesting that the technique is highly sensitive and selective and like other electrochemical techniques, ECL can be quantified.

9.4 Lab-on-chip devices

The need for more sensitive yet inexpensive and rapid analysis applications has led to the evolution of microfluidics technology [66, 67]. Microfluidics technology is considered a division of MEMS technologies, handling fluids in sub-milliliter (i.e. mostly microliter) environments. The platforms used in the fabrication of microfluidic devices enable the mixing, separation, and manipulation of fluids for various applications. The provision of a total solution (sample-to-answer) in systems that are inexpensive and rapid has been the main reason behind the fabrication of microfluidic devices. Microfluidic devices are the miniaturized, portable representatives of the traditional complex laboratory devices that are realizing the fabrication of point-of-care (POC) testing. These devices benefit from higher sensitivity, and an improved resolution compared with the benchtop laboratory devices. Andreas Manz was the first to come up with the phrase ‘micro-total analysis system’ in 1990 which then was expanded to ‘lab-on-a-chip’ (LOC) [68].

The ranges at which microfluidic devices are fabricated are between the submillimeter to less than 100 micrometers; however, it is possible to reach under 1 micrometer channels as well. Laminar flow, in which the fluid particles follow a smooth path and do not undergo any mixing or fluctuations, is of great importance while working in these dimensions. While designing an LOC system, one should consider the existence of a controlling laminar flow diffusion-based transport mechanism. The transportation of fluids in microfluidic devices takes place mainly by the impelling of bulk aqueous solution in the enclosed channels of the system. Although the evolution in microfabrication techniques has led to the improved reliability of the microfluidic systems in which one can concern the bulk flow, droplet actuation still has plain advantages over bulk. Actuation of droplets would lead to a decrease in dead-volume spaces while working with limited-volume samples.

In addition, working with pico- to microliter samples provides a suitable environment for, in this case, biomolecular assays.

9.4.1 LOC components

The architecture of an LOC device must enable the handling of untreated samples, mixing with reagents, separation and subsequently and most importantly, target detection. To address all these challenges, different components should be installed on a chip, each of which plays a different role. So generally speaking, an LOC device consists of a power supply, injector, preparator, transporter, mixer, reactor, separator, detector, and controller. These components are briefly discussed here (figure 9.2).

9.4.2 Injector

To ensure a proper and exact amount of the sample and reagents are introduced to the LOC device in the orders of micro/nanoliter, an injector is employed (figure 9.2). An injector can either be an external component delivering the samples and reagents to the system or be an internal component of the LOC system. Two of the most used injectors are syringe pumps and robotic pipettes.

9.4.3 Preparator

The preparator part deals with isolation of the analyte of interest from the rest of the sample leading to a fluid with less matrix complexity (figure 9.2). The pretreatment of the samples is often an inescapable step in bioanalysis. This shows its importance

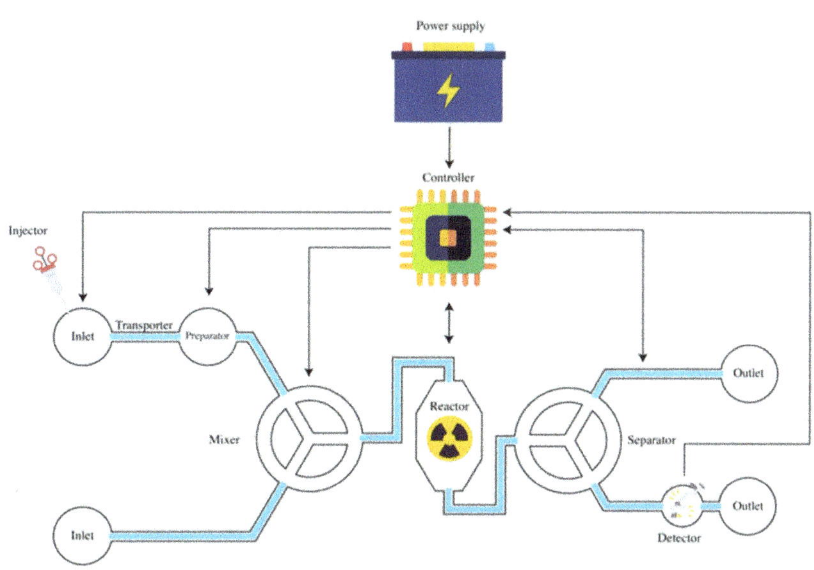

Figure 9.2. Schematic illustration of the components of an LOC device.

mostly in PCR-assisted nucleic acid amplifications since first the nucleic acids need to be extracted from the cells and second, the presence of unwanted biological parts in the PCR sample can lessen the efficiency of the process. In the aptamer-based diagnoses, which is also the main focus of this chapter, sample pretreatment, e.g. lysis of RBC, helps with a higher efficiency of the assay. Here, we discuss filtration, preconcentration, and cell lysis.

9.4.3.1 Filtration

One of the most common methods of analyte isolation is filtration. Microfilters are often used in these systems. To selectively isolate the desired analytes, different filter designs have been introduced. RBC filtration is achieved through the employment of hydrophoretic methods on LOC devices [69]. Acoustic focusing is another highly efficient method used in the manipulation of particles larger than 2 μm in fluids. The waves are generated through the implementation of a piezoelectric transducer in the device [70].

9.4.3.2 Preconcentration

The target of interest can be found at very low concentrations in untreated samples. This would often make the detection process challenging. Thus, sample enrichment can play a crucial role in enhancing the sensitivity of the assay. The mixture separation can be achieved through a process called solid-phase extraction (SPE) involving a mobile and stationary phase. The target of interest collected at the stationary phase can be obtained through rinsing with appropriate solutions. Aptamer-modified magnetic beads can be employed as solid-phase extraction probes and selectively bind to the analyte of interest following a rinsing step for further purification of the process [71, 72]. Elimination of RBCs is also carried out through the employment of a centrifugal field achieved by the specific design of the microfluidic channels on LOC devices [73].

9.4.3.3 Cell lysis

Cell lysis can be performed either when the cells are unwanted in the detection process and interfere with it or when the analyte of interest is an intracellular component. In this method the cell membrane is disrupted through various approaches (e.g. mechanical, chemical, optical, acoustic, etc) [74].

9.4.3.4 Transporter

The transporter part regulates the flow sequence, its duration as well as direction, and the rate of the flow for fluid manipulations (figure 9.2). Fluid transport can be categorized into two main groups; active and passive. The former requires the need for an outside driving force whereas the latter does not.

9.4.3.4.1 Active transport

Fluidic control is often achieved through the employment of pneumatically-driven peristaltic micropumps on LOC devices [75, 76]. The introduction of the spider-web peristaltic micropump by Wang [77] has improved the pumping rate uniformity compared to conventional linear micropumps. To simplify the fabrication process, much attention has been drawn to the fabrication of valveless pumps [78, 79]. Piezo disks are used in the fabrication of peristaltic, diffuser or nuzzle pumps as actuators. The pump's membrane is a brass disc on which a piezoelectric ceramic layer is glued forming the piezo disc. These pneumatic, thermopneumatic, and piezoelectric micropumps require high driving voltage and high power consumption. The requirement for high voltage and power leads to the installment of oversized power supplies, which is inappropriate in the fabrication of LOC devices. Thus, electro-chemical systems that eradicate the design complexity and cut fabrication costs are more preferable [80].

9.4.3.4.2 Passive transport

Diffusion-mediated transporters are highly considered in the studies because of their simplicity and no need for external power supplies. In these systems, different geometries are employed to achieve suitable flow rates. Melin *et al* introduced a liquid-triggered valve consisting of a Y-junction that acted as a stop valve [81]. Surface tension and gravity have been used as the driving force in an LOC device independent of the fluid in the reservoir [82]. Studies have shown that absorption and capillary forces can also be used in passive transport systems [83].

9.4.3.5 Mixer

The mixer component is responsible for the appropriate mixing of different streams of fluid of an LOC (figure 9.2). The mixing process often occurs based on laminar diffusion as the Reynolds number is low in the microfluidic channels. Like the transporter part, mixers are also divided into two groups, active and passive.

9.4.3.5.1 Active mixers

Active mixers require an external force for the mixing of fluids. This type of mixer provides a faster mixing of the fluids in a much shorter time compared with the passive mixers, yet they are more expensive and add to the complexity of the fabricated device. One example is the external magnetic field applied in the presence of magnetic particles in the microfluidic channel. The mixing is achieved when the movement of the magnetic particles is altered with the magnetic field. The turbulent flow can also be generated through ultrasonic vibrations. However, this approach suffers from a non-uniform turbulent flow through the channel and requires high voltage [84–86].

9.4.3.5.2 Passive mixers

Passive mixers make use of characteristics of the flow to mix different fluids in microfluidic channels. The use of these mixers eliminates the need for the utilization of expensive and complex external forces; however, it elongates the mixing duration. Mixing can be attained through the use of different geometries and designs in the microfluidic channels. Increasing channel length and incorporation of spiral designs has led to excellent mixing of the fluids.

9.4.3.6 Reactor

The reactor is the part where a chemical or biological reaction takes place in a controlled manner. There are sensors, heaters, and actuators placed in the reaction to regulate and keep an eye on the reaction process (figure 9.2). Considering the scaling laws, miniaturization of the reactor component has gained much attention as it improves heat sync and mass transfer properties resulting in a highly efficient device. Not only has the efficiency improved but also due to the lessened consumption of samples and reagents the cost of failure has dramatically decreased [87].

9.4.3.7 Separator

The separator component separates the sample and reagents after the mixing or reaction steps (figure 9.2). This component can isolate the analyte of interest and in the cases where there is no pre-decided target of interest provide the user with a set of analytes to choose from. Micro-separation technique is one of the most vital parts in the study of biological systems, characterization of biomolecules, and bioanalysis [88]. Capillary electrophoresis (CE), magnetic, chromatography, optical tweezers, and filters based on laminar flow are among the approaches used in separations. To perform CE on LOC devices, two electrodes are placed in a microfluidic channel and through the application of an appropriate potential the particles can be separated with respect to their charge. The optical tweezers employ highly focused laser beams to enable the isolation and manipulation of micro-/nanometer-sized particles. There are reports of using optical tweezers in conjunction with capillary electrophoresis on LOC devices resulting in a much better separation of the analytes [89]. Aptamer-assisted separation of the analytes has been made possible through the application of a magnetic field and in the presence of aptamer-functionalized magnetic particles. Through this, the user is able to selectively isolate the cancer biomarkers from the rest of the sample [90, 91].

9.4.3.8 Detector

After the complete isolation of the analytes, a detector is used to identify the presence of the analytes and also measure them quantitatively (figure 9.2). Detectors are the transducers used in the LOC devices that alter physiochemical signals into other detectable signals (e.g. electrical, optical, electrochemical, capacitance, etc).

9.4.3.9 Controller

The controller is in charge of all that is happening on a LOC device including data gathering, signal processing, managing the initiators, and external devices (figure 9.2). A user-friendly interface on the controller helps with a better understanding of what is happening on the chip and a better control on what should be done.

9.4.3.10 Power supply

The power supply generates the power needed by the electrical components used in LOC devices. On portable systems, a battery does the job of the power supply (figure 9.2). However, in the cases where the system uses electrophoresis, a high voltage and the ability to manipulate it accordingly is needed and is achievable through the employment of high voltage programmable power supplies [92, 93].

9.5 Aptamer-based microfluidic biosensors

Wide-concentration range detection of biomarkers has been made possible through the usage of aptamer-based microfluidic biosensors. Microfluidics is perfect in biosensing detections since they consume low amounts of sample and reagent, and enable multiplex detection of analytes; hence, lowering the failure risk and cost of bioassays [94]. While working with microfluidic systems, one can design the channels with respect to the desired flow rate, velocity, and even binding capacity [95, 96]. As mentioned previously, microfluidic systems enable a variety of sample manipulations so that the user can more easily detect their desired analyte [97]. Also, aptamers are excellent candidates for microfluidic-based biosensors due to their small size and high durability thus they can be used at large in the channels.

9.5.1 Electrochemical detection

Electrochemical detection is the employment of the 3-electrode system (i.e. work, counter, and reference) for the detection of the analyte. A voltage is applied to the working electrode (WE) that assists the electron transfer between the electrochemically active species and the WE. The reference electrode is used as a reference to measure and regulate the WE while the counter electrode balances the current observed at the WE. An electrolyte is added to the system providing a conductive environment. While using EC detectors, one can employ various techniques including; cyclic voltammetry (CV), chronoamperometry, differential pulse voltammetry (DPV), and anodic stripping voltammetry (ASV).

Revzin and colleagues have reported the use of micropatterned aptamer-modified electrodes for the sensitive detection of TNF-α and INF-γ (figure 9.3). The electrodes were embedded in microfluidic channels and incubated with immune cells. Biomarker detection was done by performing a square wave voltammetry (SWV) [98].

Hu and colleagues reported the development of an aptamer-based photoelectrochemical sensor for CA-125 detection. A GaN surface was modified with the

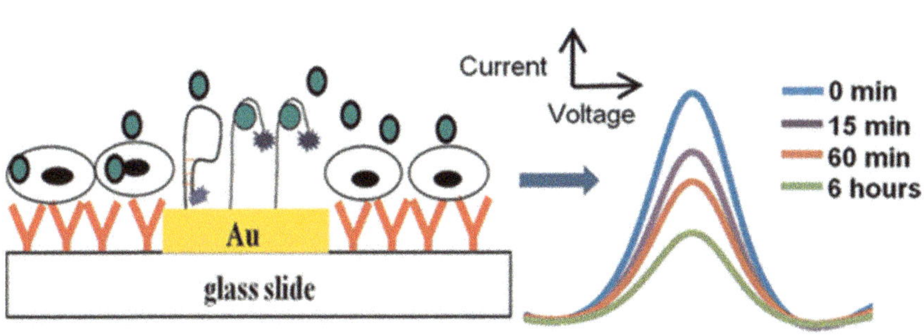

Figure 9.3. Schematic illustration of the principle of TNF-α detection. Reproduced with permission from [98]. Copyright (2011) American Chemical Society.

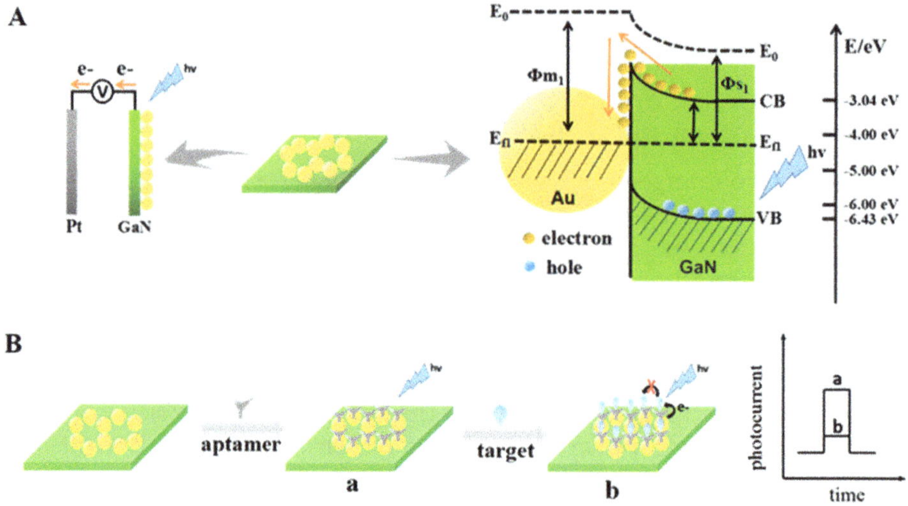

Figure 9.4. Schematic illustration of the photoelectrochemical detection of CA-125. Reproduced with permission from [99]. Copyright (2020) American Chemical Society.

aptamer-modified gold nanoparticles, which in the presence of the target reduces the current with respect to the protein concentration (figure 9.4) [99].

9.5.2 Capacitance

Field-effect transistors work on the basis of bioreceptor immobilization on a semi/conductive channel between drain and source electrodes [35]. Regulated by the gate-source voltage, the conductivity of the channel is then measured after the introduction of the target [100]. Based on the FET channel's type (i.e. N/P-type) and the charge of the analyte (i.e. positive or negative) the conductivity can either decrease or increase [101]. The FET-based biosensors benefit from label-free detection approaches and offer real-time analysis of targets. Low fabrication cost, simple sample preparation, and high sensitivity of these devices are among the many reasons for their use in sensing systems. Employing nanostructures (e.g. CNTs, SNWs) in the construction of FET-based biosensors has highly improved their sensing ability.

The team of Salimi has reported the use of a FET-based aptasensor for sensitive detection of CA-125. The specific aptamers for CA-125 were non-covalently bonded to the MWCNTs decorated on rGO nanosheets [102].

Sinha and colleagues have reported the fabrication of a FET-based aptasensor embedded in a microfluidic system for multiplex detection of 4 biomarkers including C-RP and cTnI (figure 9.5). The AlGaN/GaN high electron mobility transistor (HEMT) was able to sensitively detect CRP and cTnI in a linear range of 0.1–50 mg l^{-1} and 1–10 000 pg ml^{-1}, respectively [103].

In another study by Lee's team, a FET-based microfluidic system was developed using aptamers as bioreceptors for the selective capturing of CTCs in blood samples

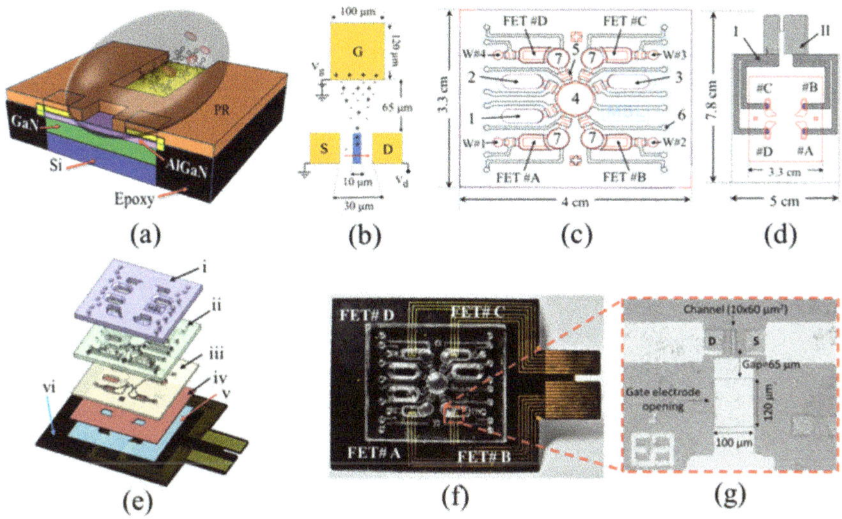

Figure 9.5. High electron mobility transistor (HEMT)-microfluidic chip design: (a) Schematic representation of HEMT sensor and its layers. (b) Source, drain, and gate contacts and their distances. (c) The fabricated microfluidic chip. (d) The microfluidic chip's detection chamber where the FET is located. (e) Schematic illustration of each layer. (f), (g) Photographed image of the fabricated sensor. Reproduced with permission from [103] Copyright (2019) Elsevier.

(figure 9.6). Each FET sensor array could trap 0–3 cells making it a maximum of 42 cells in total [104].

9.6 Challenges and future perspective

The establishment of fast and sensitive methods that are highly selective toward specific targets seems to be the trend of future detection systems. In reaching this goal, the appropriate development of microfluidic-based aptasensors promises the development of fully integrated and automated devices capable of multiplex detection of cancer biomarkers. The challenges that remain in reaching these ideals could be categorized into two main groups; aptamer challenges and microfluidic challenges. The high sensitivity and selectivity of these devices mainly rely on the development and enrichment of aptamers. Aptamer selection procedures should be improved to not only lower the costs of their synthesis but also increase their affinity to a specific target. Regarding microfluidic devices, the design of each component could have a direct impact on the efficiency of the whole system. These components (e.g. microchannels and microvalves) should be appropriately designed to their full extent to enable flexible control over the samples in the separation and detection phases. Also, the necessity of complex equipment needed for their readout systems reduces the portability of these devices. Thus, developing LOC systems that feature highly selective aptamers with a rational design of the components that benefit from simple handheld readout systems should be the focus of research in the early diagnosis of cancer biomarkers.

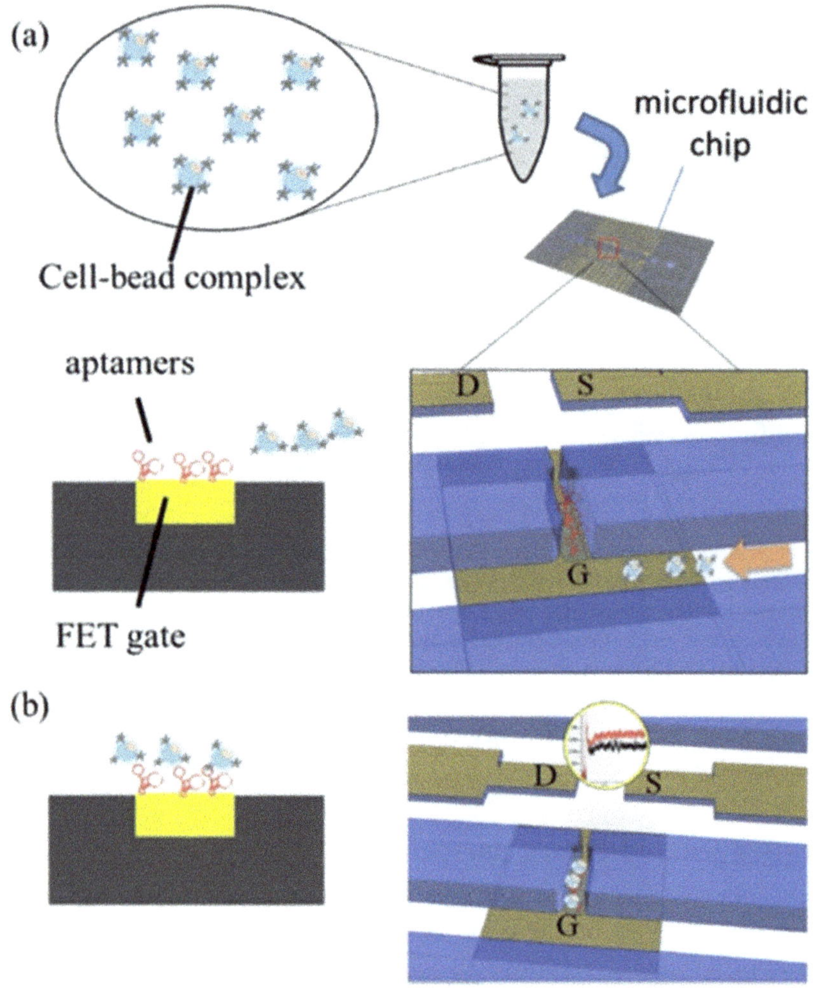

Figure 9.6. Schematic representation of the FET-based aptasensor for the diagnosis of circulating tumor cells in blood sample. Reproduced with permission from [104]. Copyright (2019) Royal Society of Chemistry.

9.7 Conclusion

Cancer as one of the leading causes of death is often diagnosed at late stages where the rate of mortality highly increases, due to the presence of non-specific signs of the disease. Another considerable challenge is the detection of its recurrence. Often at the end of treatment, the remaining cancer cells lead to the recurrence of the disease indicating that the treatment had been unsuccessful. Hence, much effort has been put into the development of sensitive assays for the early detection of cancer. Aptamer-based sensing systems offer high sensitivity, stability, and selectivity while cutting much on the expenses compared to traditional cancer detection assays. The repetitive complex laboratory tasks are simplified and automated on miniaturized devices called lab-on-a-chip. With the improvements and advancements in the fabrication of micro/nano devices and the development of their electromechanical systems, it is now believed that a variety of components can be integrated into a single device that helps with the realization of POC diagnostics. With the help of nanotechnology, non-invasive sensitive detection of small amounts of the analyte has been made possible in real time, which not only cuts on the expenses of the assay but also offers rapid yet accurate results.

References

[1] International Agency for Research on Cancer (https://gco.iarc.fr)

[2] World Health Organization (https://who.int)

[3] Chattaraj R, Mohan P, Livingston C M, Besmer J D, Kumar K and Goodwin A P 2016 Mutually-reactive, fluorogenic hydrocyanine/quinone reporter pairs for in-solution biosensing via nanodroplet association *ACS Appl. Mater. Interfaces* **8** 802–8

[4] Tong Q H, Tao T, Xie L Q and Lu H J 2016 ELISA-PLA: a novel hybrid platform for the rapid, highly sensitive and specific quantification of proteins and post-translational modifications *Biosens. Bioelectron.* **80** 385–91

[5] Zhao S, Yang W and Lai R Y 2011 A folding-based electrochemical aptasensor for detection of vascular endothelial growth factor in human whole blood *Biosens. Bioelectron.* **26** 2442–7

[6] Bettazzi F, Enayati L, Sánchez I C, Motaghed R, Mascini M and Palchetti I 2013 Electrochemical bioassay for the detection of TNF-α using magnetic beads and disposable screen-printed array of electrodes *Bioanalysis* **5** 1

[7] Eletxigerra U, Martinez-Perdiguero J, Merino S, Villalonga R, Pingarrón J M and Campuzano S 2014 Amperometric magnetoimmunoassay for the direct detection of tumor necrosis factor alpha biomarker in human serum *Anal. Chim. Acta* **838** 37–44

[8] Liu Y, Liu Y, Matharu Z, Rahimian A and Revzin A 2015 Detecting multiple cell-secreted cytokines from the same aptamer-functionalized electrode *Biosens. Bioelectron.* **64** 43–50

[9] Florea A, Taleat Z, Cristea C, Mazloum-Ardakani M and Săndulescu R 2013 Label free MUC1 aptasensors based on electrodeposition of gold nanoparticles on screen printed electrodes *Electrochem. Commun.* **33** 127–30

[10] Li Y, Zhong Z, Chai Y, Song Z, Zhuo Y, Su H, Liu S, Wang D and Yuan R 2012 Simultaneous electrochemical immunoassay of three liver cancer biomarkers using distinguishable redox probes as signal tags and gold nanoparticles coated carbon nanotubes as signal enhancers *Chem. Commun.* **48** 537–9

[11] Giovannitti A *et al* 2016 Erratum: N-Type organic electrochemical transistors with stability in water *Nat. Commun.* **7** 13066

[12] Nielsen C B *et al* 2016 Molecular design of semiconducting polymers for high-performance organic electrochemical transistors *J. Am. Chem. Soc.* **138** 10252–9

[13] Li F, Li Y, Feng J, Dong Y, Wang P, Chen L, Chen Z, Liu H and Wei Q 2017 Ultrasensitive amperometric immunosensor for PSA detection based on $Cu_2O@CeO_2$–Au nanocomposites as integrated triple signal amplification strategy *Biosens. Bioelectron.* **87** 630–7

[14] Benvidi A, Banaei M, Tezerjani M D, Molahosseini H and Jahanbani S 2018 Impedimetric PSA aptasensor based on the use of a glassy carbon electrode modified with titanium oxide nanoparticles and silk fibroin nanofibers *Microchim. Acta* **185** 50

[15] Costello L C, Franklin R B and Narayan P 1999 Citrate in the diagnosis of prostate cancer *Prostate* **38** 237–45

[16] Abarghoei S, Fakhri N, Borghei Y S, Hosseini M and Ganjali M R 2019 A Colorimetric paper sensor for citrate as biomarker for early stage detection of prostate cancer based on peroxidase-like activity of cysteine-capped gold nanoclusters *Spectrochim. Acta* A **210** 251–9

[17] Kumada T, Toyoda H, Tada T, Kiriyama S, Tanikawa M, Hisanaga Y, Kanamori A, Tanaka J, Kagebayashi C and Satomura S 2014 High-sensitivity lens culinaris agglutinin-reactive alpha-fetoprotein assay predicts early detection of hepatocellular carcinoma *J. Gastroenterol.* **49** 555–63

[18] Gao T, Liu F, Yang D, Yu Y, Wang Z and Li G 2015 Assembly of selective biomimetic surface on an electrode surface: a design of nano-bio interface for biosensing *Anal. Chem.* **87** 5683–9

[19] Malaguarnera G, Giordano M, Paladina I, Berretta M, Cappellani A and Malaguarnera M Serum markers of hepatocellular carcinoma *Dig. Dis. Sci.* **55** 2744–55

[20] Zhou H, Gan N, Li T, Cao Y, Zeng S, Zheng L and Guo Z 2012 The sandwich-type electrochemiluminescence immunosensor for α-Fetoprotein based on enrichment by Fe_3O_4–Au magnetic nano probes and signal amplification by CdS–Au composite nanoparticles labeled anti-AFP *Anal. Chim. Acta* **746** 107–13

[21] Vasudev A, Kaushik A and Bhansali S 2013 Electrochemical immunosensor for label free epidermal growth factor receptor (EGFR) detection *Biosens. Bioelectron.* **39** 300–5

[22] Arkan E, Saber R, Karimi Z and Shamsipur M 2015 A novel antibody–antigen based impedimetric immunosensor for low level detection of HER2 in serum samples of breast cancer patients via modification of a gold nanoparticles decorated multiwall carbon nanotube-ionic liquid electrode *Anal. Chim. Acta* **874** 66–74

[23] Arya S K and Estrela P 2017 Electrochemical immunosensor for tumor necrosis factor-alpha detection in undiluted serum *Methods* **116** 125–31

[24] Arya S K, Kongsuphol P and Park M K 2017 On-chip electrochemical immunoassay platform for specific protein biomarker estimation in undiluted serum using off-surface membrane matrix *Biosens. Bioelectron.* **91** 721–7

[25] Aydın E B, Aydın M and Sezgintürk M K 2017 A highly sensitive immunosensor based on ITO thin films covered by a new semi-conductive conjugated polymer for the determination of TNFα in human saliva and serum samples *Biosens. Bioelectron.* **97** 169–76

[26] Kavosi B, Salimi A, Hallaj R and Moradi F 2015 Ultrasensitive electrochemical immunosensor for PSA biomarker detection in prostate cancer cells using gold nano-particles/PAMAM dendrimer loaded with enzyme linked aptamer as integrated triple signal amplification strategy *Biosens. Bioelectron.* **74** 915–23

[27] Bin Liang W, Yang M Z, Zhuo Y, Zheng Y N, Xiong C Y, Chai Y Q and Yuan R 2016 Competitive method-based electrochemiluminescent assay with protein-nucleotide conversion for ratio detection to efficiently monitor the drug resistance of cancer cells *Chem. Sci.* **7**

[28] Rauf S, Mishra G K, Azhar J, Mishra R K, Goud K Y, Nawaz M A H, Marty J L and Hayat A 2018 Carboxylic group riched graphene oxide based disposable electrochemical immunosensor for cancer biomarker detection *Anal. Biochem.* **545** 13–9

[29] Chang Y, Li M, Wu Z, Zhuo Y, Chai Y, Xiao Q and Yuan R 2018 Homogeneous entropy catalytic-driven DNA hydrogel as strong signal blocker for highly sensitive electrochemical detection of platelet-derived growth factor *Anal. Chem.* **90** 8241–7

[30] Bruni D, Angell H K and Galon J The immune contexture and immunoscore in cancer prognosis and therapeutic efficacy *Nat. Rev. Cancer* **20** 662–80

[31] Dinarello C A Why not treat human cancer with interleukin-1 blockade? *Cancer Metastasis Rev.* **20** 317–29
[32] Elinav E, Nowarski R, Thaiss C A, Hu B, Jin C and Flavell R A Inflammation-induced cancer: crosstalk between tumours, immune cells and microorganisms *Nat. Rev. Cancer* **13** 759–71
[33] Yazdanparast S, Benvidi A, Banaei M, Nikukar H, Tezerjani M D and Azimzadeh M 2018 Dual-aptamer based electrochemical sandwich biosensor for MCF-7 human breast cancer cells using silver nanoparticle labels and a poly(glutamic Acid)/MWNT nanocomposite *Microchim. Acta* **185** 405
[34] Marquette C A, Bouteille F, Corgier B P, Degiuli A and Blum L J 2009 Disposable screen-printed chemiluminescent biochips for the simultaneous determination of four point-of-care relevant proteins *Anal. Bioanal. Chem.* **393** 1191–8
[35] Firoozbakhtian A, Rezayan A H, Hajghassem H, Rahimi F, Ghazani M F, Kalantar M and Mohamadsharifi A 2022 Buried-Gate MWCNT FET-based nanobiosensing device for real-time detection of CRP *ACS Omega* **7** 7341–9
[36] Zhao J and Ma Z 2018 Ultrasensitive detection of prostate specific antigen by electrochemical aptasensor using enzyme-free recycling amplification via target-induced catalytic hairpin assembly *Biosens. Bioelectron.* **102** 316–20
[37] Razmi N, Baradaran B, Hejazi M, Hasanzadeh M, Mosafer J, Mokhtarzadeh A and de la Guardia M Recent advances on aptamer-based biosensors to detection of platelet-derived growth factor *Biosens. Bioelectron.* **113** 58–71
[38] Pan L H, Kuo S H, Lin T Y, Lin C W, Fang P Y and Yang H W 2017 An electrochemical biosensor to simultaneously detect VEGF and PSA for early prostate cancer diagnosis based on graphene oxide/SsDNA/PLLA nanoparticles *Biosens. Bioelectron.* **89** 598–605
[39] American Cancer Society (https://cancer.org)
[40] Montagnana M, Danese E, Giudici S, Franchi M, Guidi G C, Plebani M and Lippi G 2011 HE4 in ovarian cancer: from discovery to clinical application *Adv Clin Chem.* **55** 1–20
[41] Zhao L, Han H and Ma Z 2018 Improved screen-printed carbon electrode for multiplexed label-free amperometric immuniosensor: addressing its conductivity and reproducibility challenges *Biosens. Bioelectron.* **101** 304–10
[42] Tang Z, Fu Y and Ma Z 2017 Bovine serum albumin as an effective sensitivity enhancer for peptide-based amperometric biosensor for ultrasensitive detection of prostate specific antigen *Biosens. Bioelectron.* **94** 394–9
[43] Shangguan D, Li Y, Tang Z, Cao Z C, Chen H W, Mallikaratchy P, Sefah K, Yang C J and Tan W 2006 Aptamers evolved from live cells as effective molecular probes for cancer study *Proc. Natl Acad. Sci. USA* **103** 11838–43
[44] Mendonsa S D and Bowser M T 2004 In vitro evolution of functional DNA using capillary electrophoresis *J. Am. Chem. Soc.* **126** 20–1
[45] Stoltenburg R, Reinemann C and Strehlitz B 2005 FluMag-SELEX as an advantageous method for DNA aptamer selection *Anal. Bioanal. Chem.* **383** 83–91
[46] Lai J C and Hong C Y 2014 Magnetic-assisted rapid aptamer selection (MARAS) for generating high-affinity DNA aptamer using rotating magnetic fields *ACS Comb. Sci.* **16** 321–7
[47] Hosseini M, Khabbaz H, Dadmehr M, Ganjali M R and Mohamadnejad J 2015 Aptamer-based colorimetric and chemiluminescence detection of aflatoxin B1 in foods samples *Acta Chim. Slov.* **62** 721–8
[48] Bagheri Pebdeni A, Mousavizadegan M and Hosseini M 2021 Sensitive detection of *S. aureus* using aptamer- and vancomycin-copper nanoclusters as dual recognition strategy *Food Chem.* **361** 130137

[49] Muzyka K, Saqib M, Liu Z, Zhang W and Xu G Progress and challenges in electrochemiluminescent aptasensors *Biosens. Bioelectron.* **92** 241–58

[50] Song S, Wang L, Li J, Fan C and Zhao J 2008 Aptamer-based biosensors *TrAC Trends Anal. Chem.* **27** 108–17

[51] Hori S I, Herrera A, Rossi J J and Zhou J Current advances in aptamers for cancer diagnosis and therapy *Cancers* **10** 9

[52] Kashefi-Kheyrabadi L, Mehrgardi M A, Wiechec E, Turner A P F and Tiwari A 2014 Ultrasensitive detection of human liver hepatocellular carcinoma cells using a label-free aptasensor *Anal. Chem.* **86** 4956–60

[53] Hashkavayi A B, Raoof J B, Ojani R and Kavoosian S 2017 Ultrasensitive electrochemical aptasensor based on sandwich architecture for selective label-free detection of colorectal cancer (CT26) cells *Biosens. Bioelectron.* **92** 630–7

[54] Amouzadeh Tabrizi M, Shamsipur M, Saber R and Sarkar S 2018 Isolation of HL-60 cancer cells from the human serum sample using MnO_2-PEI/Ni/Au/Aptamer as a novel nanomotor and electrochemical determination of thereof by Aptamer/gold nanoparticles-poly(3,4-ethylene dioxythiophene) modified GC electrode *Biosens. Bioelectron.* **110** 141–6

[55] Shen H, Yang J, Chen Z, Chen X, Wang L, Hu J, Ji F, Xie G and Feng W 2016 A novel label-free and reusable electrochemical cytosensor for highly sensitive detection and specific collection of CTCs *Biosens. Bioelectron.* **81** 495–502

[56] Bábelová L, Sohová M E, Poturnayová A, Buríková M, Bizík J and Hianik T 2018 Label-free electrochemical aptasensor for jurkat cells detection as a potential diagnostic tool for leukemia *Electroanalysis* **30** 1487–95

[57] Chandra P, Noh H B and Shim Y B 2013 Cancer cell detection based on the interaction between an anticancer drug and cell membrane components *Chem. Commun.* **49** 1900–2

[58] Kara P, Erzurumlu Y, Kirmizibayrak P B and Ozsoz M 2016 Electrochemical aptasensor design for label free cytosensing of human non-small cell lung cancer *J. Electroanal. Chem.* **775** 337–41

[59] Farzin L, Shamsipur M, Samandari L and Sheibani S 2018 Signalling probe displacement electrochemical aptasensor for malignant cell surface nucleolin as a breast cancer biomarker based on gold nanoparticle decorated hydroxyapatite nanorods and silver nanoparticle labels *Microchim. Acta* **185** 154

[60] Khoshfetrat S M and Mehrgardi M A 2017 Amplified detection of leukemia cancer cells using an aptamer-conjugated gold-coated magnetic nanoparticles on a nitrogen-doped graphene modified electrode *Bioelectrochemistry* **114** 24–32

[61] Cao J, Zhao X P, Younis M R, Li Z Q, Xia X H and Wang C 2017 Ultrasensitive capture, detection, and release of circulating tumor cells using a nanochannel-ion channel hybrid coupled with electrochemical detection technique *Anal. Chem.* **89** 10957–64

[62] Zhang K, Tan T, Fu J J, Zheng T and Zhu J J 2013 A novel aptamer-based competition strategy for ultrasensitive electrochemical detection of leukemia cells *Analyst* **138**

[63] Li J, Xu M, Huang H, Zhou J, Abdel-Halimb E S, Zhang J R and Zhu J J 2011 Aptamer-quantum dots conjugates-based ultrasensitive competitive electrochemical cytosensor for the detection of tumor cell *Talanta* **85** 2113–20

[64] Firoozbakhtian A, Sojic N, Xu G and Hosseini M 2023 Electrochemiluminescence sensors in bioanalysis *Encyclopedia of Sensors and Biosensors* ed R Narayan (Elsevier) pp 317–40

[65] Hosseini M *et al* 2022 Development of sandwich electrochemiluminescence immunosensor for COVID-19 diagnosis by SARS-CoV-2 spike protein detection based on Au@BSA-Luminol nanocomposites *Bioelectrochemistry* **147** 108161

[66] Whitesides G M The origins and the future of microfluidics *Nature* **442** 368–73
[67] Harrison D J, Fluri K, Seiler K, Fan Z, Effenhauser C S and Manz A 1993 Micromachining a miniaturized capillary electrophoresis-based chemical analysis system on a chip *Science* **261** 895–7
[68] Manz A, Graber N and Widmer H M 1990 Miniaturized total chemical analysis systems: a novel concept for chemical sensing *Sensors Actuators* B **1** 244–8
[69] Choi S, Song S, Choi C and Park J K 2007 Continuous blood cell separation by hydrophoretic filtration *Lab Chip* **7** 1532
[70] Jung B, Fisher K, Ness K D, Rose K A and Mariella R P 2008 Acoustic particle filter with adjustable effective pore size for automated sample preparation *Anal. Chem.* **80** 8447–52
[71] Inglis D W, Riehn R, Austin R H and Sturm J C 2004 Continuous microfluidic immunomagnetic cell separation *Appl. Phys. Lett.* **85** 5093–5
[72] Lien K Y, Lin W Y, Lee Y F, Wang C H, Lei H Y and Bin Lee G 2008 Microfluidic systems integrated with a sample pretreatment device for fast nucleic-acid amplification *J. Microelectromech. Syst.* **17** 288–301
[73] Steigert J *et al* 2005 Integrated sample preparation, reaction, and detection on a high-frequency centrifugal microfluidic platform *J. Assoc. Lab. Autom.* **10** 331–41
[74] Brown R B and Audet J Current techniques for single-cell lysis *J. R. Soc. Interface* **5** S131–8
[75] Fu A Y, Chou H P, Spence C, Arnold F H and Quake S R 2002 An integrated microfabricated cell sorter *Anal. Chem.* **74** 2451–7
[76] Tai C H, Hsiung S K, Chen C Y, Tsai M L and Bin Lee G 2007 Automatic microfluidic platform for cell separation and nucleus collection *Biomed. Microdevices* **9** 533–43
[77] Wang C H and Bin Lee G 2005 Automatic bio-sampling chips integrated with micro-pumps and micro-valves for disease detection *Biosens. Bioelectron.* **21** 419–25
[78] Nguyen N T and Huang X 2001 Miniature valveless pumps based on printed circuit board technique *Sensors Actuators* A **88** 104–11
[79] Andersson H, Van Der Wijngaart W, Nilsson P, Enoksson P and Stemme G 2001 Valve-less diffuser micropump for microfluidic analytical systems *Sensors Actuators* B **72** 259–65
[80] Suzuki H and Yoneyama R 2003 Integrated microfluidic system with electrochemically actuated on-chip pumps and valves *Sensors Actuators* B **96** 38–45
[81] Melin J, Roxhed N, Gimenez G, Griss P, Van Der Wijngaart W and Stemme G 2004 A liquid-triggered liquid microvalve for on-chip flow control *Sensors Actuators* B **100** 463–8
[82] Cho B S, Schuster T G, Zhu X, Chang D, Smith G D and Takayama S 2003 Passively driven integrated microfluidic system for separation of motile sperm *Anal. Chem.* **75** 1671–5
[83] Schulte T, Bardell R and Weigl B H 2000 Sample acquisition and control on-chip microfluidic sample preparation *J. Assoc. Lab. Autom.* **5** 83–8
[84] Suzuki H, Ho C M and Kasagi N 2004 A chaotic mixer for magnetic bead-based micro cell sorter *J. Microelectromech. Syst.* **13** 779–90
[85] Wang Y, Zhe J, Chung B T F and Dutta P 2008 A rapid magnetic particle driven micromixer *Microfluid. Nanofluidics* **4** 375–89
[86] Grumann M, Geipel A, Riegger L, Zengerle R and Ducrée J 2005 Batch-mode mixing on centrifugal microfluidic platforms *Lab Chip* **5** 560–5
[87] Doku G N, Verboom W, Reinhoudt D N and Van Den Berg A On-microchip multiphase chemistry—a review of microreactor design principles and reagent contacting modes *Tetrahedron.* **61** 2733–742

[88] Liu B F, Xu B, Zhang G, Du W and Luo Q Micro-separation toward systems biology *J. Chromatogr.* A **1106** 19–28

[89] Munce N R, Li J, Herman P R and Lilge L 2004 Microfabricated system for parallel single-cell capillary electrophoresis *Anal. Chem.* **76** 4983–9

[90] Pamme N and Wilhelm C 2006 Continuous sorting of magnetic cells via on-chip free-flow magnetophoresis *Lab Chip* **6** 947–80

[91] Ramadan Q, Samper V, Poenar D P and Yu C 2006 An integrated microfluidic platform for magnetic microbeads separation and confinement *Biosens. Bioelectron.* **21** 1693–702

[92] Erickson D, Sinton D and Li D A miniaturized high-voltage integrated power supply for portable microfluidic applications *Lab Chip* **4** 87–90

[93] Tsai C H, Wang Y N, Lin C F, Yang R J and Fu L M 2006 Experimental and numerical investigation into leakage effect in injectors of microfluidic devices *Electrophoresis* **27** 4991–8

[94] Huang L, Bian S, Cheng Y, Shi G, Liu P, Ye X and Wang W 2017 Microfluidics cell sample preparation for analysis: advances in efficient cell enrichment and precise single cell capture *Biomicrofluidics* **11** 011501

[95] Selmi M, Gazzah M H and Belmabrouk H 2017 Optimization of microfluidic biosensor efficiency by means of fluid flow engineering *Sci. Rep.* **7** 5721

[96] Liu Y J, Guo S S, Zhang Z L, Huang W H, Baigl D, Xie M, Chen Y and Pang D W 2007 A micropillar-integrated smart microfluidic device for specific capture and sorting of cells *Electrophoresis* **28** 4713–22

[97] Ferguson B S *et al* 2013 Real-time, aptamer-based tracking of circulating therapeutic agents in living animals *Sci. Transl. Med.* **5** 213ra165

[98] Liu Y, Yan J, Howland M C, Kwa T and Revzin A 2011 Micropatterned aptasensors for continuous monitoring of cytokine release from human leukocytes *Anal. Chem.* **83** 8286–92

[99] Hu D, Liang H, Wang X, Luo F, Qiu B, Lin Z and Wang J 2020 Highly sensitive and selective photoelectrochemical aptasensor for cancer biomarker CA125 based on AuNPs/GaN schottky junction *Anal. Chem.* **92** 10114–20

[100] Byon H R and Choi H C 2006 Network single-walled carbon nanotube-field effect transistors (SWNT-FETs) with Increased schottky contact area for highly sensitive biosensor applications *J. Am. Chem. Soc.* **128** 2188–9

[101] Vu C A and Chen W Y Field-effect transistor biosensors for biomedical applications: recent advances and future prospects *Sensors (Switzerland)* **19** 4214

[102] Mansouri S, Majd A and Salimi A 2018 Ultrasensitive flexible FET-type aptasensor for CA 125 cancer marker detection based on carboxylated multiwalled carbon nanotubes immobilized onto reduced graphene oxide film *Anal. Chim. Acta* **1000** 273–82

[103] Sinha A *et al* 2019 An integrated microfluidic system with field-effect-transistor sensor arrays for detecting multiple cardiovascular biomarkers from clinical samples *Biosens. Bioelectron.* **129** 155–63

[104] Chen Y H, Pulikkathodi A K, Ma Y D, Wang Y L and Bin Lee G 2019 A microfluidic platform integrated with field-effect transistors for enumeration of circulating tumor cells *Lab Chip* **19** 618–25

IOP Publishing

Chapter 10

Nanotechnology in cancer diagnosis: challenges and opportunitiesn

Arpana Parihar, Kritika Gaur and Raju Khan

The cancer is one of the main causes of mortality and low life expectancy worldwide. Cancer continues to be among the primary causes of death despite developments in novel therapy techniques. The main cause of this is the difficulty to identify malignancies at the very initial stages. The disease may have spread by the time the tumor is detected making therapy challenging, if not impossible. Thus, to spot cancer in its earliest or perhaps even pre-syndromic phases, it's indeed crucial to develop novel diagnostic methods. The recent advancement in the field of nanotechnology has tremendous potential to enhance the sensitivity of diagnostic modalities. Due to their outstanding sensitivity, specificity, and multiplexed measuring capability, nanomaterial-enabled advanced biosensors have gained much attention and are being investigated for the detection of extrinsic cancer biomarkers and cancer cells, as well as for *in vivo* imaging. The most current developments in nanotechnology applications for cancer diagnosis are summarised in this chapter.

10.1 Introduction

Cancer is a blanket term for a collection of disorders characterized by unregulated, unpredictable cellular division and intrusiveness (Zeps and Hemmings 2015). Attempts had been obligated for several years to identify various cancer risk factors. Cancer mortality and occurrence are rising steadily worldwide (Nonaka *et al* 2021). In 2020, there were 18 094 716 million cancer cases diagnosed worldwide. In 2020, the maturity level incidence including all malignancies (except non-melanoma skin cancer) was 190 per 100 000 for men and women. Men had a higher rate (206.9 per 100 000) than women (178.1 per 100 000) (Sung *et al* 2021). According to the International Agency for Research on Cancer (IARC), about one in 5 people suffered with carcinoma throughout their lifespan, and about one in 8 men to one out of every 11 women will die from disease. The latest data showed that over fifty

doi:10.1088/978-0-7503-5012-9ch10

million individuals die in the following 5 years after being diagnosed with cancer (Miller *et al* 2019). Global population aging and socioeconomic risk factors continue to be major drivers of this increase in disease condition. Early detection is critical for successful cancer treatment and combatting cancer disease. Early detection reduces cancer-related mortality significantly (Balata *et al* 2022). Breast carcinoma, for instance, has an overall 5-year chance of survival in over 90% cases, but individuals with other metastatic diseases have a five-year survival rate in just 27% cases (Giaquinto *et al* 2022). Imaging methods and morphology study of tissue taken via biopsy from a diseased person using histopathology or cells (cytology) are being employed usually for tumour identification. Most regularly utilized imaging techniques, such as x-rays, MRI, computed tomography (CT), endoscopy, and ultrasonography, and may identify malignancy only whenever a visible alteration in the diseased tissue/organ is present, hence failing to detect it early (Frangioni 2008). Additionally, existing imaging technologies are unable to distinguish between benign and malignant tumors. Thousands of cancerous cells might well have grown and perhaps spread due to delayed diagnosis (Entenberg *et al* 2023). Moreover, the inherent limitations of conventional cancer diagnostic methods have hampered early cancer detection.

Nanotechnology, an interdisciplinary discipline comprising chemistry, biology, physics, and materials engineering, has found widespread applications in several clinical and medical fields (Shanmugam 2019). These include nanoparticle-based imaging, hyperthermia, drug delivery, and biosensing applications (Khan *et al* 2021), Within the last century, some of these nanomaterial-enabled techniques have indeed been transmitted into therapeutic and clinical interventions (Babu *et al* 2013). Some of the applications of nanomaterials in imaging, drug delivery and cancer therapeutics are illustrated in figure 10.1. Because of both active and passive targeting, nanostructures have now been widely used for the treatment of various malignancies (Ranjan *et al* 2020). Various conventional medications that are being used to treat tumors typically lead to poor performance and could have a number of severe consequences, including damage to healthy cells. Several nanomaterials, such as quantum dots and gold nanoparticles are used to diagnose disease at the molecular level (Hutter and Maysinger 2011). Nanotechnology-based molecular diagnostics, which include biosensor-based detection of biological markers, can indeed detect cancers accurately and quickly.

Nano-enabled diagnostics approaches have been designed as prospective genuine, easy, and cost-effective tools for carcinoma detection and treatment (Dessale *et al* 2022). This chapter summarises recent advances in the field of nanotechnology and development of nanomaterial in cancer diagnosis. The challenges and perspectives in the field of nano-enabled diagnostics have also been discussed herein.

10.2 Conventional diagnostic techniques for cancer

Early detection of cancer typically provides better opportunity for a speedy recovery and enhanced survival (Zhao *et al* 2022). In this context, cancer screening guidelines and information are available from several medical and patient advocacy

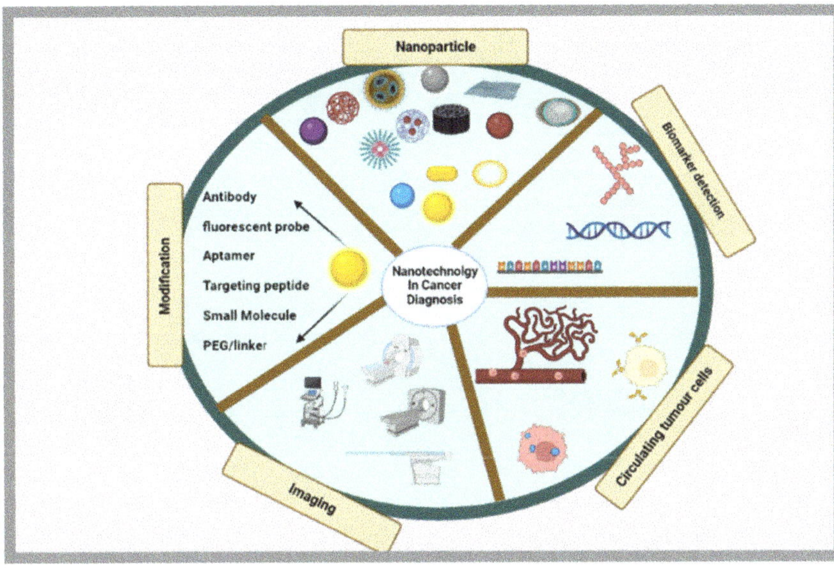

Figure 10.1. Role of nanotechnology in cancer diagnostics and therapeutics.

organizations (Pushparajah 2018). Studies demonstrated that screening could save people's lives by detecting cancer early in a few malignancies. Screening tests for various malignancies are generally advised to the persons who are at high risk. The initial stage of cancer diagnosis is a physical examination and laboratory testing (Cardoso *et al* 2019). A physical examination extensively examines a lump, enlargement, and change in skin color, whereas laboratory procedures, such as urine and blood tests, may assist to uncover anomalies that might have been triggered by cancer (Yan and Huang 2021, Ginsburg *et al* 2020, D'Souza *et al* 2021). A non-invasive way of diagnosis is used to know the cancer location and size by imaging tests that provides detailed images of inside organs. In imaging tests, x-rays (high-energy radiation), radio waves, ultrasound (high-energy sound waves), and radioactive substances-based imaging techniques have been employed (Drost *et al* 2020). They may be used to aid in illness diagnosis, treatment planning, or determining how well treatments are working. Examples of imaging tests are magnetic resonance imaging (MRI), ultrasonography, computed tomography (CT), mammography (Kasivisvanathan *et al* 2019), positron emission tomography (PET), nuclear scans, and bone scans. A biopsy is usually performed to diagnose a type of cancer and its stage (Chen and Zhao 2019). A pathologist examines the tissue underneath a microscope and does additional tests to determine whether it is cancerous or not (Crocetto *et al* 2022).

Clinical tests are critical in tumor diagnosis and therapy (Wilson *et al* 2018). There are several limitations of using conventional techniques such as delayed diagnosis, low sensitivity and having the potential to lose valuable information about the disease. Recent advances in the field of nanotechnology enabled us with the nanomaterial-enabled novel diagnostic approaches that have the potential to

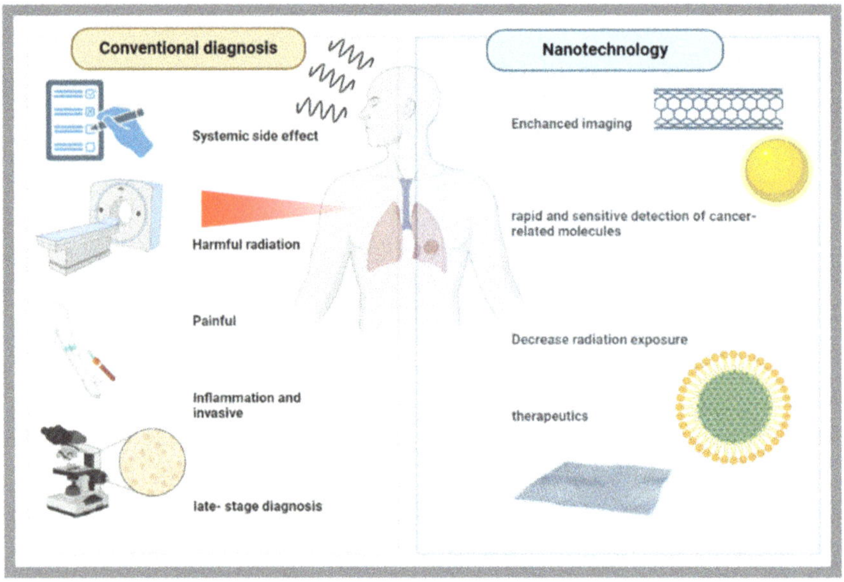

Figure 10.2. Conventional versus nanotechnology-based diagnostic methods for detection of cancer.

overcome these limitations. Some conventional and nanotechnology-based approaches are illustrated in figure 10.2. The pros and cons of these approaches are discussed in table 10.1.

10.3 Advanced cancer diagnostic approaches

Early detection is critical in the battle against cancer for successful therapeutic intervention (Wang *et al* 2019). However, the inherent limitations of traditional cancer diagnostic technologies have hampered early cancer identification. Point-of-care diagnostic devices are a promising alternative for detecting and analysing cancer markers in a timely and sensitive manner. In this context, biosensor-based approaches have proven to be beneficial over conventional diagnostic techniques in terms of quick results, cost-effectiveness, sensitivity and selectivity (Soler *et al* 2019). Recently, several diverse, effective, and accurate biosensing methods for cancer diagnostics have been investigated. The efficiency and sensitivity of biosensors can be significantly improved using nanomaterials, which enhances the signal readouts due to their excellent electrical and optical properties. The advanced nano-enabled biosensor-based approaches for cancer biomarker detection are presented in table 10.2.

10.3.1 Nano-enabled biosensor-based diagnostic approaches

With an increasing number of malignant cases being identified worldwide and an increase in mortality rate due to delayed cancer identification, there is urgent need for sensitive early diagnostic approaches. Biosensors hold potential in terms of early

Table 10.1. Advantages and disadvantages of conventional diagnostic methods.

Diagnosis type	Diagnostic tool	Advantages	Disadvantages	References
Physical examination	Morphology	Timely detection of disease	False assurance, narrow differential diagnoses	Feig and Schwartz (1981)
Lab test	Blood chemistry analysis Testing for cancer gene mutations Total blood count (CBC) Cytogenetic investigation Immunophenotyping Cytology of sputum (also called sputum culture) Tests for tumour markers Cytology of urine	To aid in cancer diagnosis, quantitative	Limit in detailed and trustworthy information regarding specific health issues, cancer and other disorders cannot be diagnosed only by laboratory tests and potential loss of spatial information	Pruthi (2019)
Imaging test	CT scan MRI Nuclear scanning Scan of the bones PET examination Ultrasound\x-rays	Provide information about type of cancer and its stage, if a malignancy is responding to therapy, identify a tumour's recurrence	Expensive, inconvenient, and uncomfortable. Also, exposing patients to quite high levels of ionizing radiation, may cause adverse effect	Mower (2008)
Biopsy	Endoscopy using a needle colonoscopy/ bronchoscopy Surgical intervention	Fast and easy	Painful. Inflammation and invasive	Ripamonti *et al* (2014)

tumor detection (Hasan *et al* 2021). Individuals' genetic patterns are being investigated utilizing novel molecular tools such as genomic and proteomic methods (Huizar *et al* 2020). Whenever combined with computational methods, such techniques provide new data that may be utilized to uncover novel disease biomarkers. Identifying specific and sensitive biomarkers associated with specific

Table 10.2. Nano-enabled biosensor-based approaches for cancer diagnosis.

Nanomaterial	Purpose	Studied target	Linear range	LOD	References
Gold nanoparticle	Detection	Correlation of cancer antigen 15–3 (CA15–3)	from 1.1 to 5.0 mU ml^{-1}	0.9 μU ml^{-1}	Mohammadi *et al* (2018)
Gold nanoparticles	Detection	MCF-7 breast cancer cell	—	—	Chinen *et al* (2015)
Gold nanorod	Detection	MCF-7 cells	10^2–10^5 cells ml^{-1}	100 cells ml^{-1}	Li *et al* (2016)
Graphene quantum dots	Detection	EpCAM	0.2–10 μmol l^{-1}	0.08 μmol l^{-1}	Bingdi Wang *et al* (2018)
Silica nanoparticle	Detection	Interleukin-6 (IL-6)	0.1 to 10 ng ml^{-1}	0.1 ng ml^{-1}	Wu *et al* (2008)
Gold nanocluster	Detection	HER2-positive	10–1000 cells	—	Li *et al* (2019)
Gold nanocluster	Detection	Breast cancer cells	5–1000	5 cells	Tao *et al* (2017)
Silver nanoparticles	Detection	Sialic acid (SA) levels in saliva	—	7 mg dl^{-1}	Hernandez *et al* (2009)
Silver nanoparticles	Detection	BRCA1	0.015 65–10 and 0.625–20 pg ml^{-1}	0.003 pg ml^{-1}	Hasan *et al* (2021)
Silver nanoclusters	Detection	Breast cancer gene 1	5×10^{-13}–1×10^{-9} M	1.2×10^{-13} M	Borghei *et al* (2016)
Carbon nanotubes	Detection	HRP-Ab_2	0.05–5 and 5–200 ng ml^{-1}	0.018 ng ml^{-1}	Yang *et al* (2014)

cancer diseases is a challenging task. Likewise, biomarker concentrations in body fluids may vary depending on cancer stages and phases (Broza *et al* 2019).

Biomarkers are molecules whose level significantly changes throughout malignancy and have high diagnostic value (Wadowska *et al* 2020). Proteins, metabolites, isoenzymes, hormones or nucleic acids are examples of biomarkers, which can be prognostic, predictive, or diagnostic. Biomarkers for diagnosis are used to detect the illness, whereas prognostic biomarkers provide information regarding the disease's path of recurrence (Tang *et al* 2020). In contrast, prediction biomarkers are being used to aid in the optimization of appropriate therapies and frequently indicate the chance of benefitting from a given therapy. The presence or absence of certain biomarkers in a cell is typically a sign of cancer progression. The detection and classification of cancer-specific biomarkers may assist in presymptomatic screening and treatment of the disease (Oh and Joo 2020). To detect cancer, biomarkers (Zahavi and Weiner 2020), overexpressed receptors (Varty *et al* 2021), and antigens (Perera *et al* 2020) specific biorecognition (BRE) elements such as enzymes, antibodies, and aptamers have been used. When BREs interact with a specific analyte, a desired signal produces which get transformed to an electric signal by the transducer. A good transducer provides low noise signals and exhibit outstanding reliability, high resolution, and gives consistent results. The transducers can be optical (luminescence, fluorescence, interferometry, and colorimetric), calorimetric (thermistors), electrochemical (amperometry, potentiometry, and conductometry/ impediments), or based on mass changes (acoustic waves/ piezoelectric) (Filice *et al* 2021).

10.3.1.1 Tumor cell detection using an electrochemical biosensor

The electrochemical technique provides the benefits of rapid diagnosis, excellent sensitivities (single-cell detection), and malignant cell selectivity (Topkaya *et al* 2016), which is not only effective in separating tumour cells from healthy cells, but also offers selective identification of cancerous cells and circulatory tumour cells. In precision research, electrochemical sensors have been employed for early cancer detection, grading, and prediction. An electrochemical biosensor (Cui *et al* 2017) based on a cell impedance was developed to detect cell layer resistivity caused by cell structure, mobility, or interaction. It was used for quantitative monitoring of cell dynamic movement instantaneously without any inflicting cell injury (Ranjan *et al* 2020).

In the study by Wang *et al* (2019) fabricated a simple direct plasmon-enhanced electrochemistry (DPEE) based biosensor, to identify circulating tumour cells in ultra-sensitive manner (CTCs). The sensor was fabricated using the plasmonic gold nanostars (AuNSs) on the glassy carbon (GC) electrodes and immobilized using the aptamer probe, which allows it to selectively capture CTCs in samples. The developed technique enables ultra-sensitive and label-free monitoring of CTCs with high specificity. The results showed a detection limit as low as 5 cells ml^{-1}. Further, the developed sensor possesses future technology's potential for CTC identification. The schematic of this sensor is depicted in figure 10.3(A).

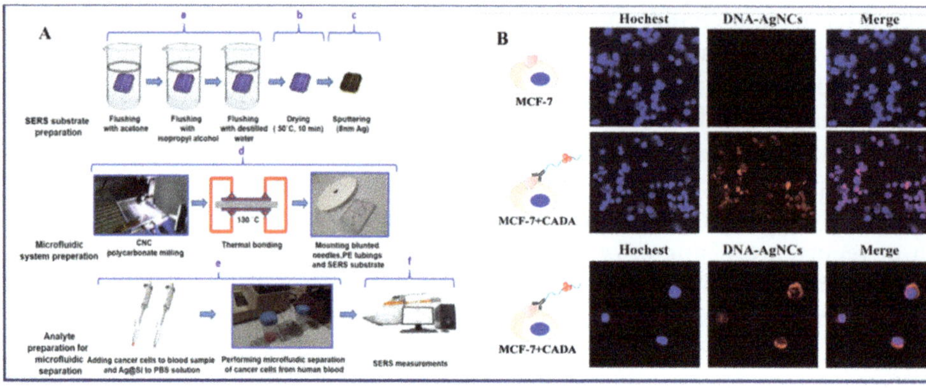

Figure 10.3. (A) SERS substrates preparations, microfluidic system, analyte preparation, and measurement, Reproduced with permission from (Nicinski *et al* 2019). CC BY 4.0. (B) Cross-linking of Anti-MUC1 and DNA-AgNCs; Synthesis of DNA-AgNCs qualitative imaging and quantitative detection mechanisms using DNA-AgNCs as fluorescent and electrochemical probes. Reproduced with permission from (Cao *et al* 2019). Copyright (2019) Elsevier.

The over-expression of CD44 over HeLa cells were experimented by Liu *et al* (2018). They developed a sandwich-type electrochemical cytosensor for measuring CD44-overexpressing HeLa cells. It was fabricated using hyaluronic acid (HA), which functions as a targeted molecule and it was *in situ* introduced into the sensor using an indium-tin oxide (ITO) electrode modified using multi-walled carbon nanotubes (MWCNTs). The 3D-MWCNT structure improves the electrical characteristics and surface area significantly. The HA-modified sensor was extremely sensitive to HeLa cells.

An integrated system developed by Cao *et al* used for cancerous cell imaging qualitatively as well as quantitatively (Cao *et al* 2019). As dual signal probes, DNA-templated silver nanoclusters (DNA-AgNCs) with distinct fluorescence and electrochemical characteristics was fabricated. AS1141 aptamer preferentially binds to nucleolin, which is abundantly expressed on the membrane of a breast cancer cell line, MCF-7 immobilized on the indium-tin-oxide electrode. The anti-MUC1 antibody and DNA-AgNCs complex subsequently binds to MUC1 on the surface of the MCF-7 cell, producing a sandwich-like structure. As a result, this technology enables intraoperative fluorescence scanning and magnified electrochemical detection on the same substrate, providing a biocompatible and incredibly specific approach for adequate cancerous cell identification with a limit of detection of three cells as demonstrated in figure 10.3(B).

10.3.1.2 Tumor cell detection using an optical biosensor

Optical biosensors are quick, legitimate, and accessible, with a low limit of detection and great specificity, and displayed tremendous promise for detecting a variety of cancer types (Kaur *et al* 2022). Optical biosensors can identify malignancy in a million cell groups as opposed to standard detection procedures that need at least 1 billion cells in tumour tissue with a diameter of 7–10 nm (Arshad *et al* 2022). Light wavelength/intensity fluctuations are measured using optical biosensors. Colorimetric, fluorescent, interferometric, or luminescent transducers types are being used to fabricate optical biosensors (Damborský *et al* 2016). Variations in wavelengths/intensity in response to analyzing specific analyte binding are transformed by optical transducers, and converted into electrical interpretations as digital signal output. A biosensor using photonic crystals is a novel form of sensor that uses an optical transducer. Such sensors are intended for detecting very limited quantities of analyte or signal regions, allowing measurements at a greater sensitivity and displaying good selectivity. For optical sensors, several energy conversion processes such as Forster resonance energy transfer (FRET), fluorescence energy transfer, resonance energy transfer, or electronic energy transfer are playing crucial role.

A FRET approach using quantum dots for treatment of ovarian cancer has been explored (Stanisavljevic *et al* 2015). The FRET technology transmits energy from the quantum dot (QD) to the drug molecule doxorubicin (DOX) while it is bonded to graphene. The fluorescence emission was monitored, and suppression had been observed when DOX released from the QD. A novel nanocomposite displays great anticancer efficacy using DOX-conjugated QDs, which is coupled with a glycoprotein specific to the MUC1 cancer biomarker, allowing for targeted administration of the drug. According to some findings, a graphene or graphene oxide-based FRET sensor with an antibody-DNA-AuNP combination can be utilized to identify cancer cells (Kattke *et al* 2011).

Chemiluminescence resonance energy transfer (CRET) procedures ignite an acceptor in a CRET pair using luminescent organic compounds. The graphene-based CRET sensor has been created to detect the interaction between anti-CRP and C-reactive protein (CRP). This type of immunological sensor can specifically detect C-reactive protein levels. CRP levels are frequently less than 3 mg L^{-1} when compared to normal values. When there is an infection associated with cardiovascular disease, the concentration of CRP significantly increases. Moreover, CRP levels are higher in the lung, pancreas, breast, ovary, esophagus, liver, biliary tract, stomach, and multiple myeloma (Balaji and Zhang 2017).

A non-invasive screening device demonstrated by Al Ahmad *et al* (2018) relies heavily on label-free discriminating techniques to distinguish between normal and malignant cells. The cells (both malignant and normal) communicate more information via liver, lung, and breast. They distinguish and identify many cell types, including BEAS-2B, HCC-827, THLE2, Hep G2, MCF 10A, and MDA MB231, as well as HeLa and HEK-293T, all suspended in a homogenous solution and employing an optical absorption-based technique as illustrated in figure 10.4(B).

A fluorescence turn-on biosensor was developed for epithelial adhesion molecule (EpCAM) detection based on graphene quantum dots (GQDs) and molybdenum disulfide (MoS_2) nanosheets (Shi *et al* 2016). PEGylated GQDs was attached to EpCAM aptamer which was adsorbed onto the MoS_2 sheets via van der Waals forces. This sensing platform was used for EpCAM proteins detection. Functionalized GQDs act as the donor molecule in this FRET approach, while MoS_2 serves as the responder. Adsorption among these two portions via FRET decreases the fluorescence intensity of GQDs. Nevertheless, the existence of

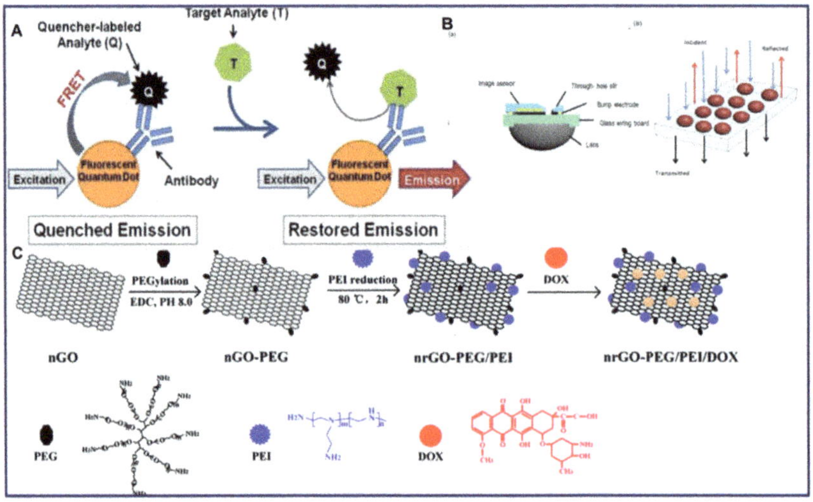

Figure 10.4. (A) schematic representation of the QD-FRET-based immunoassays for *Aspergillus amstelodami* spores. CdSe/ZnS QDs with amine-derivatized (PEG) coatings. Reproduced with permission from (Kattke *et al* 2011). CC BY 3.0. (B) Illustrations of the optical sensor for BEAS-2B, HCC-827, THLE2, Hep G2, MCF 10A, and MDA MB231, as well as HeLa and HEK-293T detection. Reproduced with permission from (Ahmad *et al* 2018). Copyright (2018) IEEE. (C) The steps of synthesis of nrGO-PEG/PEI/DOX. Reproduced with permission from (Li *et al* 2016). Copyright (2016) Royal Society of Chemistry.

targeted, sophisticated and highly specific binding between the aptamer and EpCAM proteins separates the GQD-labelled aptamer from the MoS_2 surface and GQDS fluorescence intensity restoration happens. The FRET assays exhibit a linear response from 3 nM to 54 nM with a detection limit of about 450 pM (figure 10.4(C)). Most previous studies have primarily focused on determining a single BC biomarker, whereas incorporating many capturing molecules integrated into a sensor (all-in-one) can show the differentially expressed quantities of multiple targets molecule simultaneously.

10.3.2 CRISPR/Cas systems

Current cancer diagnostic approaches for molecular analysis are expensive and need specialized equipment. Furthermore, specialized cancer therapies, such as monoclonal Abs and limited drugs, may have non-specific consequences while only being available to a percentage of tumor tissue. As a result, there is still a need for diverse, efficient, and precise approaches for cancer diagnosis and therapy. Over recent times, the CRISPR-based genomic and transcriptomic manipulation toolkit has expanded considerably (Palaz *et al* 2021). CRISPR-mediated targeted enzymatic digestion can be used as a diagnostic tool to discover cancer-specific sequence alterations. To detect miRNA biomarkers, Duan *et al* (2013) used hairpin-mediated quadratic enzymatic amplification (HQEA) in conjunction with molecular beacon (MB) probes. A primer, Bst DNA polymerase, Nb.BbvCI nicking endonuclease, and Lambda exonuclease are involved in the synthesis of HQEA. When the target miRNA is recognized by a complementary strand in the MB probe's loop region, the MB stem undergoes a structural shift, leading to the emission of a fluorescent signal from the open MB stem. When Bst polymerase starts constructing a DNA duplex based on the MB probe, the primer anneals with open stems, expelling the miRNA. As a consequence, the miRNA is ready to engage new MB probes and begin the process all over again. Duan *et al* demonstrate its effectiveness by detecting miR-21 in isolated compounds of breast carcinoma tissues. The study revealed the ratio of healthy to carcinoma cells from 1:1 to 10:1 and they found very minor fluorescence changes over prior studies (figure 10.5(A)) (Duan *et al* 2013).

Microsatellites, a cancer diagnostic marker, can be identified sensitively utilising CRISPR-mediated digesting of microsatellites and other short tandem repeats (STRs) (Yin *et al* 2019). These have been proven as strong diagnostic possibilities, owing to their recognized actions in cancer cells, such as immunoevasion, tumour development, and angiogenesis, whilst miRNAs are dysregulated by cancer cells and supplied by cancer-derived exosomes (CEx). Although quantitative polymerase chain reactions (qPCR) have shown promising findings in identifying cancer-derived exosome micro-RNAs (CEx-miRNAs) linked to CRC, it has major drawbacks, particularly mobility and responsiveness concerns in research study and material integrity. Based on recent findings (Aman *et al* 2020), a direct CRISPR/Cas13-based diagnosis using a poly-A/T universal tag for CEx-miRNAs with a theoretical two-step procedure was developed. This method was found to be appropriate for detection of expanding CEx-miRNAs as shown in figure 10.5(B). The resultant DNA fragments were high-throughput sequenced (STR-seq), which revealed improved quality and sensitivity for microsatellite identification (Shin *et al* 2017). Using Cas9-mediated digestion, Bennett-Baker and Mueller (2017) shown the controlled drug release of megabase-sized pieces from genomic DNA. When paired with duplex sequencing and integrated with double-stranded DNA barcodes, it avoid reading mistakes, Cas9-mediated disintegration enables targeted genetic analysis of genomic areas that require relatively little DNA input (termed CRISPR-DS) (Nachmanson *et al* 2018). CRISPR-DS is being tested in a clinical

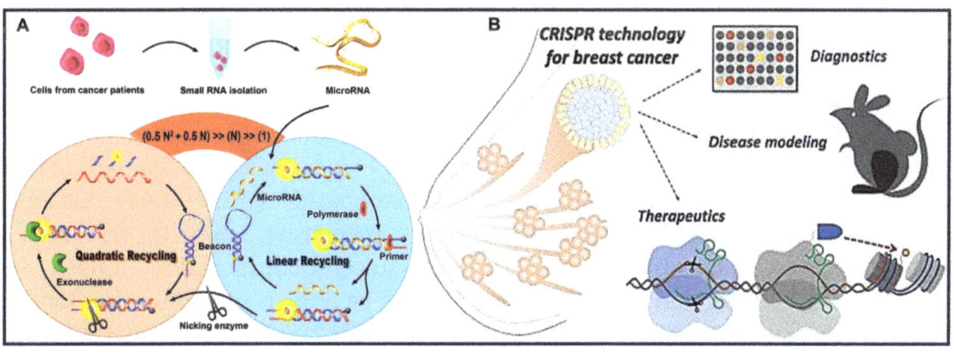

Figure 10.5. (A) Within the recycling process, a schematic diagram of HQEA with MB probes. Reprinted with permission from (Duan *et al* 2013). Copyright 2013 American Chemical Society. (B) Applications of CRISPR technology for breast cancer. Reproduced with permission from (Mintz *et al* 2018). Copyright (2018) Wiley-VCH.

trial to detect p53 mutations in ovarian tumors. Furthermore, Cas12 and Cas13-mediated nucleic acid detection using selective high-sensitivity enzymatic reporter unlocking (SHERLOCK) or DNA endonuclease-targeted CRISPR trans reporter (DETECTR) has just been utilised to discover cancer-associated mutations in carcinoma biopsies samples (figure 10.5(C)).

10.4 Nanoparticles for improving cancer diagnosis

Early diagnosis represents half of the battle in the cure for cancer. Nanotechnology allows for the creation of new molecular contrast agents and materials that can be used for advanced and traditional diagnostics as well as therapy of cancer (Kemp and Kwon 2021). Nanodevices are being employed for detection of biomarkers such as cancer-associated proteins, circulating tumour cells and DNA, with tumor-shed exosomes that are present in blood samples (Guerrini *et al* 2018). Nanobiosensors have great sensitivity, specificity, and multiplexing capabilities (Singhal *et al* 2022). Next-generation technologies combine both capture probes with genetic analysis to better understand a type of malignancy, prospective therapies, and disease progression. Recent discoveries in proteomics and genomics have resulted in significant development in this field (Sallam 2015). These emerging approaches have revealed a number of biomarkers whose aberrant regulation is directly linked to carcinogenesis and its progression. The development and manufacture of magnetic nanoparticles, quantum dots, and gold nanoparticle-based diagnostics approaches, together with their prospective advantages in cancer diagnostic imaging, are described in detail in the following section.

10.4.1 Nanoparticle use for the detection of cancer biomarkers

Identifying and detecting biomarkers in the blood or other physiological fluids that are correlated with the presence of cancer is one potential strategy in the early diagnosis of cancer. Biomarkers are molecules that are connected with malignant cells and they can be proteins (either cell surface glycoproteins or secreted proteins), polysaccharides, or nucleic acids (i.e. genome sequences or RNA transcripts) (Parihar *et al* 2021). Nonetheless, the use of biomarkers has been hampered by a number of obstacles, including low biomarker quantities in physiological fluids, individual heterogeneity in biomarker quantity and timings, and the challenge of performing predictive research. Nanoparticles have high specificity and sensitivity, in addition to the ability to evaluate several objectives at the same time. Nanomaterials have the potential to improve the sensitivity of biosensors and provide selective targeting (Dessale *et al* 2022). Additionally, the use of nanoparticles raises their surface-to-volume ratio, rendering biosensors increasingly responsive towards the needs of particular biomolecular investigations. For instance, quantum dots (QDs), gold nanoparticles (AuNPs), and polymer dots (PDs) can be used as probes for development of effective cancer diagnostics methods (Liu *et al* 2013).

Protein biomarkers are generally divided into three groups depending on where they're found: intracellular, extracellular, and cytoplasmic membrane. Diverse biomarkers are sought for different purposes in nanoparticle-enabled diagnostics

(Parihar *et al* 2022). It is more frequent in imaging to identify cellular membrane protein indicators, and it is more practical in *in vitro* diagnostics to address soluble proteins which are lost into the bloodstream. Intracellular protein, in contrast, receive less attention due to the fact that nanoparticles are comparatively large in size, and as a result they are unable to pass through cell membranes.

Thousands of biomarker candidates have indeed been identified via research aimed at identifying cancer biomarkers, but only a few have received FDA approval (Khleif *et al* 2010). The preponderance of FDA-approved biomarkers is used to track the course of cancer instead of its early detection. Despite the significance of early detection and the significant research resources dedicated toward it, the application of these tests for early cancer diagnosis is restricted. In fact, no early cancer biomarker test has been approved or certified by the FDA, highlighting the difficulties in designing sensors for cancer biomarkers (Ranjan *et al* 2020).

Studies are being conducted perfectly to explore various nanomaterials to address these difficulties as particular features of some classes of nanoparticle probes provide the opportunity to construct speedy, affordable, tailorable, high-throughput tests with excellent sensitivity and selectivity. A sandwich-type test is a typical approach for detecting protein biomarkers and it consists many components, including a biomarker, a capture antibody, and a secondary antibody that binds to the capture antibody. The secondary antibody is used in a variety of traditional techniques, including staining and fluorescence (Hosu *et al* 2018).

10.4.2 Gold nanoparticles for cancer biomarker detection

Because of their high absorbance, AuNPs are used as fluorescence quenchers in the fabrication of many biosensors, resulting in detectors having reduced backscatter compared to organic fluorophore quenchers. Conventionally, Raman spectroscopy could not identify cancer biomarkers at ultralow levels since the Raman scattering intensity (biological recognition interface and Raman reporter) can be insufficient. The amplitude of the Raman probe molecule can be enhanced by 10^8–10^{14} orders of magnitude as they are immobilized on the plasmonic surface of a noble metal nanoparticle such as gold. The limit of detection of prostate-specific antigen (PSA) has been achieved at the femtomolar level by employing this SERS property of AuNPs (Devi *et al* 2015).

Cho and colleagues (Cho *et al* 2012) detected vascular endothelial growth factor (VEGF) using AuNPs and Cyanine 3B (Cy3B), an organic fluorophore in a 'on–off' probe. Specifically, employing positively charged poly-L-lysine, VEGF-targeting aptamers tagged with Cy3B were electrically charged coupled to 80 nm AuNPs. When the aptamer bound to VEGF, the emission intensity decreased as measured by a fluorescence microscope. In a study, the tumor-homing penetrating peptides iRGD (9-amino acid cyclic peptide) allows anticancer medications to enter tumorigenic blood vessels. It improves diagnostic sensitivities and treatment efficacy by increasing permeability to tumour arteries, triggering internalisation, and penetrating deep into tumour tissues. It was co-administered with a legumain-responsive gold nanoparticle to create an iRGD (CRGDKGPDC)-mediated enzyme-induced precise targeting of gold nanoparticles (iRGD/AuNPs-A&C). In four T1 mammary tumours, iRGD/AuNPs-A&C demonstrated significant penetration.

An optical enzyme-linked immunosorbent assay (ELISA) for measuring CA15–3 antigen, a critical biomarker of breast cancer found in blood samples, was developed by Ambrosi *et al* (2010). To produce an amplified optical signal, gold nanoparticles (AuNPs) were utilised as carriers of the signalling antibody anti-CA15–3-HRP (horseradish peroxidase). When compared to traditional ELISA techniques, the assay using AuNPs as an enhancer resulted in greater sensitivity and shorter assay time in the range of 0 to 60 U ml^{-1}. The addition of AuNPs into the commercially available ELISA test can help to enhance essential immunoanalysis techniques.

10.4.3 Quantum dots for cancer biomarker detection

QD-based biosensors have been utilised to detect cancer biomarkers in several recent investigations. QDs have a high quantum yield and appropriate molar extinction coefficient, as well as a broad absorbance band, and offer maximum sensitivity. Multiplexed QD-conjugated antibodies against neuron-specific enolase (NSE) and carcinoembryonic antigen (CEA) were utilised to detect two biomarkers, with the limit of detection (LOD) of each 1.0 ng ml^{-1} (figure 10.6(A)). Using ZnO nanowire substrates, which possess high surface area and multiple binding sites for the analyte, a sandwich immunoassay based on zinc oxide (ZnO) QDs was fabricated. The most

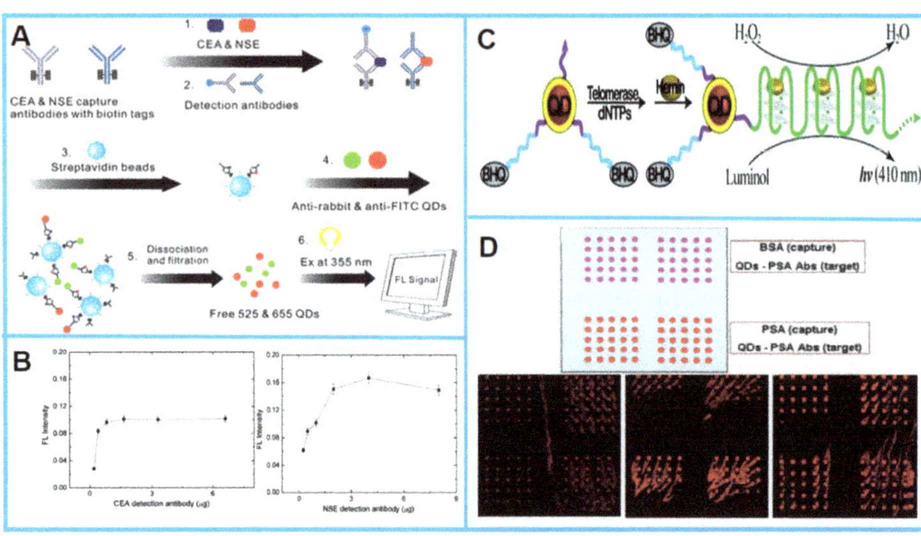

Figure 10.6. (A) Multiplexed QD-based detection of two lung cancer biomarkers. Reproduced with permission from (Li *et al* 2011). Copyright (2011) Royal Society of Chemistry. (B) FL intensity in relation to CEA and NSE capture antibodies. Reproduced with permission from (Li *et al* 2011). Copyright (2011) Royal Society of Chemistry. (C) The biochip showing protein–protein interactions in PSA and BSA microarrays with and without any blocking layer. Reproduced with permission from (Jou *et al* 2015). Copyright (2015) Royal Society of Chemistry. (D) Telomerase-stimulated telomerization of a primer associated with the QDs increased detection of miR-141. Reproduced with permission from (Gokarna *et al* 2008). Copyright (2008) Wiley-VCH.

widely studied cancer biomarker CEA could predict cancerous conditions, help to monitor anticancer therapy response, and predict tumour recurrence. NSE is an enzyme that converts 2-phosphoglycerate to phosphoenolpyruvate and has been associated to carcinoma such as small cell lung cancer and islet cell cancer. Following secretion, they were detectable at quantities greater than 15 ng ml^{-1}, with a LOD of 1.0 ng ml^{-1} for each (Li *et al* 2011). The detection procedure is shown in figure 10.6(B).

A sensing platform for sensitive detection of miR-141, a prostate cancer biomarker, was fabricated by using CdSe/ZnS QDs modified with FRET quencher-functionalized nucleic acids including a telomerase primer sequence as well as a recognition sequence for the miR-141 recognition sequence (figure 10.6(C)) (Jou *et al* 2015).

Gokarna and colleagues (Gokarna *et al* 2008) created QD-based protein micro- and nanoarrays for PSA detection in order to assess biomarkers in a high-throughput manner. Dip pen nanolithography (DPN) was used to create the PSA micro- and nanoarrays, which were then introduced to PEGylated QDs functionalized with an anti-PSA antibody (figure 10.6(D)). A microarray scanner was used to detect the presence of PSA (detected by QD fluorescence). Because these micro- and nanoarrays enable quick screening of numerous chemicals, they may enable high-throughput multiplexed clinical screening.

10.4.4 Nanoparticles for detection of cancer cells

Early cancer identification improves patient survival dramatically. Metastasis can occur when cancer progresses, which reduces the prognosis of cancer disease. Current clinical approaches for detecting cancer metastasis involves imaging techniques such as computed tomography imaging. A cancerous cell comes out from the primary tumour and invades the nearby tissue before moving into the blood and lymphatic system's microvasculature (intravasation) (Scully *et al* 2012). The cancerous cell moves forward through the bloodstream to microvessels in distant tissues (extravasation), continuing to reside inside the microenvironment of tissues, which offers a favourable foreign environment for growth and advancement (Catalano *et al* 2013). Thus, it is possible to detect the type of cancer via identifying circulating tumour cells (CTCs), also referred to as metastatic tumor cells in the circulation. The immunogenic separation based on the affirmation of cellular membrane antigens like epithelial cell adhesion molecule (EpCAM), a membrane-spanning molecule associated with cell signalling, migration, and propagation of cells and thus connected to tumor growth, is indeed the basis for current CTC sensing technologies (Riethdorf *et al* 2007, Yu *et al* 2011). Although this method has received FDA approval and has been marketed by Janssen Diagnostics' Cell Search technology, it is really constrained by the requirement to identify cell surface antigens, which makes it difficult to distinguish CTC populations whose protein expression level is inadequate for separation and thus is not permissible to estimate the gene expression (Yu *et al* 2011).

The high specific surface area of nanoparticles enables the binding of highly effective targeting ligands with the capacity to identify specific receptors over cancerous cells. The CTC detection method offers good selectivity, reproducibility, and sensitivity. Different nanoparticles, such as magnetic particles (MNPs), gold nanoparticles (AuNPs), quantum dots (QDs), nanowires, silicon nanopillars, carbon nanotubes, dendrimers, graphene oxide, and polymers have all been investigated for CTC detection.

10.4.5 Gold nanoparticles for cancer cell detection

Shen *et al* (2011) used multifunctional nanoparticles (MFNPs) that were conjugated with monoclonal anti-HER2 antibodies for the detection of HER2-positive cells. The fabricated sensor demonstrated that the MFNPs had a good sensing ability for breast cancer BT474 cells (biomarker HER2-positive). The MFNPs comprise a clear core–shell structure made of UCNP@ Fe3O4@Au coated with anti-HER2 antibodies and poly(ethylene glycol). The researchers showed an innovative high property of a photothermal effect at the single-cell level using a near-IR laser. The nanocrystals were employed to produce a photothermal impact at the single-cell level. The authors employed AuNPs capped with various hydrophobic ligands and coated with green fluorescent protein to differentiate cell types and cancer stages. Because the capping ligands utilised had distinct chemical structures, each AuNP-GFP complex was associated with cancer cells to varying degrees, taking into account cell membrane composition changes.

A novel, homogeneous SERS-based cellular tracking method was devised to quickly and precisely quantify circulatory cancerous cells in the bloodstream. In less than an hour, cells were detected50 tumour cells ml^{-1} in the presence of whole blood using magnetic beads and SERS tags attached to EpCAM and HER2 antibodies (Sha *et al* 2008). Furthermore, noble metal nanoparticles, particularly AuNPs, are frequently utilised in conjunction with organic fluorophores to create 'off–on' probes for intracellular gene expression measurement. Because of the effective quenching capabilities of AuNPs, compared to conventional molecular techniques, these tags have much less detection sensitivity.

10.5 Imaging *in vivo*

Currently available imaging techniques can only detect cancer at later stages after it has significantly altered the tissues and many hundreds of cells have already been grown and perhaps spread (Ho *et al* 2021). Recently, *ex vivo* detection and biomarkers in liquid biopsy samples have addressed the presence of malignant tissues and offered various benefits in order to diagnose and treat cancer (Huang *et al* 2020). The effective nanoparticle probe for detection must circulate slowly and should be specific towards malignant cells, but also harmless to normal cells. Numerous nanoparticles, including iron oxide nanoparticles, have optical, magnetic, acoustical, and structural characteristics which can significantly enhance visualisation and detection processes (Werner *et al* 2020). Conventional scanning technologies like magnetic resonance imaging (MRI), positron emission tomography (PET), and computed tomography (CT) offer the ability to specifically target and significantly enhance the identification of tumours *in vivo* employing nanotechnology-based imaging contrast agents that are now being developed and translated (Pichler *et al* 2008). Additionally, innovative detection methods, such as photoacoustic tomography (PAT), Raman spectroscopic imaging, and multimodal imaging, have shown promise towards early cancer detection but have not yet been exploited for clinical cancer therapy and diagnostics. However, contemporary nanoscale imaging systems (i.e. contrast agents specific to several imaging modalities simultaneously) above channels have been made possible by nanotechnology's ability to transport multiple components at once (such as cancer cell-specific targeting agents or common imaging contrast agents), as well as nanoscopic substances that seem to be contrast agents themselves, resulting in a noticeably improved signal (Novoselova *et al* 2021).

The enhanced extradural ability of 10–150 nm nanoparticles is referred to as passive targeting. Nanoparticles can disproportionately concentrate in tumour tissue because strong connections among endothelial cells in new blood vessels in tumours don't really develop correctly (Patel and Patel 2019). Recently, nanoparticles have been used which showed enhanced permeability and retention (EPR) effects, which help in tumor imaging and can be used for positron emission tomography (PET)-based imaging systems. Active tumour targeting outperforms passive targeting, which depends on the EPR effect, identification of cancers at an early stage by utilising images with high resolution (Acharya and Sahoo 2011).

10.5.1 Nanoparticles involved in imaging tests

Recent interventions of nanotechnology introduced several nanoparticles that were used in imaging-based diagnostics of cancer. The details of some of these important nanoparticles are discussed in this section.

10.5.2 Magnetic nanoparticles

Several main applications of magnetic nanoparticles, mostly in the field of biomedicine, are the contrasting probes used throughout magnetic resonance (MRI) (Estelrich *et al* 2015). Magnetic nanoparticles, namely iron oxide nanoparticles (IONPs), are employed in imaging of the liver, lymph nodes, and cell tracking. Magnetic nanoparticles have already been used as probes in systems with extraordinarily high sensitivity (Jain 2003). Magnetic nanoparticle-based tumour imaging probes composed of ferromagnetic materials were combined with targeting motifs and investigated for tumour homing and imaging. RGD, for example, has been conjugated to silica (Barreto *et al* 2011), triblock-copolymers (Miki *et al* 2009), polyaspartic acid (Cowger and Xie 2013), and dextran (Tassa *et al* 2011) coated IONPs and tested as MRI contrast probes. Gao *et al* used paramagnetic NP probes including an anti-epidermal growth factor receptor monoclonal antibody (mAb) to image tiny tumours. Thawani *et al* (Thawani *et al* 2017) created ICG-coated superparamagnetic iron oxide NP clusters (about 97 nm in diameter) for presurgery

MRI identification of the tumour location and intraoperative excision under photoacoustic guidance in mice.

10.5.3 Quantum dot nanoparticles

Through combination of the EPR effect and passive aggregation, QDs can be used for fluorescence imaging of tumour tissue (Subhan *et al* 2021). The fluorescence spectra possess distinct absorption and emission patterns in semiconductor nanoparticles made of elements from groups II and VI (e.g. CdSe and CdTe) (Song *et al* 2016) or groups III and V (e.g. InP and InAs). Hong *et al* (2012) synthesized silver sulphide (Ag_2S) QDs for *in vivo* imaging of tumour tissues in a 4T1 metastatic breast cancer cell xenograft mice model. For a long time (up to 24 h post-injection (p.i.), they noticed NIRII fluorescence of 6PEG-Ag_2S QDs grew firmly in tumour site and diminished in other organs and the skin between 30 min and 24 h p.i. The EPR action resulted in remarkable accumulation of 6PEG-Ag_2S QDs in tumours (>10% ID gram^{-1}, where % ID gram^{-1} signifies a proportion of the probe's concentration over injected dosage (ID) percentage per gram of tissue). They claim that using these NIR-II QDs for imaging provided deep inner organ registration, dynamic tumour contrast, and quick tumour identification. The influence of nanoparticle size on tumour tissue accumulation was investigated using silica-coated QDs of varying thicknesses (Popović *et al* 2010). The 12 nm QDs quickly penetrated into cancerous tissues, whereas the 60 nm QDs extravasated but stayed in 10 m blood arteries. The 120 nm QDs, on the other hand, showed no discernible extravasation.

10.5.4 Gold nanoparticles

GNPs perform well in optical coherence tomography (OCT), photoacoustic imaging (PA), surface-enhanced Raman scattering (SERS), and computed tomography imaging (CT) (Gao and Li 2016). OCT is a non-intrusive biomedical imaging technology with micron-level resolution (Mu *et al* 2019). OCT can help with real-time diagnosis and surgical planning. However, if incident field coherence of inelastic dispersed light is absent, OCT is unable to detect it. Many studies have recently demonstrated that the magnitude of OCT might vary depending upon the NPs' motion state. GNRs, GNSs, and GNCs in particular appear promising in terms of both scattering and absorbance mostly in the NIR area (Jelveh and Chithrani 2011). GNCs with 800 nm SPR are used for imaging techniques. Investigation proves that GNRs with maximum SPR at 775 nm can be used for OCT imaging. In the study by Mallidi *et al* (2016) when gold nanoparticles were conjugated with antibodies that specifically bind to receptors on cell surfaces, they undergo molecular aggregation, resulting in a red shift in their plasmon resonance frequency. They show the effectiveness of the molecular-specific photoacoustic imaging using systemic tumor-imitating gelatin implanted in *ex vivo* rat tissue. According to research, it could possibly be able to identify cancerous cells in a very precise and selective manner by using a combination of molecular-specific gold nanoparticles and multiwavelength photoacoustic imaging. Another study by Zhang *et al* (2009) focused into the potential of systematically synthesized poly(ethylene glycol)-coated (PEGylated) gold nanoparticles as a contrast material for *in vivo* tumour imaging using PAT (Mallidi *et al* 2011). Researchers demonstrated that when comparing to *ex vivo* mouse tissue, gold nanoparticles (20 and 50 nm) had a strong photoacoustic contrast. In rats the presence of gold nanoparticles *in vivo* after receiving PAT subcutaneously was observed. Following intravenous injection of PEGylated gold nanoparticles to tumor-bearing mice, PAT can successfully monitor accumulated gold nanoparticles within the tumor. While utilising gold nanoparticles as a contrast agent, PAT offers substantial potential in image-guided treatment of superficial cancers such as lobular carcinoma, melanosarcoma and trabecular cancer (Mehrmohammadi *et al* 2013). GNPs have piqued the interest of researchers since they have a higher x-ray absorbance value than iodine (such as Ultravist), which is frequently also used to increase contrast and employed in this field (W. Li and Chen 2015). CT has always been viewed as structural scanning technology which is unsuitable for diagnosing early-stage tumours. GNPs enable cellular scanning on the CT platform using targeted compounds (Popovtzer *et al* 2008).

10.5.5 Nanoparticles use in cancer therapy

The utilisation of tiny biomolecules and nanoparticles as means of administration of drugs is indeed the foundation of nanotechnology advancement. Quantum dots, nanotubes, lipid membranes, micelles, dendritic macromolecules, and dendritic nanoparticles are a few forms of nanocarriers being extensively employed for treatment of cancer (Mir *et al* 2017). The vascular system, micro metastases, and angiogenesis in cancerous conditions can be cured using targeted therapy (Zhang *et al* 2009). The carbon nanotubes have the capacity to absorb light in the near-infrared (NIR) range. This allows them to target tumour cells by heating up owing towards the thermo impact (Kam *et al* 2005). In their own natural condition, carbon nanotubes encourage non-invasive biofilm penetration and are thought to be extremely capable transporters for such delivery of different therapeutic compounds inside human tissue (Jin *et al* 2020). Because of the suitability of carbon nanotubes for cancer treatment, drugs such as paclitaxel are assembled with them and administered both *in vitro* and *in vivo*. Moreover, the size of nanocarriers such as liposomes has shown to affect their half-life in the patient body. Bigger liposomes have a shorter half-life since the mononuclear phagocytic cells systems are able to recognize and eliminate them more quickly than smaller lipid vesicles up to 100 nanometers in size. Additionally carbon-based materials have also been employed for cancer diagnostics; for instance Chen *et al* (2009) successfully detected BC using quantum-dot-based probes, demonstrating that, unlike traditional immunohistochemistry (IHC), quantum dot (QD) IHC can detect very low levels of Human Epidermal Growth Factor Receptor 2 (HER2) expression as well as multichannel detection.

10.6 Challenges in clinical translation

As nanotechnology has evolved, there has been a sharp increase in the quantity of information gathered through several studies done upon nanostructures. However, only a small number of nanomaterials reach the clinical testing level. Most of them failed during their *in vivo* and *in vitro* efficacy testing phase (Ruiz *et al* 2014). Clinical manifestations of nanomaterials present distinct limitations for every nanoemulsion (Younis *et al* 2021). Nanomaterials offer tailored efficacy in diseased tissues with lower cellular toxicity in normal tissues due to their selectivity. However, several drawbacks that hinder their usage include general and organ-specific toxicities that have a negative impact on the outcomes (Jin *et al* 2020). Considering the limitation of nanomaterials, greater advancements are required to enhance therapeutic administration, potency, and reduce normal cell damage. The nanostructured material can be used for detection and therapies that are more efficient and safer and offers tuneable physical and chemical characteristics.

NPs have still not been employed as first-line cancer treatments, despite of various successful authorised nanoformulations (Gavas *et al* 2021). They are being used only when the majority of cancerous conditions become drug resistant and worse due to repetition of traditional treatment approaches. Apart from this, several biological challenges, including a lack of route of administration, tempering bioavailability, NPs passing through biological barriers, degeneration, and toxic effects to normal tissue, needs special attention (Nguyen 2011). Notably, NPs when typically injected intravenously directly into the blood get removed through clearance processes making it difficult for them to stay and interact with the target site (Bakhtiary *et al* 2016). This issue can be resolved by using 3D magnetic fields that regulate the motion of NPs and prevent their clearance via blood circulation. This approach has been employed in several *in vivo* and *in vitro* investigations, which suggests that magnetic NPs could be utilised to resolve the issue of blood NPs clearance (Cardoso *et al* 2018). Nevertheless, it is necessary to look at the impact of magnetic fields over the human organ processes in addition to the interaction among magnetic fields and NPs.

The protein corona (PC) is a structure formed when NPs enter a biological system. It is made up of cell and serum proteins. Avoiding the 'mononuclear phagocytic system (MPS)' is another challenging event as NPs are adsorbed on proteins in bodily fluids to create PC, which then induces the MPS process to engulf NPs. However, this could be resolved by covering NPs with substances that inhibit the formation of the PC (Farshbaf *et al* 2022).

The development of nanoparticle-based POC (point of care) technologies may substantially improve the field of diagnostics in terms of enhanced device sensitivities, simplicity of operation, and cheaper cost (Parihar *et al* 2020). Although several nanoparticle probe-based assays have been developed for the fluorescence-based determination of cancer biomarkers, no specific assay has been designated as the 'gold standard' within healthcare settings (Ranjan *et al* 2020). This is another challenging issue to compare data obtained from various test setups. Moreover, some of the nanomaterial-based formulations to treat and detect cancerous conditions that are under clinical trials are listed in table 10.3.

Table 10.3. Nanomaterial used in clinical trials for disease treatment and diagnostics

Name	Material	Application	Clinical trial.gov identifier
AuroLase®	Silica–gold nanoshells coated with PEG	Laser responsive thermal ablation of solid tumors: head/neck cancer, primary and/or metastatic lung tumors	NCT00848042, NCT01679470
Ferumoxytol	Iron oxide nanoparticle	Ferumoxytol-iron oxide nanoparticle magnetic resonance dynamic contrast-enhanced MRI Head and neck cancer	NCT01895829
Location and Biopsy of Axillary Lymph Nodes	Carbon Nanoparticles	Targeted biopsy of carbon NPs labelled axillary node for cN+breast cancer	NCT04482803
Prostate cancer	64Cu-NOTA-PSMA-PEG-Cy5.5-C'	The use of NPs to guide the surgical treatment of prostate cancer	NCT04167969
MagProbe (TM)	Iron oxide nanoparticles	A novel magnetic needle using iron oxide NPs for the detection of leukemia	NCT01411904
Head and neck cancer melanoma Breast cancer Colorectal cancer	Silica nanoparticles	Targeted silica nanoparticles for real-time image-guided intraoperative mapping of nodal metastases	NCT02106598
Diagnosing Cancers From Healthy From Human Exhaled Breath With Na-nose	Metallic Nanoparticles	Volatile organic compounds/cancer/diagnoses disease	NCT03967652

10.7 Conclusion

The recent developments in cancerous disease detection methods that employed nanotechnology are outlined in this chapter. Over the past ten years, several initiatives have begun to develop assays relying on nanotechnology-generated nanomaterials for cancer diagnostics, especially in comparison to traditional cancer diagnostics methods. A number of nanoparticle-based assays provide heightened sensitivity as well as specificity and open new possibilities to replace or overcome drawbacks of the conventional methods. The effective diagnostics improve cancer patients' survival by allowing earlier detection and timely therapeutic management. Furthermore, these advancements are possibly useful for tracking cancer progression in response to treatment, and also helps to evaluate efficacy of new treatment regimes. Nanostructures have the potential to transform a variety of imaging modalities. Magnetic nanoparticles, for example, can be used as contrast probes in MRI, and QDs can be used as probes in fluorescence imaging. GNPs can be used in OCT imaging, PA imaging, or CT imaging depending on their nanostructure. Extensive testing on small animal models confirms the benefits of the nanoparticle-based probe. On considerations of multi-modality scanning, numerous imaging functionalities may be included into a composition of nanoparticles, and the resultant conjugates can serve as reporters for various imaging modalities. Current imaging methods all have advantages and disadvantages that make multi-modal imaging intriguing. Nano-based biosensors are more likely to receive immediate regulatory approval than *in vivo* imaging. Unlike imaging, which involves the systematic administration of nanoparticles, nanobiosensors are used *in vitro* and do not involve complications such as toxic effects and altered biodistribution. Moreover, with close cooperation between scholars, designers, and physicians, nanotechnology-based cancer diagnostics is expected to revolutionize the field of cancer diagnostics, despite the fact that merely a small number of NP-based assays have progressed to clinical testing. Among its high precision, selectivity, or combinatorial measuring capability, nanotechnology presents a number of options to enhance cancer detection, resulting in an increased patient's survival rate.

Acknowledgments

The authors appreciate the direction and inspiration provided by the CSIR-AMPRI director for this research. Arpana Parihar thankfully acknowledged the fellowship provided by DST under the DST/WOS-B/HN-4/2021 scheme. RK would like to thank SERB for funding the IPA/2020/000130 project with their support.

References

Acharya S and Sahoo S K 2011 PLGA nanoparticles containing various anticancer agents and tumour delivery by EPR effect *Adv. Drug Deliv. Rev.* **63** 170–83

Ahmad A, Mahmoud M, Najar A, El Moutaouakil A, Nasir N, Hussein M, Raji S and Hilal-Alnaqbi A 2018 Label-free cancer cells detection using optical sensors *IEEE Access* **6** 55807–14

Aman R, Mahas A and Mahfouz M 2020 Nucleic acid detection using CRISPR/Cas biosensing technologies *ACS Synth. Biol.* **9** 1226–33

Ambrosi A, Airo F and Merkoçi A 2010 Enhanced gold nanoparticle based ELISA for a breast cancer biomarker *Anal. Chem.* **82** 1151–56

Arshad F, Nabi F, Iqbal S and Khan R H 2022 Applications of graphene-based electrochemical and optical biosensors in early detection of cancer biomarkers *Colloids Surf.* B **212** 112356

Babu A, Templeton A K, Munshi A and Ramesh R 2013 Nanoparticle-based drug delivery for therapy of lung cancer: progress and challenges *J. Nanomater.* **2013** 863951

Bakhtiary Z, Saei A A, Hajipour M J, Raoufi M, Vermesh O and Mahmoudi M 2016 Targeted superparamagnetic iron oxide nanoparticles for early detection of cancer: possibilities and challenges *Nanomed. Nanotechnol. Biol. Med.* **12** 287–307

Balaji A and Zhang J 2017 Electrochemical and optical biosensors for early-stage cancer diagnosis by using graphene and graphene oxide *Cancer Nanotechnol.* **8** 1–12

Balata H, Quaife S L, Craig C, Ryan D J, Bradley P, Crosbie P A J, Murray R L and Evison M 2022 Early diagnosis and lung cancer screening *Clin. Oncol.* **34** 708–15

Barreto J A, O'Malley W, Kubeil M, Graham B, Stephan H and Spiccia L 2011 Nanomaterials: applications in cancer imaging and therapy *Adv. Mater.* **23** H18–40

Bennett-Baker P E and Mueller J L 2017 CRISPR-mediated isolation of specific megabase segments of genomic DNA *Nucleic Acids Res.* **45** e165

Borghei Y S, Morteza Hosseini M D, Saman Hosseinkhani M R G and Sheikhnejad R 2016 Visual detection of cancer cells by colorimetric aptasensor based on aggregation of gold nanoparticles induced by DNA hybridization *Anal. Chim. Acta* **904** 92–7

Broza Y Y, Zhou X, Yuan M, Qu D, Zheng Y, Vishinkin R, Khatib M, Wu W and Haick H 2019 Disease detection with molecular biomarkers: from chemistry of body fluids to nature-inspired chemical sensors *Chem. Rev.* **119** 11761–817

Cao Y, Yuhao Dai H C, Yingying Tang X C, Ying Wang J Z and Zhu X 2019 Integration of fluorescence imaging and electrochemical biosensing for both qualitative location and quantitative detection of cancer cells *Biosens. Bioelectron.* **130** 132–8

Cardoso F, Kyriakides S, Ohno S, Penault-Llorca F, Poortmans P, Rubio I T, Zackrisson S and Senkus E 2019 Early breast cancer: ESMO clinical practice guidelines for diagnosis, treatment and follow-up *Ann. Oncol* **30** 1194–220

Cardoso V F, Francesko A, Ribeiro C, Bañobre-López M, Martins P and Lanceros-Mendez S 2018 Advances in magnetic nanoparticles for biomedical applications *Adv. Healthc. Mater.* **7** 1700845

Catalano V, Turdo A, Di Franco S, Dieli F, Todaro M and Stassi G 2013 Tumor and its microenvironment: a synergistic interplay *Semin. Cancer Biol.* **23** 522–32

Chen C, Peng J, Xia H S, Yang G F, Wu Q S, Chen L D, Zeng L B, Zhang Z L, Pang D W and Li Y 2009 Quantum dots-based immunofluorescence technology for the Quantitative determination of HER2 expression in breast cancer *Biomaterials* **30** 2912–8

Chen M and Zhao H 2019 Next-generation sequencing in liquid biopsy: cancer screening and early detection *Hum. Genet* **13** 1–10

Chinen A B, Guan C M, Ferrer J, Barnaby S N, Merkel T J and Mirkin C A 2015 Nanoparticle probes for the detection of cancer biomarkers, cells, and tissues by fluorescence *Chem. Rev.* **115** 10530–74

Cho H, Yeh E-C, Sinha R, Laurence T A, Bearinger J L and Lee L P 2012 Single-step nanoplasmonic VEGF165 aptasensor for early cancer diagnosis *ACS Nano* **6** 7607–14

Cowger T and Xie J 2013 Polyaspartic acid coated iron oxide nanoprobes for PET/MRI Imaging *Nanomaterial Interfaces in Biology* (Springer) pp 225–35

Crocetto F, Russo G, Zazzo E D, Pisapia P, Mirto B F, Palmieri A, Pepe F, Bellevicine C, Russo A and Civita E L 2022 Liquid biopsy in prostate cancer management—current challenges and future perspectives *Cancers* **14** 3272

Cui H, Margaret Nowicki J P and Fisher L G Z 2017 3D bioprinting for organ regeneration *Adv. Healthc. Mater.* **6** 1601118

Damborský P, Švitel J and Katrlík J 2016 Optical biosensors *Essays Biochem.* **60** 91–100

Dessale M, Mengistu G and Mengist H M 2022 Nanotechnology: a promising approach for cancer diagnosis, therapeutics and theragnosis *Int. J. Nanomed.* **17** 3735–49

Devi R V, Doble M and Verma R S 2015 Nanomaterials for early detection of cancer biomarker with special emphasis on gold nanoparticles in immunoassays/sensors *Biosens. Bioelectron.* **68** 688–98

Drost F-J H, Osses D, Nieboer D , Bangma C H, Steyerberg E W, Roobol M J and Schoots I G 2020 Prostate magnetic resonance imaging, with or without magnetic resonance imaging-targeted biopsy, and systematic biopsy for detecting prostate cancer: a cochrane systematic review and meta-analysis *Eur. Urol* **77** 78–94

D'Souza N, Delisle T G, Chen M, Benton S and Abulafi M 2021 Faecal immunochemical test is superior to symptoms in predicting pathology in patients with suspected colorectal cancer symptoms referred on a 2WW pathway: a diagnostic accuracy study *Gut* **70** 1130–8

Duan R, Zuo X, Wang S, Quan X, Chen D, Chen Z, Jiang L, Fan C and Xia F 2013 Lab in a tube: ultrasensitive detection of MicroRNAs at the single-cell level and in breast cancer patients using quadratic isothermal amplification *J. Am. Chem. Soc.* **135** 4604–7

Ruiz M E, Gantner M E and Talevi A 2014 Applications of nanosystems to anticancer drug therapy (part II. dendrimers, micelles, lipid-based nanosystems) *Recent Pat. Anticancer Drug Discov.* **9** 99–128

Entenberg D, Oktay M H and Condeelis J S 2023 Intravital imaging to study cancer progression and metastasis *Nat. Rev. Cancer* **23** 25–42

Estelrich J, Sánchez-Martín M J and Busquets M A 2015 Nanoparticles in magnetic resonance imaging: from simple to dual contrast agents *Int. J. Nanomed.* **10** 1727

Farshbaf M, Valizadeh H, Panahi Y, Fatahi Y, Chen M, Zarebkohan A and Gao H 2022 The impact of protein corona on the biological behavior of targeting nanomedicines *Int. J. Pharm.* **614** 121458

Feig S A and Schwartz G F 1981 Advantages and limitations of physical examination and mammography in breast cancer screening *Cancer Detect Prev* **4** 553–63

Filice M, Marchal J A and Gamiz F 2021 Biosensors based on two-dimensional materials *2D Materials for Nanophotonics* (Elsevier) pp 245–312

Frangioni J V 2008 New technologies for human cancer imaging *J. Clin. Oncol.* **26** 4012

Gao Y and Li Y 2016 Gold nanostructures for cancer imaging and therapy *Advances in Nanotheranostics* I (Springer) pp 53–101

Gavas S, Quazi S and Karpiński T M 2021 Nanoparticles for cancer therapy: current progress and challenges *Nanoscale Res. Lett.* **16** 1–21

Giaquinto A N, Sung H, Miller K D, Kramer J L, Newman M A, Minihan A, Jemal A and Siegel R L 2022 Breast cancer statistics, 2022 *CA: Cancer J. Clin* **72** 524–41

Ginsburg O, Yip C H, Brooks A, Cabanes A, Caleffi M, Yataco J A D, Gyawali B, McCormack V, Anderson M M L and Mehrotra R 2020 Breast cancer early detection: a phased approach to implementation *Cancer* **126** 2379–93

Gokarna A, Jin L H, Hwang J S, Cho Y H, Lim Y T, Chung B H, Youn S H, Choi D S and Lim J H 2008 Quantum dot-based protein micro-and nanoarrays for detection of prostate cancer biomarkers *Proteomics* **8** 1809–18

Guerrini L, Garcia-Rico E and Alvarez-Puebla R 2018 The role of nanoscience in cancer diagnosis *Handbook of Nanomaterials for Cancer Theranostics* (Elsevier) pp 177–97

Hasan M R, Ahommed M S, Mahbuba Daizy M S, Bacchu M R, Ali M R, Al-Mamun M, Aly Saad Aly M Z H K and Imdadul Hossain S 2021 Recent development in electrochemical biosensors for cancer biomarkers detection *Biosens. Bioelectron.: X* **8** 100075

Hernandez F J, Kalra N, Wengel J and Vester B 2009 Aptamers as a model for functional evaluation of LNA and 2′-Amino LNA *Bioorg. Med. Chem. Lett.* **19** 6585–87

Ho Y J, Huang C C, Fan C H, Hao-Li L and Chih-Kuang Y 2021 Ultrasonic technologies in imaging and drug delivery *Cell. Mol. Life Sci.* **78** 6119–41

Hong G, Joshua T R, Zhang Y, Diao S, Antaris A L, Wang Q and Dai H 2012 *In vivo* fluorescence imaging with Ag_2S quantum dots in the second near-infrared region *Angew. Chem. Int. Ed.* **51** 9818–21

Hosu O, Selvolini G, Cristea C and Marrazza G 2018 Electrochemical immunosensors for disease detection and diagnosis *Curr. Med. Chem.* **25** 4119–37

Huang S, Jie Yang S F and Zhao Q 2020 Artificial intelligence in cancer diagnosis and prognosis: opportunities and challenges *Cancer Lett.* **471** 61–71

Huizar C C, Raphael I and Forsthuber T G 2020 Genomic, proteomic, and systems biology approaches in biomarker discovery for multiple sclerosis *Cell. Immunol.* **358** 104219

Hutter E and Maysinger D 2011 Gold nanoparticles and quantum dots for bioimaging *Microsc. Res. Tech.* **74** 592–604

Jain K K 2003 Nanodiagnostics: application of nanotechnology in molecular diagnostics *Expert Rev. Mol. Diagn.* **3** 153–61

Jelveh S and Chithrani D B 2011 Gold nanostructures as a platform for combinational therapy in cancer therapeutics *Cancers* **3** 1081–110

Jin A, Wang Y, Lin K and Jiang L 2020 Nanoparticles modified by polydopamine: working as 'drug' carriers *Bioact. Mater.* **5** 522–41

Jin C, Wang K, Oppong-Gyebi A and Hu J 2020 Application of nanotechnology in cancer diagnosis and therapy: a mini-review *Int. J. Med. Sci.* **17** 2964

Jou A, Fang-ju C H, Lu Y C, Ou S S, Wang S L, Hsu I, Willner and Ho J A 2015 Diagnosing the MiR-141 prostate cancer biomarker using nucleic acid-functionalized CdSe/ZnS QDs and telomerase *Chem. Sci.* **6** 659

Kam N W S, O'Connell M, Wisdom J A and Dai H 2005 Carbon nanotubes as multifunctional biological transporters and near-infrared agents for selective cancer cell destruction *Proc. Natl Acad. Sci.* **102** 11600–5

Kasivisvanathan V *et al* 2019 Magnetic resonance imaging-targeted biopsy versus systematic biopsy in the detection of prostate cancer: a systematic review and meta-analysis *Eur. Urol* **76** 284–303

Kattke M D, Gao E J, Sapsford K E, Stephenson L D and Kumar A 2011 FRET-Based quantum dot immunoassay for rapid and sensitive detection of *Aspergillus amstelodami Sensors* **11** 6396–410

Kaur B, Kumar S and Kaushik B K 2022 Recent advancements in optical biosensors for cancer detection *Biosens. Bioelectron.* **197** 113805

Kemp J A and Kwon Y J 2021 Cancer nanotechnology: current status and perspectives *Nano Converg.* **8** 1–38

Khan R, Parihar A, Kaushik A K and Kumar A (ed) 2022 *Advanced Biosensors for Virus Detection: Smart Diagnostics to Combat SARS-CoV-2* (Academic)

Khan R, Parihar A and Sanghi S K (ed) 2021 *Biosensor Based Advanced Cancer Diagnostics: From Lab to Clinics* (Academic)

Khleif S N, James H D and Hait W N 2010 AACR-FDA-NCI cancer biomarkers collaborative consensus report: advancing the use of biomarkers in cancer drug developmentadvancing biomarker use in cancer drug development *Clin. Cancer Res* **16** 3299–318

Li H, Cao Z, Zhang Y, Lau C and Lu J 2011 Simultaneous detection of two lung cancer biomarkers using dual-color fluorescence quantum dots *Analyst* **136** 1399–405

Li M, Lao Y H, Mintz R L, Chen Z, Shao D, Hu H, Wang H X, Tao Y and Leong K W 2019 A multifunctional mesoporous silica–gold nanocluster hybrid platform for selective breast cancer cell detection using a catalytic amplification-based colorimetric assay *Nanoscale* **11** 2631–36

Li W and Chen X 2015 Gold nanoparticles for photoacoustic imaging *Nanomedicine* **10** 299–320

Li Y, Zhang Y, Zhao M, Zhou Q, Wang L, Wang H, Wang X and Zhan L 2016 A simple aptamer-functionalized gold nanorods based biosensor for the sensitive detection of MCF-7 breast cancer cells *Chem. Commun.* **52** 3959–61

Liu M, Xu Y, Huang C, Jia T, Zhang X, Yang D P and Jia N 2018 Hyaluronic acid-grafted three-dimensional MWCNT array as biosensing interface for chronocoulometric detection and fluorometric imaging of CD44-overexpressing cancer cells *Microchim. Acta* **185** 1–8

Liu Q, Yeh Y C, Rana S, Jiang Y, Guo L and Rotello V M 2013 Differentiation of cancer cell type and phenotype using quantum dot-gold nanoparticle sensor arrays *Cancer Letters* **334** 196–201

Mallidi S, Anbil S, Bulin A L, Obaid G, Ichikawa M and Hasan T 2016 Beyond the barriers of light penetration: strategies, perspectives and possibilities for photodynamic therapy *Theranostics* **6** 2458–87

Mallidi S, Luke G P and Emelianov S 2011 Photoacoustic imaging in cancer detection, diagnosis, and treatment guidance *Trends Biotechnol.* **29** 213–21

Mehrmohammadi M, Soon Joon Y, Yeager D and Stanislav Y E 2013 Photoacoustic imaging for cancer detection and staging *Curr. Mol. Imaging* **2** 89–105

Miki K, Kuramochi Y, Oride K, Satoru I, Hiroshi H, Masahiro H and Kouichi O 2009 Ring-opening metathesis polymerization-based synthesis of ICG-containing amphiphilic triblock copolymers for *in vivo* tumor imaging *Bioconjug. Chem.* **20** 511–17

Miller K D, Nogueira L, Mariotto A B, Rowland J H, Yabroff K R, Alfano C M, Jemal A, Kramer J L and Siegel R L 2019 Cancer treatment and survivorship statistics *CA: Cancer J Clin* **69** 363–85

Min Y, Stott S, Toner M, Maheswaran S and Haber D A 2011 Circulating tumor cells: approaches to isolation and characterization *J. Cell Biol.* **192** 373–82

Mintz R L, Gao M A, Lo K, Lao Y H, Li M and Leong K W 2018 CRISPR technology for breast cancer: diagnostics, modeling, and therapy *Advanced Biosyst.* **2** 1800132

Mir M, Ishtiaq S, Rabia S, Khatoon M, Zeb A and Majid Khan G 2017 Nanotechnology: from *in vivo* imaging system to controlled drug delivery *Nanoscale Res. Lett.* **12** 1–16

Mohammadi S, Abdollah S, Somayeh H G, Fardin F and Soleimani F 2018 A FRET immunosensor for sensitive detection of CA 15-3 tumor marker in human serum sample and breast cancer cells using antibody functionalized luminescent carbon-dots and AuNPs-dendrimer aptamer as donor-acceptor pair *Anal. Biochem.* **557** 18–26

Mower W R 2008 Radiation doses among blunt trauma patients: assessing risks and benefits of computed tomographic imaging *Ann. Emerg. Med.* **52** 99–100

Mu N, Gao W and Zhou Y 2019 Non-invasive observation of human tissue samples with full field optical coherence tomography *Chin. J. Electron.* **28** 987–2

Nachmanson D *et al* 2018 Targeted genome fragmentation with CRISPR/Cas9 enables fast and efficient enrichment of small genomic regions and ultra-accurate sequencing with low dna input (CRISPR-DS) *Genome Res.* **28** 1589–99

Nguyen K T 2011 Targeted nanoparticles for cancer therapy: promises and challenge *J. Nanomedic Nanotechnol.* **2** 5

Niciński K, Krajczewski J, Kudelski A, Witkowska E, Trzcińska-Danielewicz J, Girstun A and Kamińska A 2019 Detection of circulating tumor cells in blood by shell-isolated nano-particle–enhanced Raman spectroscopy (SHINERS) in microfluidic device *Sci. Rep.* **9** 9267

Nonaka M, Hosoda H and Uezono Y 2021 Cancer treatment-related cardiovascular disease: current status and future research priorities *Biochem. Pharmacol.* **190** 114599

Novoselova M *et al* 2021 Multifunctional nanostructured drug delivery carriers for cancer therapy: multimodal imaging and ultrasound-induced drug release *Colloids Surf.* B **200** 111576

Oh H H and Joo Y E 2020 Novel biomarkers for the diagnosis and prognosis of colorectal cancer *Intest. Res.* **18** 168

Palaz F, Kalkan A K, Can O, Demir A N, Tozluyurt A, Ozcan A and Ozsoz M 2021 CRISPR-Cas13 system as a promising and versatile tool for cancer diagnosis, therapy, and research *ACS Synth. Biol.* **10** 1245–67

Parihar A, Jain S, Parihar D S, Ranjan P and Khan R 2022 Biomarkers associated with different types of cancer as a potential candidate for early diagnosis of oncological disorders *Biosensor Based Advanced Cancer Diagnostics* (Elsevier) pp 47–57

Parihar A, Malviya S and Khan R 2021 Identification of biomarkers associated with cancer using integrated bioinformatic analysis *Cancer Bioinformatics*

Parihar A, Ranjan P, Sanghi S K, Srivastava A K and Khan R 2020 Point-of-care biosensor-based diagnosis of COVID-19 holds promise to combat current and future pandemics *ACS Appl. Bio Mater.* **3** 7326–43

Parihar A, Kumar A, Panda U, Khan R, Parihar D S and Khan R 2023 Cryopreservation: A Comprehensive Overview, Challenges, and Future Perspectives *Adv. Biol.* **7** 2200285

Parihar A, Yadav S, Sadique M A, Ranjan P, Kumar N, Singhal A, Khare V, Khan R, Natarajan S and Srivastava A K 2023 Internet-of-medical-things integrated point-of-care biosensing devices for infectious diseases: toward better preparedness for futuristic pandemics *Bioeng. Transl. Med.* e10481

Parihar A, Pandita V and Khan R 2022 3D printed human organoids: high throughput system for drug screening and testing in current COVID-19 pandemic *Biotechnol. Bioeng.* **119** 2669–88

Parihar A, Khan R, Kumar A, Kaushik A K and Gohel H (ed) 2022 *Computational Approaches for Novel Therapeutic and Diagnostic Designing to Mitigate SARS-CoV2 Infection: Revolutionary Strategies to Combat Pandemics* (Academic)

Parihar A, Choudhary N K, Sharma P and Khan R 2022 MXene-based aptasensor for the detection of aflatoxin in food and agricultural products *Environ. Pollut.* **316** 120695

Parihar A, Choudhary N K, Parihar D S and Khan R 2023 Tumor-on-a-chip: microfluidic models of hypoxic tumor microenvironment. *Hypoxia in Cancer: Significance and Impact on Cancer Therapy* (Springer) pp 297–328

Patel J K and Patel A P 2019 Passive targeting of nanoparticles to cancer *Surface Modification of Nanoparticles for Targeted Drug Delivery* (Springer) pp 125–43

Perera M, Papa N, Roberts M, Williams M, Udovicich C, Vela I, Christidis D, Bolton D, Hofman M S and Lawrentschuk N 2020 Gallium-68 prostate-specific membrane antigen positron emission tomography in advanced prostate cancer—updated diagnostic utility, sensitivity, specificity, and distribution of prostate-specific membrane antigen-avid lesions: a systematic review and meta-analysis *Eur. Urol.* **77** 403–17

Pichler , Bernd J, Wehrl H F, Kolb A and Judenhofer M S 2008 Positron emission tomography/magnetic resonance imaging: the next generation of multimodality imaging? *Semin. Nucl. Med.* **38** 199–208

Popović Z, Liu W, Chauhan V P, Lee J, Wong C, Greytak A B, Insin N, Nocera D G, Fukumura D and Jain R K 2010 A nanoparticle size series for *in vivo* fluorescence imaging *Angew. Chem.* **122** 8831–34

Popovtzer R, Agrawal A, Kotov N A, Popovtzer A, Balter J, Carey T E and Kopelman R 2008 Targeted gold nanoparticles enable molecular CT imaging of cancer *Nano Lett.* **8** 4593–96

Pruthi M D S 2019 Cancer blood tests: lab tests used in cancer diagnosis *Mayo Clin.*

Pushparajah D S 2018 Making patient engagement a reality *Patient* **11** 1–8

Ranjan P, Arpana P, Surbhi J, Neeraj K, Chetna D, Murali S and Deepti M *et al* 2020 Biosensor-based diagnostic approaches for various cellular biomarkers of breast cancer: a comprehensive review *Anal. Biochem.* **610** 113996

Riethdorf S, Fritsche H, Müller V, Rau T, Schindlbeck C, Rack B, Janni W, Coith C, Beck K and Jänicke F 2007 Detection of circulating tumor cells in peripheral blood of patients with metastatic breast cancer: a validation study of the cell search system *Clin. Cancer Res.* **13** 920–28

Ripamonti C I, Bossi P, Santini D and Fallon M 2014 Pain related to cancer treatments and diagnostic procedures: a no man's land? *Ann. Oncol* **25** 1097–106

Sallam R M 2015 Proteomics in cancer biomarkers discovery: challenges and applications *Dis. Markers* **2015** 321370

Scully O J, Boon-Huat Bay G Y and Yu Y 2012 Breast cancer metastasis *Cancer Genom. Proteom* **9** 311–20

Sha M Y, Xu H, Natan M J and Cromer R 2008 Surface-enhanced raman scattering tags for rapid and homogeneous detection of circulating tumor cells in the presence of human whole blood *J. Am. Chem. Soc.* **130** 17214–5

Shanmugam S 2019 *Nanotechnology* (MJP Publisher)

Shen W, Tian D, Cui H, Yang D and Bian Z 2011 Nanoparticle based electrochemiluminescence immunosensor with enhanced sensitivity for cardiac troponin I using N-(aminobutyl)-N-(ethylisoluminol)-functionalized gold nanoparticles as labels *Biosens. Bioelectron.* **27** 18–24

Shi J, Wang B, Chen Z, Liu W, Jingjing P, Lin H and Zhenzhong Z 2016 A multi-functional tumor theranostic nanoplatform for MRI guided photothermal-chemotherapy *Pharm. Res.* **33** 1472–85

Shin G W, Grimes S M, Lee H J, Lau B T, Xia L C and Ji H P 2017 CRISPR–Cas9-targeted fragmentation and selective sequencing enable massively parallel microsatellite analysis *Nat. Commun.* **8** 1–13

Singhal A, Arpana P, Neeraj K and Khan R 2022 High throughput molecularly imprinted polymers based electrochemical nanosensors for point-of-care diagnostics of COVID-19 *Mater. Lett.* **306** 130898

Soler M, Huertas C S and Lechuga L M 2019 Label-free plasmonic biosensors for point-of-care diagnostics: a review *Expert Rev. Mol. Diagn.* **19** 71–81

Song G, Jiali Hao C L, Teng Liu M G, Liang Cheng J H and Liu Z 2016 Degradable molybdenum oxide nanosheets with rapid clearance and efficient tumor homing capabilities as a therapeutic nanoplatform *Angew. Chem. Int. Ed.* **55** 2122–6

Stanisavljevic M, Krizkova S, Vaculovicova M, Kizek R and Adam V 2015 Quantum dots-fluorescence resonance energy transfer-based nanosensors and their application *Biosens. Bioelectron.* **74** 562–74

Subhan Md A, Satya Siva Kishan Y, Nina F, Farzana P and Vladimir P T 2021 Recent advances in tumor targeting via EPR effect for cancer treatment *J. Pers. Med.* **11** 571

Hyuna S, Ferlay J, Siegel R L, Laversanne M, Soerjomataram I, Jemal A and Bray F 2021 Global cancer statistics 2020: GLOBOCAN estimates of incidence and mortality worldwide for 36 cancers in 185 countries *CA: Cancer J. Clin.* **71** 209–49

Tang J, Shaozhe Cai C Y and Dong L 2020 Biomarkers in IgG4-related disease: a systematic review *Seminars in Arthritis and Rheumatism* (Elsevier) pp 354–59

Tao Y, Li M, Kim B and Debra T A 2017 Incorporating gold nanoclusters and target-directed liposomes as a synergistic amplified colorimetric sensor for HER2-positive breast cancer cell detection *Theranostics* **7** 899

Tassa C, Stanley Y S and Weissleder R 2011 Dextran-coated iron oxide nanoparticles: a versatile platform for targeted molecular imaging, molecular diagnostics, and therapy *Acc. Chem. Res.* **44** 842–52

Thawani J P, Amirshaghaghi A, Yan L, Stein J M, Liu J and Tsourkas A 2017 Photoacoustic-guided surgery with indocyanine green-coated superparamagnetic iron oxide nanoparticle clusters *Small* **13** 1701300

Topkaya S N, Azimzadeh M and Ozsoz M 2016 Electrochemical biosensors for cancer biomarkers detection: recent advances and challenges *Electroanalysis* **28** 1402–19

Varty K, O'Brien C and Ignaszak A 2021 Breast cancer aptamers: current sensing targets, available aptamers, and their evaluation for clinical use in diagnostics *Cancers* **13** 3984

Wadowska K, Bil-Lula I, Trembecki Ł and Śliwińska-Mossoń M 2020 Genetic markers in lung cancer diagnosis: a review *Int. J. Mol. Sci.* **21** 4569

Wang B, Yang Y, Jiang Z, Zhao J, Mao Y, Liu J and Zhang J 2019 Clinicopathological Characteristics, diagnosis, and prognosis of pregnancy-associated breast cancer *Thorac. Cancer* **10** 1060–8

Wang B, Shen J, Huang Y, Liu Z and Zhuang H 2018 Graphene quantum dots and enzyme-coupled biosensor for highly sensitive determination of hydrogen peroxide and glucose *Int. J. Mol. Sci.* **19** 1696

Wang Q, Liyuan Zou X Y, Xiaofeng Liu W N, Yan Zheng Q C and Wang K 2019 Direct quantification of cancerous exosomes via surface plasmon resonance with dual gold nano-particle-assisted signal amplification *Biosens. Bioelectron.* **135** 129–36

Werner R A, Thorsten D, Constantin L, Sara S, Takahiro H, Giesel F L, Behr S, Drzezga A, Kimura H and Buck A K 2020 18F-Labeled, PSMA-targeted radiotracers: leveraging the advantages of radiofluorination for prostate cancer molecular imaging *Theranostics* **10** 1

Wilson M L, Fleming K A, Kuti M A, Looi L M, Lago N and Ru K 2018 Access to pathology and laboratory medicine services: a crucial Gap *Lancet* **391** 1927–38

Wu H, Huo Q, Varnum S, Wang J, Liu G, Nie Z, Liu J and Lin Y 2008 Dye-doped silica nanoparticle labels/protein microarray for detection of protein biomarkers *Analyst* **133** 1550–5

Yan L and Huang Z 2021 Application value and feasibility analysis of humanistic health management for cancer screening in physical examination *Am. J. Transl. Res* **13** 14229

Yang P, Li X, Wang L, Wu Q, Chen Z and Lin X 2014 Sandwich-type amperometric immunosensor for cancer biomarker based on signal amplification strategy of multiple enzyme-linked antibodies as probes modified with carbon nanotubes and concanavalin A *J. Electroanal. Chem.* **732** 38–45

Yin H, Xue W and Anderson D G 2019 CRISPR–cas: a tool for cancer research and therapeutics *Nat. Rev. Clin. Oncol.* **16** 281–95

Younis M A, Hesham M T, Abdellatif A A H, Abdel-Aleem J A and Harashima H 2021 Clinical translation of nanomedicines: challenges, opportunities, and keys *Adv. Drug Delivery Rev.* 114083

Zahavi D and Weiner L 2020 Monoclonal antibodies in cancer therapy *Antibodies* **9** 34

Zeps N and Hemmings C 2015 Rare cancers *Rare Diseases* (Berlin: Springer) pp 109–30

Zhang Q, Iwakuma N, Sharma P, Moudgil B M, Wu C, McNeill J, Jiang H and Grobmyer S R 2009 Gold nanoparticles as a contrast agent for *in vivo* tumor imaging with photoacoustic tomography *Nanotechnology* **20** 395102

Zhao M, Mi D, Ferdows B E, Li Y, Wang R, Li J, Patel D, Kong N, Shi S and Tao W 2022 State-of-the-art nanotechnologies for the detection, recovery, analysis and elimination of liquid biopsy components in cancer *Nano Today* **42** 101361

Chapter 11

Current perspectives on aptasensors as diagnostic tool for cancer screening

Shagun Gupta, Deepak Kala, Nkurunziza Florien, Surbhi Sharma and Ankur Kaushal

Cancer diagnosis at its early stages is a lifesaving step in its treatment and disease management. However, the asymptomatic manifestation of cancers at the initial stages affects its diagnosis as well as ability to treat it. The limitations in cancer diagnosis either in terms of asymptomatic manifestations or the limitations of existing diagnosis methods need improvements. The current scenario of cancer diagnosis demands the new diagnosis methods with higher accuracy and sensitivity in cancer detection at untimely stages. In this sense, aptasensors are becoming a noticeable reliable tool for the detection of different cancer biomarkers including exosomes, circulating tumors, proteins, cell free DNA and miRNA. Aptamers are mostly referred to as the nucleic acid sequences (DNA or RNA) that bind particularly to targeted antigens like proteins, peptides and cells. Systematic Evolution of Ligands by Exponential Enrichment, also known as the SELEX technique, is used to decipher DNA–protein interaction specificity for aptamer designing. Aptamer research is in the limelight in the last three decades due to their excellence, specificity, wide range of target molecules, binding affinity, stability, ease of synthesis, less toxicity and immunogenicity. Their ability to specifically bind with a wide range of molecules with simple to complex structures makes it a suitable tool for diagnostics application. This chapter illustrates the current issues of aptasensors in diagnosis of cancer as well as their possible future expectations.

11.1 Introduction

Changes in the lifestyle altered the dietary patterns like high intake of saturated fats, less vegetables and fruits, environmental pollutants, stress, etc, are all factors that have a negative impact on human health and increase the risk of various non-transmissible illnesses like cardiovascular disease, diabetes, neurological disease and

doi:10.1088/978-0-7503-5012-9ch11

cancer. [1–6]. Cancer is challenging and global disease caused by viruses, genetic predeposition and also interconnected with the risk factors like poor food habits, few physical activities, smoking, chemicals, radiation, and poor lifestyle [7–10]. Every year reports reveal million cases of cancer and more than half of that number dies as a result [11]. The lack of facility for untimely stage cancer detection is among the major difficulties with its treatment [12–17]. Delay in cancer diagnosis causes its advancement to the metastasis stage, resulting into a huge obstacle to solve in the path of cancer treatment [18–21]. Besides behindhand detection, cancer occupies other tissues as well as organs that lead to its treatment process being complex [20, 21].

Recognizing noble biomarkers expressed at early stages in cancerous cells can be the major role player in the development of assays with the ability for early-stage cancer diagnosis [22–24]. Normally, a biomarker means the indicator of a biological condition [25, 26]. The biomarkers commonly identify the diseased condition and reveal the result to a particular therapy. In prior decades various biomarkers were identified for the identification of several diseases and proven to be an asset in the area of diagnostics.

The most important features for an idle biomarker include sensitivity, specificity, non-invasiveness and identification at early stages even before onset of symptoms [27, 28]. In the previous three decades, the significance of nucleic acid aptamers has been enlarged in the area of diagnosis and medicine due to their higher specificity, stability, and sensitivity [29–31]. The aptamers have higher binding affinity and particularity with their target molecules [32, 33]. The aptasensors use aptamers as a biorecognition layer for the detection of targeted analyte in the sample [34, 35]. Since aptamers are synthetic, their features like affinity and specificity toward the targeted molecules can be adjusted [36, 37]. The higher sensitivity of aptasensors helps them to identify even the smallest concentration of analyte in the sample, which is not possible with most of the existing diagnostic methods [38, 39]. Further significances connected with the aptasensors are their low cost, portability, point-of-care diagnosis and rapid detection at early stages [40–42].

11.2 Cancer diagnosis

The cancer diagnosis at early stages is a crucial requisite for its suitable treatment. Present diagnosis of cancer depends on oncological imaging such as magnetic resonance imaging (MRI) and computed tomography (CT) with other methods like biopsy, flow cytometry and cancer biomarkers-based assays (figure 11.1). However, they have limitations of being expensive and time consuming. One of the great limitations of the existing methods is their unavailability in remote areas, which leads to a delay in cancer diagnosis and occurrence of metastasis, making its treatment difficult. Consequently, novel methods need to be improved that can detect cancer at early stages by identifying the biomarkers.

Biological markers, usually known as cancer biomarkers (CB), exhibit marvelous genetic features of malignant cells. Each molecule, activity or structure that can be noticed in the body that predicts the existence of any disease is known as a

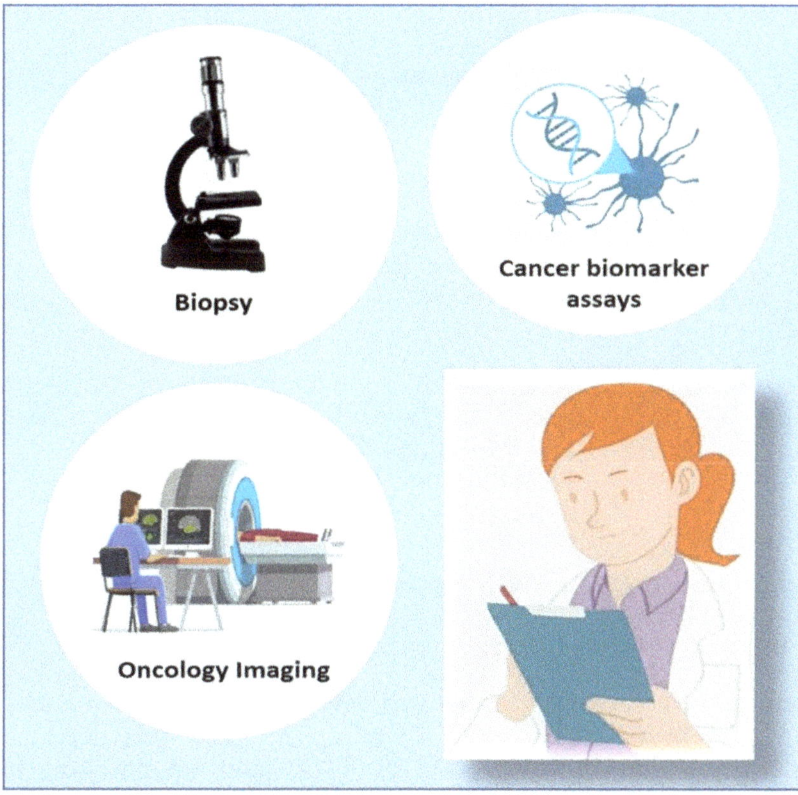

Figure 11.1. Common diagnostic tests of cancer.

biomarker. Nevertheless, the interference of other proteins in the sample and lower concentrations of a target protein makes it difficult to diagnose at early stages. Besides, these techniques could need more workforces and take too much time [43, 44]. Consequently, aptamers provide the solution with their lower detection limit (LOD) abilities of the target molecules [45, 46]. The study even reported the detection limit of 10 cancer cells, which shows its excellence in terms of detection limits [47]. Moreover, aptamers can detect biomarkers and metabolites of cancers, tumor behavior affecting molecules and differentiating cells.

11.2.1 Aptamers in cancer diagnosis

Aptamers coupled with nanoparticles is one of the most-often utilized cancer detection technologies. These complexes can be deployed for screening of cancer cells in complex samples like serum and blood. Cancer-specific aptasensors can be attached to the nanoparticles or nanocomposite surface for diagnostics or therapeutic purposes. These conjugates will facilitate the selection with sensitive identifications of targeted cells using aptamers, whereas stability and protection from DNA degradative enzymes like nucleases will be provided by the

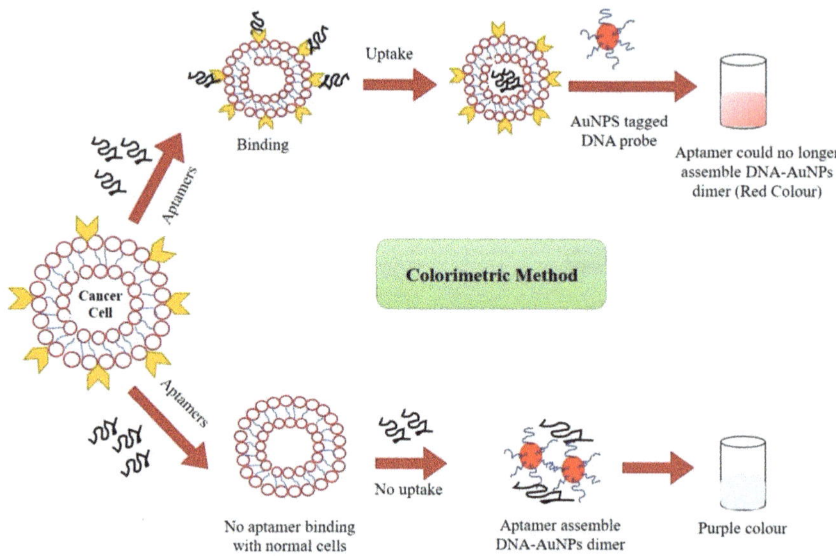

Figure 11.2. Colorimetric method of cancer detection using aptamers.

nanomaterials. A colorimetric assay was invented by Borghei *et al* [47], for identification of breast cancer (MCF-7) cells. The assay was developed using nucleolin receptor-specific aptamers (AS 1411) and aptamer-complimentary ssDNA-coated gold nanoparticles (ssDNA-AuNPs) (figure 11.2). The aptamers (AS 1411) binding with the targeted cancer cells cause its intake and clearance from the solution [47]. As the aptamers were sequestered by the cancer cells, no complementary binding sites were available for ssDNA-AuNP probes, resulting in a red solution. Aptamers were available for binding with ssDNA-AuNP conjugates causing their aggregation and formation of a unique purple color in the absence of cancer cells. Recently, an orthotopic xenograft mouse model was used to detect aptamers for identification refractory prostate cancer hormone of hormone-refractory prostate cancer [48]. Aptamers that target specifically androgen-independent prostate cancers within living mice was identified by the help of a random DNA library. Aptamers that target various tumors were found using recurring SELEX cycles, with the D3P-21 aptamer having great specificity and affinity for *in vivo* prostate tumor identification.

11.2.1.1 Interaction between aptamer and tumor cell

Interaction between aptamers and tumor cells was predicted based on the addition of a polyethylene glycol to the S5′-end of the oligonucleotide. The aptamer-fluorescent silica nanoparticle (FSNP) conjugate method created by Tan *et al* (2016) and used for identifying blood cancer or leukemia cells (figure 11.3).

Carboxyl-modified FSNPs together with Sgc8 amine-labeled aptamers were used to identify leukaemia cells [49].

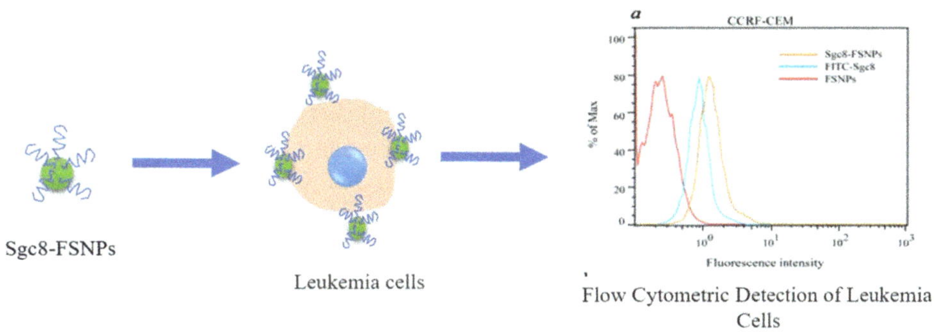

FSNPs: fluorescent silica nanoparticles; Sgc8: Sc8 aptamer

Figure 11.3. Fluorescent silica nanoparticles tagged aptamer-based leukemia cells identification.

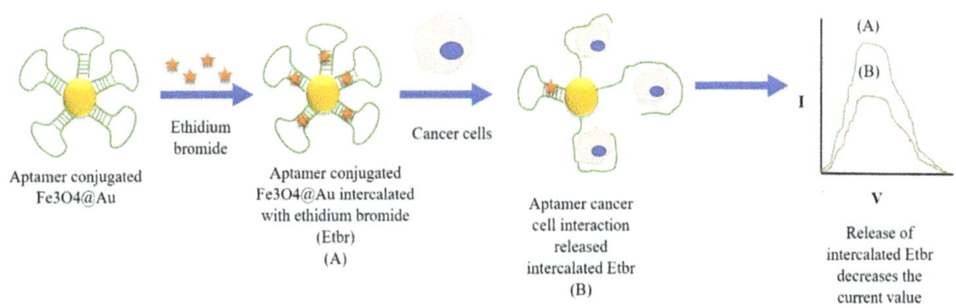

Fe3O4@Au: gold nanoparticles-coated magnetic nanoparticles

Figure 11.4. Electrochemical identification of cancer cells by gold-coated magnetic NP-aptamer conjugate-based approach.

The Sgc8 aptamer, another sensitive biosensor for T-cell leukaemia detection, was described [50]. Magnetic Fe_3O_4 NPs coated with gold nanoparticle (Apt-GMNPs) combined with the Sgc8 aptamer. Furthermore, the stem of the aptamer hairpin was intercalated with ethidium bromide (EB), which was released after the hairpin was damaged due to the presence of cancer cells. A decrease in the electrochemical signal was found (figure 11.4). Leukemia cells at concentrations ranging from 10 to 1×10^6 cells per ml of the tested sample was identified by this method. Hu *et al* [51] designed another method using streptavidin-modified fluorescent silica nanoparticles and biotin-labeled aptamers (TLS11a) specific to the hepatoma cells. The biotin-labeled aptamers bind with the purposed cells and give the binding site at streptavidin-modified silica nanoparticles for fluorescent tagging [51].

The developed assay takes advantage of the strong and specific interaction of biotin–streptavidin to detect the hepatoma cancer cells more precisely and accurately. The fluorescent quantum dot nanoparticles have been deployed for the development of cancer biomarkers such as nucleolin, tenascin-C, and protein tyrosine kinase 7. The aptamers can be designed for different target sites for detecting multiple biomarkers simultaneously in different cancer cell lines [52, 53]. In brain and spinal cord cancer cell's fluorescence-guided surgery, they use conjugated QD-aptamers [54]. On the surface of glioma cancer cells, there is an aptamer (A32) which acts as a receptor of epidermal growth factor specifically and is identified by using fluorescence evaluation. The aptamer-florescent dye conjugates were also deployed in metastatic cancer cells identification. The Cy5 is used as a fluorescent tag to couple with aptamers (J3) in metastatic cancer cells bioimaging and identification [55]. Accuracy of the method was 73.9 percent in identification of metastatic colon cancer. Flow cytometry-based analysis was used in studies to investigate the affinity of an aptamer (e.g. R13) with cancer cells in clinical investigation of cancer patients (R13 aptamer for ovarian cancer) [56]. However, researchers also used confocal microscopy to investigate the binding of the R13 aptamer with ovarian cancer patients. A total of 80 samples of ovarian cancer and 10 normal samples of ovary tissues as a control were involved in study. In NOD/SCID tumor models of mice, R13 affinity was validated. The R13 aptamer demonstrated excellent binding affinity to various ovarian cancer cell lines (SKOV3, Caov3, HO8910 and A2780), and dissociation constants (KD) ranged in the nanomolar size (158 28.22, 47.48 7.15, 29.24 8.55, 37.87 4.93 nM, respectively). In a randomized 30mer RNA library, six aptamers have been discovered by Pan *et al* [57] with significant affinity towards CEA, CA72–4, and CA50 as gastric cancer biomarkers. For CEA, CA72–4 and CA50, KD was determined by fluorescence spectroscopy to be 52.7–71.2 nM, 16.5–156 nM and 30.7–38.0 nM, respectively [57]. A CEA aptamer probe added the potential of RNA aptamers in gastric cancer bio-sensing and bioimaging upon the use of a positive fluorescent signal from a gastric adenocarcinoma (AGS) cell line. Four highly specific aptamers (Seq-3, Seq-54, Seq-19 and Seq-6) were found in another study published in 2019 with exceptional binding capacity to stomach cancer serum using SELEX as the whole-serum subtractive approach. These particular aptamers have KDs of 149 23.6 nM 202 25.6 nM, 128 26.3 nM and 232 44.2 nM, respectively. Because of their great target specificity, these oligonucleotides were used to construct a quantitative PCR methodology in timely identification of stomach cancer. These aptamers were utilized to find Importin subunit alpha-1, APOA4, PARD3 and APOA1 biomarkers of gastric cancer, where Importin subunit alpha-1 became most promising option for future gastric cancer detection. One of the most regular malignancies is colorectal cancer and there are no effective treatments available presently.

Aptamers on an SBA-15–3-aminopropyltriethoxysilane (SBA-15-pr-NH2) and Au nanoparticle-modified graphite screen-printed electrode (GSPE) had been used by Hashkavayi *et al* [58] in creating an electrochemical diagnostic platform for CT26 cancer cell identification. Diagnosis was very specific, with no cross-reactivity with other cancer cell lines including AGS, VERO, or SKOV-3. The devised diagnostic test exhibited a limit of detection of 2 cells ml^{-1}, according to impedance spectroscopy and cyclic voltammetry results [58]. Aptamers are used together with clinical devices like ultrasonography and magnetic resonance imaging to detect cancer. Ultrasound-propelled gold nanowire motors (FAM-AIB1-apt) coated with graphene oxide together with fluorescein-labeled aptamers were employed, for example, for standard detection of AIB1 oncoproteins in breast cancer cells (MCF-7) when overexpressed.

11.2.1.2 Nanomotors and nanoprobes

In an ultrasonic field, the nanomotor movement resulted in quicker aptamer uptake and binding to the target, resulting in fluorescence [59]. When nanomotors are combined with a driven aptamer, fluorescence intensity increased when compared to the fixed circumstances. Correspondingly, partnership between T-acute leukemia cells (CCRF-CEM) and the Sgc8 aptamer under different flow parameters in microfluidic instruments was surveyed. Furthermore, impacts of apparatus design and rate of flow affinity on aptamer–leukemia cells was studied [60]. MRI technology harnesses action in magnetic field protons to create three-dimensional pictures of biological systems and body parts for bioimaging and diagnostics. MRI therapy capability for many medical situations, such as cancer diagnosis, has been developed. The TLS11a aptamer, for example, was coupled with magnetite nanoparticles with a fluorescent silicon dioxide shell, for identification and bioimaging of human hepacellular carcinoma, cancer cells of the liver (figure 11.5). MRI and fluorescence demonstrated that HepG2 cells specifically ingest aptamers that were not found in other types of cancer cell (SGC-7901, MCF-7, 4T1). It was further supported by MRI of animals and tumors of the liver, although excellent biocompatibility and minimal toxicity was demonstrated from nanoprobes [61], demonstrating the system's treatment possibility. Correspondingly, AS1411 magnetite-gold NPs aptamer-conjugated were employed in the prognosis and imaging of nucleolin-expressing cancer cells of the breast. The relationship of aptamer–

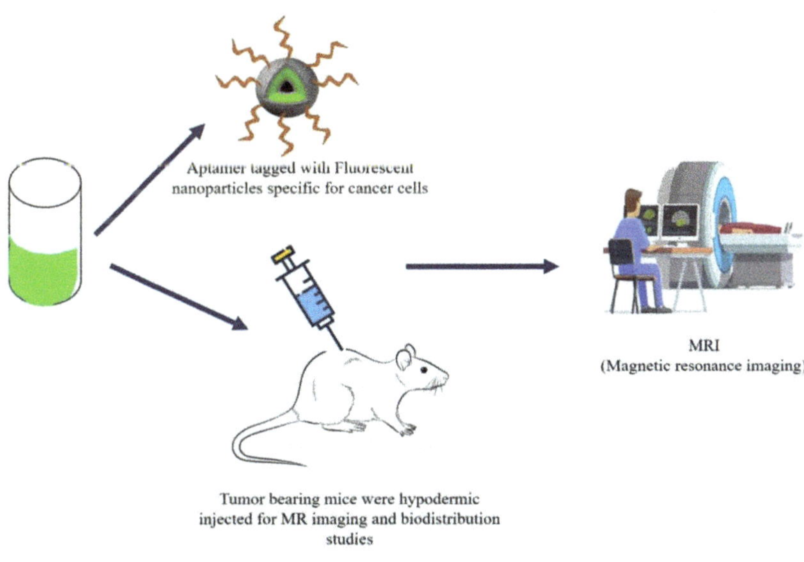

Figure 11.5. Improvement of the cancer diagnosis capacity of MRI using cancer biomarkers specific fluorescent tagged aptamer sequences.

nanoparticle conjugates with several cancer cells of the breast resulted in a notable increase in signal intensity as measured by MRI [62].

This nanoprobe has a greater selectivity and affinity for 4T1 cancer cells of the breast and used as an MRI contrast agent. The ability of the aptamer to precisely adhere to tissues, living cells, and their non-toxicity with more cohesiveness in comparison with proteins on the basis of affinity reagents makes them an important technology in cancer cells as targeted drug delivery. Currently, C8 is being delivered by an AS1411 aptamer, an acridine ligand based on G-quadruplex, to HeLa or cervical cancer cells [63], demonstrating their medicinal value. Massive RNA payloads (175–250 nt) can be delivered to various cancer lines of human B cells by aptamers. Aptamers coupled to fluorogenic RNA reporters particularly bound with B cell lines for leukemia, resulting in persistence of fluorescence for 2 h [64], demonstrating the system's substantial application of medicinal carriage toward cells of cancer. In another work, an aptamer of LC09 was functionalized with a PEG-PEI-cholesterol lipopolymer that encased CRISPR/Cas9 and Cas9 plasmids, which code for VEGFA gRNA to specifically target VEGFA (the vascular endothelial growth factor A) of osteosarcoma cancer cells. The specific binding of LC09 allowed CRISPR/Cas9 to be delivered to orthotopic osteosarcoma and metastasis in the lung [65], resulting in suppressing both types of malignancies and effective VEGFA genome editing in cancer cells.

Finally, a DNA aptamer with 59 bases, named AB3, was employed to be targeted on a receptor protein of immature laminin in AML cancer cells. Doxorubicin medication molecules were delivered to AML cells by aptamers. The aptamer binded to OFA/iLRP with a KD of 101 nM but not to ovalbumin trypsin, albumin or OFA/iLRP-negative control cells [66]. Apt-Dox (Aptamer-doxorubicin) combination was created by inserting doxorubicin into the DNA structure of the aptamer, which enabled delivery of Dox to OFA/iLRP-positive tumor cells of AML, thereby successfully demolishing cells of AML. Aptamer–nanoparticle conjugates and aptamers had eventually come out as a robust technology for treating practically every kind of tumor and quickly used in timely healthcare investigations for speedy and dependable diagnostics and bioimaging. Table 11.1 lists some aptamers used in identification of cancer.

11.3 Conclusions

Numerous malignancies have been found at their late stages, as a result of the insufficiency of detection mechanisms. Cancer biomarker detection in body fluids and plasma is kinder with a more effective approach used in therapeutic settings. Nonetheless, biomarkers derived from fluids physiologically in early phases of cancer can't be identified, potentially leading to a false-negative cancer diagnosis. As a result, developing a high-efficiency identification technique to identify minute levels of an antigen in physiological fluids might result in a huge potential for early cancer diagnosis. Electrochemical/optical biosensors, SomaScan^{TM} tests, and microfluidic chips (aptamer detection methods) have risen in popularity in the detection of CTCs, proteins, free DNA, miRNA, and exosomes (oncomarkers) in cancer.

Table 11.1. Aptamers used *in vivo* and *in vitro* SELEX cancer identification.

Analyte	Aptamer's sequence (5′–3′)	Method	Binding affinity	Reference
Breast cancer cells (MCF-7)	GGTGGTGGTGGTT-GTGGTGGTGGTGG	SELEX (cell)	30–50 nM	[47]
Prostate cancer cells	GGAGGCAACGGAG-CGGAGACATTGAC-TGAGTGAACGTGT-AGTG	*In vivo* SELEX	2–100 nM	[48]
Blood cancer or leukemia cells	TTTTTTTTTTATCT-AACTGCTGCGCCG-CCGGGAAAATACT-GTACGGTTAGA	Live cell-SELEX	—	[49]
Leukemia cells	TTTTTTTTTTATCT-AACTGCTGCGCCG-CCGGGAAAATACT-GTACGGTTAGA	SELEX (Live cell)	5.16 nM	[50]
Liver cancer cells (HepG2)	ACAGCATCCCCAT-GTGAACAATCGCA-TTGTGATTGTTAC-GGTTTCCGCCTCA-TGGACGTGCTG	SELEX (Live cell)	—	[51]
Tenascin-C and Nucleolin cancer biomarkers	TTGGTGGTGGTGG-TTGTGGTGGTGGT-GG and CCTGCACTTGGCT-TGGATTTCAGAAG-GGAGACCC	SELEX (Cell)	—	[52]
Cancer cells of Glioma	GCAATGGTACGGT-ACTTCCTGAATGT-TGTTTTTTCTCTT-TTCTATAGTACAA-AAGTGCACGCTAC-TTTGCTAA	SELEX (Cell)	—	[54]
Ovarian cancer Cells	TCTCTAGTTATTG-AGTTTTCTTTTAT-GGGTGGGTGGGG-GGTTTTT	SELEX (Cell)	29.24–158 nM	[56]
Gastric cancer cells	GGATCCGACACGA-CCCTATAGTGAGT-CGTATTA	SELEX (Cell)	16.5–156, 52.7–71.2, 30.7–38 nM	[57]
Gastric cancer cells	CCTCGGCACGTTC-TCAGTAGCGCTCG-CTGGTCATCCCAC-A	Whole-serum subtractive SELEX	128 nM	[45]
4T1 and MCF-1 breast cancer cells	GGTGGTGGTGGTT-GTGGTGGTGGTGG	SELEX (Cell)	30–50 nM	[59, 62]
Leukemia cells	ATCTAACTGCTGC-GCCGCCGGGAAAA-TACTGTACGGTTA-GATTTTTTTTTT	SELEX (Cell)	0.04 Hz	[60]
HepG2 liver cancer cells	ACAGCATCCCCAT-GTGAACAATCGCA-TTGTGATssTGTTAC-GGTTTCCGCCTCA-TGGACGTGCTG	SELEX (Cell)	—	[61]
Cancer cells of AML	TGCGTGTGTAGTG-TGTCTGTTGTTTG-TATTGTTGTCTAT-CCTCTTAGGGATT-TGGGCGG	SELEX (*in vitro*)	101 nM	—

Furthermore, research must be undertaken to improve specificity as well as selectivity of the developed aptasensors. Extensive research should be conducted on aptamer's choice and outline (like pH, ionic strength, etc) to provide a solid platform for the early identification of malignancy and boosting patient health.

References

[1] Kunst A E, Stronks K and Agyemang C 2011 Non-communicable diseases *Migration and Health in the European Union* **1** 116

[2] McQueen D V (ed) 2013 *Global Handbook on Noncommunicable Diseases and Health Promotion* (Springer)

[3] Priyadarsini R V, Nagini S, Shankar S and Srivastava R K 2012 *Nutrition, Diet and Cancer*

[4] Stanner S 2007 A growing issue—understanding and promoting healthy growth and development in toddlers *Nutrition Bulletin* **33** 62–6

[5] Wu S, Powers S, Zhu W and Hannun Y A 2016 Substantial contribution of extrinsic risk factors to cancer development *Nature* **529** 43–7

[6] Fedewa S A, Sauer A G, Siegel R L and Jemal A 2015 Prevalence of major risk factors and use of screening tests for cancer in the United States *Cancer Epidemiol. Prev. Markers* **24** 637–52

[7] Johnson A 2011 *Reduce Your Cancer Risk: Twelve Steps to a Healthier Life. Barbara Boughton and Michael Stefanek* (Demos Medical Publishing)

[8] Hamdi Y, Abdeljaoued-Tej I, Zatchi A A, Abdelhak S, Boubaker S, Brown J S and Benkahla A 2021 Cancer in Africa: the untold story *Front Oncol* **11** 650117

[9] Wardle J, Robb K, Vernon S and Waller J 2015 Screening for prevention and early diagnosis of cancer *Am Psychol* **70** 119

[10] Jin Z, Jiang W and Wang L 2015 Biomarkers for gastric cancer: progression in early diagnosis and prognosis *Oncol. Lett.* **9** 1502–8

[11] Barh D, Carpi A, Verma M and Gunduz M (ed) 2014 *Cancer Biomarkers: Minimal and Noninvasive Early Diagnosis and Prognosis* (CRC Press)

[12] Gearhart S and Ahuja N 2010 *Early Diagnosis and Treatment of Cancer Series: Colorectal Cancer E-Book: Expert Consult* (Elsevier)

[13] Mascarenhas L, Felgenhauer J L, Bond M C, Villaluna D, Femino J D, Laack N N and Marina N 2016 Pilot study of adding vincristine, topotecan, and cyclophosphamide to interval-compressed chemotherapy in newly diagnosed patients with localized Ewing sarcoma: a report from the Children's Oncology Group *Pediatr Blood Cancer* **63** 493–8

[14] Hayat M A (ed) 2010 *Methods of Cancer Diagnosis, Therapy, and Prognosis: Ovarian Cancer, Renal Cancer, Urogenitary Tract Cancer, Urinary Bladder Cancer, Cervical Uterine Cancer, Skin Cancer, Leukemia, Multiple Myeloma and Sarcoma*6 (Springer)

[15] Brown B J, Adeleye A O and Ibeh J N 2015 A prospective study on the causes of delayed diagnosis of childhood cancer in Ibadan, Nigeria *Pediatr Hematol Oncol* **32** 365–73

[16] Car L T, Papachristou N, Bull A, Majeed A, Gallagher J, El-Khatib M and Vincent C 2016 Clinician-identified problems and solutions for delayed diagnosis in primary care: a PRIORITIZE study *BMC Fam. Pract* **17** 1–9

[17] Seneviratne S, Campbell I, Scott N, Coles C and Lawrenson R 2015 Treatment delay for Māori women with breast cancer in New Zealand *Ethn Health* **20** 178–93

[18] Lo P C, Dahlberg S E, Nishino M, Johnson B E, Sequist L V, Jackman D M and Oxnard G R 2015 Delay of treatment change after objective progression on first-line erlotinib in epidermal growth factor receptor-mutant lung cancer *Cancer* **121** 2570–7
[19] DeSantis C E, Siegel R L, Sauer A G, Miller K D, Fedewa S A, Alcaraz K I and Jemal A 2016 Cancer statistics for African Americans, 2016: progress and opportunities in reducing racial disparities *CA. Cancer J. Clin.* **66** 290–308
[20] Siegel R L, Miller K D and Jemal A 2020 Cancer statistics *CA Cancer J. Clin.* **66** 7–30
[21] Sattarahmady N, Heli H, Mehdizadeh A R, Yarmohammadi H and Mortazavi S M J 2015 Evaluation of serum catalase activity and malondialdehyde level as stress oxidative biomarkers among Iranian welders *Galen Med. J.* **4** 62–6
[22] Walters C C and Moldowan J M 2005 *Walters and Moldowan, JM, The Biomarker Guide* (Cambridge: Cambridge University Press) 1155
[23] Sawyers C L 2008 The cancer biomarker problem *Nature* **452** 548–52
[24] Verma M 2012 Personalized medicine and cancer *J. Pers. Med.* **2** 1–14
[25] Ravelli A, Reuben J M, Lanza F, Anfossi S, Cappelletti M R, Zanotti L and Generali D 2015 Breast cancer circulating biomarkers: advantages, drawbacks, and new insights *Tumor Biol.* **36** 6653–65
[26] Hermann T and Patel D J 2000 Adaptive recognition by nucleic acid aptamers *Science* **287** 820–5
[27] Brody E N and Gold L 2000 Aptamers as therapeutic and diagnostic agents *Rev. Mol. Biotechnol.* **74** 5–13
[28] Tombelli S, Minunni M and Mascini M 2005 Analytical applications of aptamers *Biosens. Bioelectron.* **20** 2424–34
[29] Nilsen-Hamilton M 2009 Aptamers in bioanalysis *J. Am. Chem. Soc.* **131** 12018
[30] Iliuk A B, Hu L and Tao W A 2011 Aptamer in bioanalytical applications *Anal. Chem.* **83** 4440–52
[31] Mascini M 2009 *Aptamers in Bioanalysis* (Wiley)
[32] Lyons G E, Moore T, Brasic N, Li M, Roszkowski J J and Nishimura M I 2006 Influence of human CD8 on antigen recognition by T-cell receptor–transduced cells *Cancer Res.* **66** 11455–61
[33] O'Sullivan C K 2002 Aptasensors–the future of biosensing? *Anal. Bioanal. Chem.* **372** 44–8
[34] Luzi E, Minunni M, Tombelli S and Mascini M 2003 New trends in affinity sensing: aptamers for ligand binding *TrAC, Trends Anal. Chem.* **22** 810–8
[35] Hianik T and Wang J 2009 Electrochemical aptasensors–recent achievements and perspectives *Electroanalysis* **21** 1223–35
[36] Chen X, Zhang Q, Qian C, Hao N, Xu L and Yao C 2015 Electrochemical aptasensor for mucin 1 based on dual signal amplification of poly (o-phenylenediamine) carrier and functionalized carbon nanotubes tracing tag *Biosens. Bioelectron.* **64** 485–92
[37] Robati R Y, Arab A, Ramezani M, Langroodi F A, Abnous K and Taghdisi S M 2016 Aptasensors for quantitative detection of kanamycin *Biosens. Bioelectron.* **82** 162–72
[38] Cheng L, Zhang J, Lin Y, Wang Q, Zhang X, Ding Y and Fan H 2015 An electrochemical molecular recognition-based aptasensor for multiple protein detection *Anal. Biochem.* **491** 31–6
[39] Sattarahmady N, Rahi A and Heli H 2017 A signal-on built in-marker electrochemical aptasensor for human prostate-specific antigen based on a hairbrush-like gold nanostructure *Sci. Rep.* **7** 1–8

[40] Negahdary M, Behjati-Ardakani M, Sattarahmady N, Yadegari H and Heli H 2017 Electrochemical aptasensing of human cardiac troponin I based on an array of gold nanodumbbells-Applied to early detection of myocardial infarction *Sensors Actuators* B **252** 62–71

[41] Negahdary M, Behjati-Ardakani M, Sattarahmady N and Heli H 2018 An aptamer-based biosensor for troponin I detection in diagnosis of myocardial infarction *J. Biomed. Phys. Eng.* **8** 167

[42] Negahdary M, Behjati-Ardakani M and Heli H 2019 An electrochemical troponin T aptasensor based on the use of a macroporous gold nanostructure *Microchim. Acta* **186** 1–10

[43] Kurt H, Yüce M, Hussain B and Budak H 2016 Dual-excitation upconverting nanoparticle and quantum dot aptasensor for multiplexed food pathogen detection *Biosens. Bioelectron.* **81** 280–6

[44] Yüce M, Kurt H, Hussain B, Ow-Yang C W and Budak H 2018 Exploiting Stokes and anti-Stokes type emission profiles of aptamer—functionalized luminescent nanoprobes for multiplex sensing applications *Chemistry Select* **3** 5814–23

[45] Zheng Y, Zhao Y, Di Y, Xiu C, He L, Liao S and Huang B 2019 DNA aptamers from whole-serum SELEX as new diagnostic agents against gastric cancer *RSC Adv.* **9** 950–7

[46] Ruiz Ciancio D, Vargas M R, Thiel W H, Bruno M A, Giangrande P H and Mestre M B 2018 Aptamers as diagnostic tools in cancer *Pharmaceuticals* **11** 86

[47] Borghei Y S, Hosseini M, Dadmehr M, Hosseinkhani S, Ganjali M R and Sheikhnejad R 2016 Visual detection of cancer cells by colorimetric aptasensor based on aggregation of gold nanoparticles induced by DNA hybridization *Anal. Chim. Acta* **904** 92–7

[48] Civit L, Theodorou I, Frey F, Weber H, Lingnau A, Gröber C and Mayer G 2019 Targeting hormone refractory prostate cancer by *in vivo* selected DNA libraries in an orthotopic xenograft mouse model *Sci. Rep.* **9** 1–16

[49] Zhu B, Li Y, Lin Z, Zhao M, Xu T, Wang C and Deng N 2016 Silver nanoparticles induce HePG-2 cells apoptosis through ROS-mediated signaling pathways *Nanoscale Res. Lett.* **11** 1–8

[50] Saljooqi A, Shamspur T and Mostafavi A 2017 Ag-4-ATP-MWCNT electrode modified with ds DNA as label-free electrochemical sensor for the detection of daunorubicin anticancer drug *Bioelectrochemistry* **118** 161–7

[51] Hu Z, Tan J, Lai Z, Zheng R, Zhong J, Wang Y and Lu X 2017 Aptamer combined with fluorescent silica nanoparticles for detection of hepatoma cells *Nanoscale Res. Lett.* **12** 1–8

[52] Lee J, Kang H J, Jang H, Lee Y J, Lee Y S, Ali B A and Kim S 2015 Simultaneous imaging of two different cancer biomarkers using aptamer-conjugated quantum dots *Sensors* **15** 8595–604

[53] Li Z, He X, Luo X, Wang L and Ma N 2016 DNA-programmed quantum dot polymerization for ultrasensitive molecular imaging of cancer cells *Anal. Chem.* **88** 9355–8

[54] Tang J, Huang N, Zhang X, Zhou T, Tan Y, Pi J and Cheng Y 2017 Aptamer-conjugated PEGylated quantum dots targeting epidermal growth factor receptor variant III for fluorescence imaging of glioma *Int. J. Nanomed.* **12** 3899

[55] Yuan B, Jiang X, Chen Y, Guo Q, Wang K, Meng X and Wen X 2017 Metastatic cancer cell and tissue-specific fluorescence imaging using a new DNA aptamer developed by Cell-SELEX *Talanta* **170** 56–62

[56] Li F, Wang Q, Zhang H, Deng T, Feng P, Hu B and Cao L 2018 Characterization of a DNA aptamer for ovarian cancer clinical tissue recognition and *in vivo* imaging *Cell. Physiol. Biochem.* **51** 2564–74

[57] Pan Q, Law C O, Yung M M, Han K C, Pon Y L and Lau T C K 2018 Novel RNA aptamers targeting gastrointestinal cancer biomarkers CEA, CA50 and CA72-4 with superior affinity and specificity *PLoS One* **13** e0198980

[58] Hashkavayi A B, Raoof J B, Ojani R and Kavoosian S 2017 Ultrasensitive electrochemical aptasensor based on sandwich architecture for selective label-free detection of colorectal cancer (CT26) cells *Biosens. Bioelectron.* **92** 630–7

[59] Beltrán-Gastélum M, Esteban-Fernández de Ávila B, Gong H, Venugopalan P L, Hianik T, Wang J and Subjakova V 2019 Rapid detection of AIB1 in breast cancer cells based on aptamer-functionalized nanomotors *Chem. Phys. Chem.* **20** 3177–80

[60] Chen K, Georgiev T Z, Sheng W, Zheng X, Varillas J I, Zhang J and Hugh Fan Z 2017 Tumor cell capture patterns around aptamer-immobilized microposts in microfluidic devices *Biomicrofluidics* **11** 054110

[61] Wei Z, Wu Y, Zhao Y, Mi L, Wang J, Wang J and Liu S 2016 Multifunctional nanoprobe for cancer cell targeting and simultaneous fluorescence/magnetic resonance imaging *Anal. Chim. Acta* **938** 156–64

[62] Mahmoudi P, Veladi H and Pakdel F G 2017 Optogenetics, tools and applications in neurobiology *J. Med. Signals Sens.* **7** 71

[63] Carvalho J, Paiva A, Cabral Campello M P, Paulo A, Mergny J L, Salgado G F and Cruz C 2019 Aptamer-based targeted delivery of a G-quadruplex ligand in cervical cancer cells *Sci. Rep.* **9** 1–12

[64] Porciani D, Cardwell L N, Tawiah K D, Alam K K, Lange M J, Daniels M A and Burke D H 2018 Modular cell-internalizing aptamer nanostructure enables targeted delivery of large functional RNAs in cancer cell lines *Nat. Commun.* **9** 1–13

[65] Liang C, Li F, Wang L, Zhang Z K, Wang C, He B and Zhang G 2017 Tumor cell-targeted delivery of CRISPR/Cas9 by aptamer-functionalized lipopolymer for therapeutic genome editing of VEGFA in osteosarcoma *Biomaterials* **147** 68–85

[66] An Y, Hu Y, Li X, Li Z, Duan J and Yang X D 2019 Selection of a novel DNA aptamer against OFA/iLRP for targeted delivery of doxorubicin to AML cells *Sci. Rep.* **9** 1–11

[67] Tan J *et al* 2016 Aptamer-functionalized fluorescent silica nanoparticles for highly sensitive detection of leukemia cells *Nanoscale Res. Lett.* **11** 1–8

Chapter 12

Applications of nucleic acid aptamers in cancer diagnostics from the laboratory to the clinic

Enamala Manoj Kumar, Supraja Enamala, Rishibha Dixit, S M Faheem, Payal B Joshi and Murthy Chavali

Aptamers are non-coding, short, functional, single-stranded oligonucleotides (RNA or DNA) developed *in vitro* through SELEX technology. Aptamers bind to specific targets with high affinity and are considered good therapeutic agents providing stability and non-immunogenicity. Due to their small size and excellent chemical stability they are also known as 'chemical antibodies', thus widely enabling them in cancer imaging and therapy applications. Aptamers are adaptable and good recognition motifs for cancer biomarker identification due to their chemical production, structural engineering, and site-specific alterations with functional moieties. Cancer protein functions, drug design or screening can be engineered and regulated by designing aptamers. This review summarizes the development of nucleic acid aptamers, cell-SELEX technology, and clinical applications that are significant and can be promising players in cancer research.

12.1 Introduction

Aptamers (from the Latin phrase *aptus* meaning *to fit*) are functional nucleic acids that are selected *in vitro* for binding with target molecules with greater specificity. Usually, aptamers are chemically synthesized single-stranded DNA or RNA oligonucleotides that tend to fold in 3D structural conformations and exhibit binding affinity similar to that observed in antigen–antibody interactions (Ellington and Szostak 1990). Nucleic acid aptamers exhibit enhanced binding affinities and specificity towards a variety of molecular targets such as proteins, small molecules and ionic species. This property of enhanced binding capabilities is hugely exploited in diverse applications of therapeutics, diagnostics, bioinformatics and biotechnology. Aptamers can easily compete with antibody characteristics as the former has greater molecular recognition properties and can be entirely

doi:10.1088/978-0-7503-5012-9ch12

engineered chemically in a test tube or a Petri dish. The easy conjugation and biocompatibility of aptamers make it a promising anti-cancer agent. During treatment of a disease, an aptamer is either employed as an antagonist or as an activator. As an antagonist, the aptamer strongly binds with target proteins thereby disallowing interactions between proteins. As an activator, the aptamer enhances the target protein activity. Aptamers are widely used as drug delivery agents wherein it is combined with a drug molecule either through embedding or loading with nanoparticles.

Aptamers are chemically synthesized using SELEX technology that begins with synthesizing a pool of DNA or RNA oligonucleotides comprising about 100 nucleotides with conserved sequences containing primer binding sites. While selecting RNA aptamers, the T7 RNA polymerase promoter is usually present in the nucleotide sequence. The genesis of combining nucleic acids with proteins came during the emergence of adenovirus and human immunodeficiency virus (HIV). Both adenovirus and HIV consist of short RNA strands that bind to viral proteins with enhanced specificity and affinity.

In 1990, the Gold laboratory and Szostak laboratory individually demonstrated the technique of aptamers. In the Gold laboratory, SELEX technology allowed the selection of RNA ligands against T4 DNA polymerase. Similarly, Szostak's lab performed the RNA ligand selection against different organic dye molecules. Later, Gilead Sciences and the Szostak lab separately worked towards *in vitro* selection to obtain ssDNA ligands for thrombin and various organic dye molecules. There is hardly any difference between the two different nucleic acid aptamers in terms of binding capabilities, though their sequences and folding patterns are different (Ellington & Szostak 1990).

12.2 Properties of aptamers and their types

Aptamers offer a number of benefits over conventional immunological and chemical recognition molecules, including high affinity and specificity, a broad spectrum of activity, small size, good stability, low cost, and ease of synthesis and screening. Aptamers have also demonstrated a wide range of potential applications in the diagnosis and treatment of diseases. Aptamers and monoclonal antibodies (mAbs) share certain commonalities. Both aptamers and mAbs can bind target molecules with great specificity and affinity. Aptamers are referred to as 'chemical antibodies' since they can be applied in medical research, clinical diagnosis, and treatment just like mAbs can. Aptamers don't have immunogenicity or antigenicity, and they don't trigger an immunological reaction or immune rejection like mAbs do. This property makes aptamers reusable for the same patient in the diagnosis and treatment of clinical diseases (Ozalp *et al* 2015).

12.2.1 Advantages of aptamers

To develop targeted therapeutic agents, researchers modify antibodies to detect specific circulating proteins.

While aptamers have certain benefits over antibodies that can help overcome some challenging scientific problems, antibodies are still quite useful for many other applications.

1. Aptamers can be developed against molecules as small as 60 daltons, ten times smaller than the smallest antibody targets
2. Base pair biotechnologies have developed specific selection and characterization techniques for the development of aptamers to small molecules
3. Pursue toxic and non-immunogenic targets
4. Design stable molecular 'sensors' and 'switches'
5. Allosteric aptamers undergo a conformational change upon ligand binding that either alters binding to a second effector or changes the enzymatic activity of the aptamer. Allosteric aptamers can be coupled with fluorescence quenching for direct detection assays, the development of biosensors, or *in vivo* imaging
6. Direct detection eliminates wash steps and simplifies the assay design
7. Penetrate tissues and cells (typically small, ~30–80 nucleotides)—they are very efficient at penetrating tissues to reach specific targets
8. Perform simple chemical modifications—enhance affinity, stability, or solubility through sequence-specific modifications. Functional groups that increase nuclease resistance extend survival time in biofluids
9. Hydrophobic groups can be added to improve binding to hydrophobic targets
10. Superior affinity and specificity
11. Generate enzymatic aptamers
12. Aptazymes have been developed for a growing number of ligands including adenosine triphosphate (ATP), flavin mononucleotide (FMN), cyclic nucleotide monophosphates, and thiamine pyrophosphate (TPP)
13. Combining allosteric properties with selective ligand binding offers significant therapeutic potential
14. Once selected, the production of new batches of material is fast and inexpensive
15. Aptamers with fewer than ~75 bases can be chemically synthesized
16. Aptamers are chemically synthesized, simplifying scale-up and enabling a high degree of manufacturing control from batch to batch
17. Production is easily scalable to multi-gram batches
18. Produce stable products
19. Long-term storage is possible
20. Possible to transport at ambient temperature
21. Can reform to their correct 3D configuration at room temperature
22. Reduce manufacturing time and cost
23. Denaturation at high temperatures is reversible
24. Improve lot-to-lot reproducibility and simplify regulatory procedures
25. Regulatory procedures are reduced as no organisms were involved

Aptamers are single-stranded oligonucleotides that fold into defined architectures and bind to targets such as proteins. In binding proteins, they often inhibit protein–protein interactions and thereby may elicit therapeutic effects such as antagonism.

Aptamers offer significant advantages over antibodies (see table 12.1). They are in general more stable than antibodies and have a longer shelf life. Aptamers are produced through a simple and inexpensive process and the time required to generate aptamers is comparatively short.

The development of artificial molecules known as aptamers allows for the attack of any target, including hazardous or immune-neutralizing ones. They have an affinity for their target that is on par with or higher than antibodies. They are smaller (10 times) than antibodies and are capable of exact chemical manipulation. They can be reversibly heat denatured and are easy to deliver and store. The source is secured by a high level of batch-to-batch repeatability. They can be applied for analytical reasons in non-physiological settings. They can be employed *in vivo* and are non-immunogenic.

Depending on the aptamer or the target biomarker, some minor adjustments to the current IHC protocols might be required, but in the end, aptamers can replace traditional antibodies in these applications with very little additional capital investment, resources/reagents, or staff training needed.

Table 12.1. Comparison of monoclonal antibody and aptamer.

	Monoclonal antibody	Aptamer
Stability	Antibodies must be refrigerated since they are temperature-sensitive. The denaturation cannot be reversed.	Aptamers have a longer shelf life since they are stable at room temperature. Denaturation can be reversed
Size	Large molecules (~160 kDa), resist filtration by the kidneys	Small compounds, that exhibit improved target access
Development process	The immune response is needed and animals are required	Greater affinity, and increased specificity. For selection, only a few nanomoles are needed. A wide variety of molecules are screened.
Target potential	Targets must produce an immune response	Can bind to harmful, non-immunogenic, toxictargets.
Production time and cost	In several months Long and expensive *in vivo* techniques are needed for antibody synthesis.	The chosen aptamers are chemically synthesized in a few weeks, lowering the cost of production.

12.2.2 Chemical structure of aptamers

The negatively charged backbone connections of aptamers cause them to engage with positively charged protein surfaces (figure 12.1).

On observing the crystal structure of the aptamer-target protein complex, electrostatic interactions are the most common binding forces. Thrombin binds with aptamers through a negatively charged surface which is naturally wanted for the binding of heparin (Long *et al* 2008).

The conformational variety and targeted specificity of RNA aptamers are important aspects of employing them in therapy. Aptamers are excellent protein–protein interaction inhibitors for cancer therapy due to their dual properties. An ideal aptamer must be stable in the human body to function as a therapeutic agent. Since it is well known that endogenous nucleases can damage nucleic acids, changes to sugar and phosphodiester links must be taken into account. Truncation of the nucleotides is a necessary step to both minimise overall therapeutic costs and lessen toxicity. A good pharmacokinetic profile is also required for therapeutic aptamers, as seen in the case of other anti-cancer medicinal compounds.

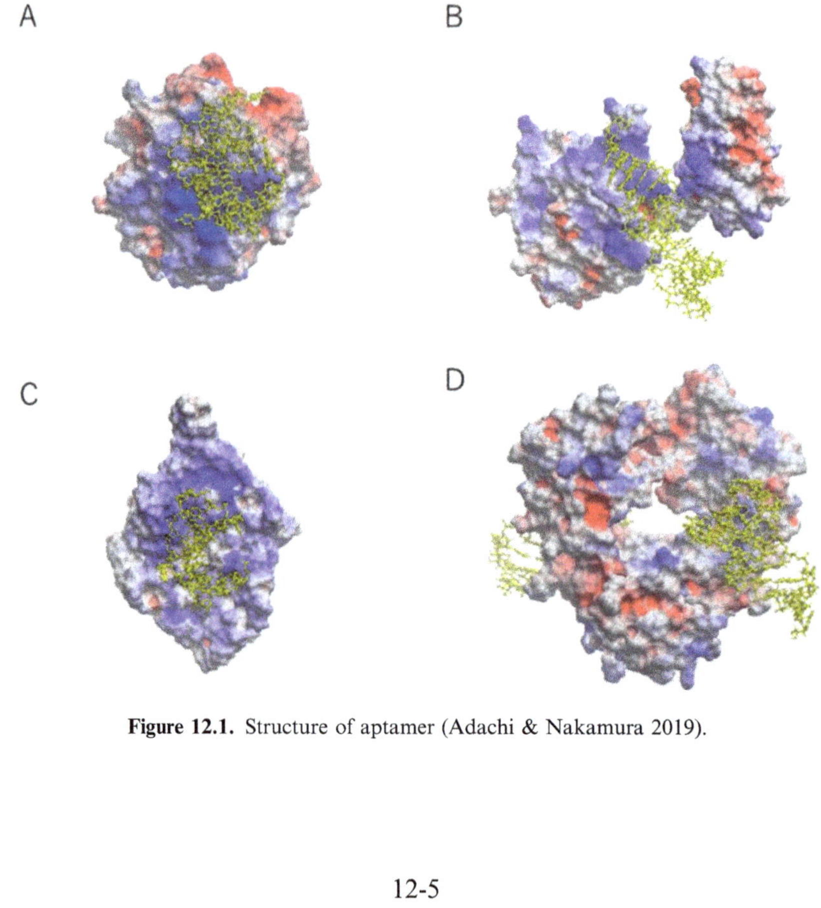

Figure 12.1. Structure of aptamer (Adachi & Nakamura 2019).

12.3 Development of nucleic acid aptamers

DNA or RNA oligonucleotides bind to their target with high affinity and specificity and can be selected due to their ability to adapt three-dimensional shapes in solution. They have structured sequence-specific ssDNA or RNA aptamers. Recently, nucleic acid-based therapy is significant in therapeutic applications. Various approaches based on the nucleic acid active component such as ribozymes, si-RNA, miRNA, antisense and aptamers can be used (Opalinska and Gewirtz 2002). To improve the aptamer stability and function we can develop nucleic acid aptamers that are modified chemically on the sugar backbone.

The nucleic acid modifications help in achieving pharmacokinetic properties of selected aptamers towards the ligands chosen chemically modified on the sugar backbone (Santosh and Yadava 2014). The various aptamers that can be generated against various targets are metal ions, organic dyes, amino acids, drugs, cofactors, aminoglycosides, nucleotides, peptides, base analogs, enzymes, growth factors, immunoglobulins, gene regulatory factors, surface receptors, several antibiotics. Aptamers can be selected against targets such as viral particles, pathogenic bacteria and whole cancer cells (Derbyshire *et al* 2012). From a large set of libraries, nucleic acid aptamers are isolated by the Systematic Evolution of Ligands by the Exponential Enrichment (SELEX) procedure. Applications of aptamers are represented in figure 12.2.

12.3.1 RNA mediated therapy

Unique RNA folds from a library of RNAs are identified by *in vitro* selection and amplification methodologies that can eventually target any target ligands with good affinities in a range of micromolar and nanomolar scales. Numerous examples of RNA aptamers can target antibiotics, co-factors, proteins, peptides, saccharides, nucleotides, and amino acids. RNA aptamers contribute to catalytic activity

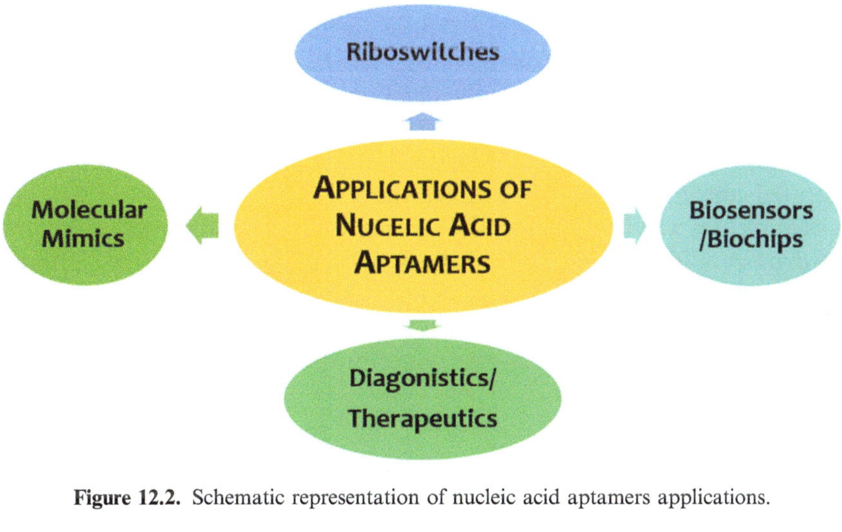

Figure 12.2. Schematic representation of nucleic acid aptamers applications.

(Ellington and Szostak 1990). The structure of RNA-aptamer (50 nucleotides in length) complexes is studied using NMR techniques. NMR-based hydrogen measurements resolve imino protons, which define the individual base and its mismatched pairings. A literature survey has reported the conjugation of RNA aptamer with flavins mononucleotide, AMP, L-citrulline, arginine, tobramycin, and HIV-1Rev peptide.

The aptamer identifies the nucleic acid binding site and occupies and mimics the natural interactions. Literature studies have reported examples of such RNA-aptamer bindings as observed in the crystal structure of human thrombin, binding to dye xanthene tetramethylrhodamine, pro-inflammatory chemokine L-CLL2 (monocyte chemoattractant protein-1) (Duchardt-Ferner *et al* 2020). Artificial RNA creates an RNA aptamer library which is generated with high affinity and selectivity through the pooling of random sequences. Through this RNA aptamer's understanding of RNA-ligand interaction, structural complexity and ligand affinity, specificity, RNA structure, and RNA folding, different random sequences are flanked to start with SELEX technology. Amplification of different sequences is done by polymerase chain reaction (PCR). 20-nucleotide long primers are usually used for PCR. For designing and developing RNA aptamers a promoter sequence of T7 RNA polymerase is required at the 5′ end of the PCR template sequence within the template design (Duchardt-Ferner *et al* 2020).

12.3.2 DNA-mediated therapy

G-quadruplexes are four-stranded DNA structures with four planar arrays of guanines in which each guanine pairs with Hoogsteen bonding (Patel *et al* 1997). Due to their unique architecture, they are promoted for drug design and aptamer development, and can be envisaged to differentiate with cationic proteins or small molecules (Dai *et al* 2007). Due to the G-quadruplex having a higher electrostatic potential per unit length, G4s can be used as DNA aptamers. RNA-based G4s are also considered to participate in mRNA turnover, translation interference in eukaryotic cells, and FMRP binding. There are literature studies on the structure of a complex between human α-thrombin and a 15-nucleotide aptamer. In the crystal structure, the G4 is sandwiched between two thrombin molecules (Padmanabhan *et al* 1993). Other such examples are guanosine-rich oligodeoxyribonucleotides (GROs) inhibiting the proliferation of human tumor cell lines. It was demonstrated through several methods that a G-rich oligonucleotide (GROs) known as nucleolin was identified in G4 structures. GROs (aptamers) are considered effective drug candidates (Xu *et al* 2001). As DNA-based aptamers exhibit high G contents they are amenable to G4 folding. In *in vitro* analysis d (GGGGTGGGAGGAGGGT) (*93del*) forms an aptamer that exhibits anti-HIV1 integrase activity *in vitro* in nanomolar concentrations (Chou *et al* 2005, Phan *et al* 2005).

12.4 Principle and designing of systematic evolution of ligands by exponential enrichment (SELEX)

12.4.1 The SELEX method

Tuerk and Gold (1990) created the procedure of Systematic Evolution of Ligands by Exponential Enrichment (SELEX). In this technique, the *in vitro* selection of nucleic acids was done based on the catalytic activity or affinity of the target. From the nucleic acid libraries with diversities of 10^{15} different molecules, secondary and tertiary structures were designed. Oligonucleotides for SELEX consist of a randomized region (15–75 bases) and conserved regions designed for primer binding sites during reverse transcription and PCR amplification. A T7 promoter site was used as a conserved region and *in vitro* transcription with T7-RNA polymerase on dsDNA was used as a template for designing a library of different sequences with 3D structures. The RNA molecules are initially pooled, purified and folded and then mixed with target molecules to be eluted by the phenol/chloroform method. The chosen RNA molecules are amplified by RT-PCR and a next-generation DNA pool has to be produced. For the next selection of the cycle *in vitro* transcription of the newly formed DNA pool provides the RNA pool. The RNA molecules are purified in the final pool, reverse-transcribed to DNA and cloned. The isolated clones are then identified by DNA sequencing (figure 12.3) representation (Ulrich 2006). The SELEX protocol is significant as it decreases the pool size of the library to the small number of binding partners (Santosh and Yadava 2014).

12.4.2 Modified SELEX method

The improved modifications, stability, affinity, or specificity in the SELEX method were developed in 1990. The modified process consists of automated SELEX, photo SELEX, toggle-SELEX, mirror-image and intramers. Parallel processes and selection cycles with automated aptamer selection to target multiple targets are used. Automated aptamers are coupled to an *in vitro* translation system for the target protein (White *et al* 2001). A list of aptamers specific for various ligands is presented in table 12.2.

12.5 Nucleic acid aptamers used in cancer diagnostics

12.5.1 Aptamers used for breast cancer

There are several specific aptamers developed for tumor treatment of various kinds of cancer, like breast cancer. The aptamers used for breast cancer targeting are enlisted in table 12.3.

12.5.2 Aptamers used for colorectal cancer

Among 10%–15% of all cancers, colorectal cancer (CRC) is the third most common cancer worldwide. It is considered a heterogeneous complex of diseases. Carcinoembryonic antigen (CEA) is used extensively to determine prognosis and monitor disease progression (Ogino and Goel 2008). For selective molecular

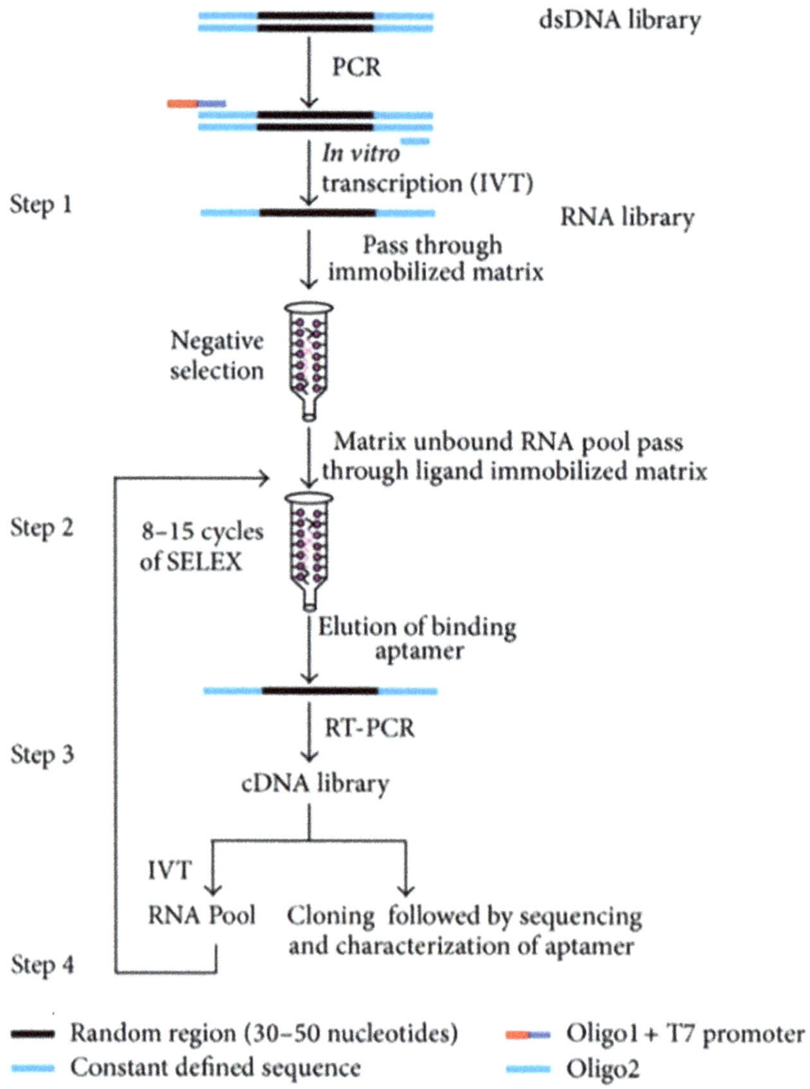

Figure 12.3. SELEX Technology with schematic representation using RNA Library (Santosh & Yadava 2014).

markers for CRC, we can specifically select cell-based aptamers that can potentially help in a short time (table 12.4). It is observed that in cancer mostly carcinoembryonic antigens such as CEA, CEACAM5, or CD66e are overexpressed, inducing tumor metastasis (Hammarström 1999, Taheri *et al* 2000). Due to liver metastasis death mostly occurs in colorectal cancer patients. Thus, the survival rate of patients can be increased if we effectively treat liver metastasis.

In literature, it was observed that induction of apoptosis causes the blocking between death receptor 5 and CEA. *In vitro* experiments on mice demonstrated that the

Table 12.2. A list of aptamers generated against various ligands (Santosh and Yadava 2014).

Nature	Ligand/target	Aptamer name	Disease	References
RNA	AFP (fetal protein)	AFP aptamer	Hepatocellular carcinoma	Lee and Lee (2012)
	RIG1 (1–925aa)	RNA aptamer	Antiviral activity via modulating IFNα/β production	Hwang *et al* (2012)
	Rev peptide	RNA aptamer	HIV	Xu and Ellington (1996)
	V3 loop of gp120, HIV-1RT	RNA aptamer S66A-C6 RNA aptamer S69A-C15	HIV	Gronewold *et al* (2009)
	Glycoprotein 120 (gp120)	Anti-gp120 aptamer chimaera	HIV	Zhou *et al* (2008)
	Glutathione	Class III GSH aptamer 8.17	Breast cancer (human breast adenocarcinoma cell line, MCF-7)	Bala *et al* (2011)
	MDA (4,4′-methylenedianiline)	MDA aptamer M1	Carcinogenic and DNA-damaging agents	Brockstedt *et al* (2004)
	Acetylcholine receptor (AChR)	Class I and Class II AChR aptamer	Neuromuscular disorder	Ulrich *et al* (1998)
	Beta-Secretase BACE1 (B1-CT)	RNAapt TH14	Alzheimer's disease	Rentmeister *et al* (2006)
	Erythrocyte membrane protein 1 (PfEMP1)	DBL1α-specific RNA aptamer Erythrocyte membrane protein 1 (PfEMP1) 33 inhibitory conc. Malaria 2-F RNA and 2-NH2 aptamer	Malaria	Barfod *et al* (2009)
	L-selectin	RNA aptamer	Inflammation	Codnnell *et al* (1996)
	NF-kB p50 homodimer	RNA aptamer	Cancer and inflammation	Huang *et al* (2003)
	Prostate-specific membrane antigen	Anti-PSMA chimaera	Prostate cancer	McNamara *et al* (2006)
	T-cell factor 1	Aptamer no. 5	Colon cancer	Lee *et al* (2005)
	Tenascin-C	TTA1	Breast cancer, Glioblastoma	—
	TGFβ type III receptor	RNA aptamer	Ovarian cancer	—
	WT1	RNA aptamer 22	Wilm's tumor	—
	VEGF 165 (vascular endothelial growth factor 165)	Pegaptanib sodium, NX1838	Age-related macular degeneration	—
	β-Catenin	RNA aptamer	Colon cancer	—
	K Ras-derived peptide	RNA aptamer G4	Oncogenic protein	—
	Amyloid β-peptide A4 (1–40)	RNA aptamer	Alzheimer's disease	—

Table 12.3. Representation of the known breast cancer aptamers and their available targets (Li *et al* 2021, Varty *et al* 2021).

Type of Cancer	Aptamers	Targets	Cell Lines	Clinical Applications	References
Breast cancer	HeA2–3 ApMNK2F ApMNK3R PNDA-3 ERaptD4 EpDT3 5TR1 S2.2 Vap7 V7t1 RNV66 Pegaptanib ARC247 SYL3 EpDT3 EpApt-siEp Clone 2 Clone 4 Clone 5	HER2 MNK Periostin Alpha estrogen receptor EpCAM Mucin 1 Vascular endothelial growth factor Epithelial cell adhesion molecule Cancer antigen 15–3	MDA-MB-231 cell, SKBR3, MCF7, MDA-MB-231, MDA-MB-231, SKOV3 cell	None	Gijs *et al* (2016) García-Recio *et al* (2016) Lee *et al* (2013) Paterni *et al* (2014) Cimino *et al* (2009) Ferreira *et al* (2007) Konecny *et al* (2004) Song *et al* (2013) Liu *et al* (2017)

Table 12.4. Representation of the known colorectal cancer aptamers and their available targets.

Cancer	Aptamers	Targets	Cell lines	References
Colorectal cancer	YJ-1 Aptamer MP7 KC2D3 KC2D4 KC2D8 KCHA10 KCHB10	CEA PDGF-BB PD-1 Cell	LS174T, SW480 cell Caco-2, SW480 cell MC38 cell DLD-1 HCT 116	Lee *et al* (2012) Sae-Lim *et al* (2019) Prodeus *et al* (2015) Sefah *et al* (2010)

transfer of human colon cancer cells to the liver was prevented by YJ-1 (Lee *et al* 2012). Using cell-SELEX technology, we can selectively target specific aptamers which can be used on colorectal cancer-cultured cell lines DLD-1 and HCT 116. The above table represents the aptamers that can be used for the selective treatment of CRC.

12.5.3 Aptamers used for lung cancer

Lung cancers are prevalent and it is observed that 85% of lung cancer patients are identified as non-small cell lung cancer (NSCLC). NSCLC can be classified as adenocarcinoma, squamous cell carcinoma, and large cell carcinoma (Alipoor *et al* 2018, Qin *et al* 2020). Genetic abnormalities are the main cause of NSCLC initiation. Such types of genes are TP53, KRAS, EGFR, ALK, ROS1, BRAF, NRAS, RET, MET, etc, genes (Inamura 2017, Smolle *et al* 2020). DNA aptamers such as apMAFG6F, apMAFG11F, and ApMAFG3F are specific to musculoaponeurotic fibrosarcoma oncogene family protein *(MAFG)*, which is engaged in chemoresistance in NSCLC and breast tumors MSAFG causes downregulation of reactive oxygen species (ROS) in the cell (Vera-Puente *et al* 2018). Aptamer AS1411 has a G-quadruplex structure responsible for the stimulation of promoter regions of various genes (e.g. c-MYC, VEGF, HIF-1_, BCL-2, K-RAS, PDGF-A, and PDGF-R_). Further, it is also involved in telomerase shortening. The aptamer binds specifically to nucleolin, a phosphoprotein highly expressed on the cell surface of different cancer sub-types (Sengupta *et al* 2019, Yang 2019). MA3 is a DNA aptamer that is used to deliver doxorubicin to lung adenocarcinoma cell line A549 and MCF-7 breast cancer cells. Osteopontins are a group of cytokines that are expressed along with integrins $\alpha v\beta 3$, PIM-3 and the stage of lung cancer (Hunter *et al* 2012).

A-P50 is an RNA aptamer with a high affinity to the NF-κB p50 subunit. It blocks DNA replication (Jin *et al* 2014). Aptamer-specific ARC126/AX102 binds to the B subunit of platelet-derived growth factor (PDGFB) on pericytes. Studies confirmed the anti-angiogenic effect of ARC126/AX102 in lung cancer (Zhou *et al* 2016). The S15 aptamer is a Cy5-labeled 85-nucleotide DNA aptamer synthesized commercially. S15-APT-PEG-PCL nanoparticle whose core consists of polycaprolactone (PCL) conjugated with hydrophilic polyethene glycol (PEG) and treated with 30 nM of S15-aptamers. After endocytosis, PTX-loaded S15-APT-PEG-PCL NPs perform enzymatic lysis and the drug paclitaxel is secreted inside the NSCLC cell (Engelberg *et al* 2019). NOX-A12 is an L-RNA aptamer involved in tumor metastasis. Two strategies can be developed for anti-NSCLC aptamers: (i) *in vivo* selection specific to cancer cell types and (ii) selection based on known molecules.

12.5.4 Aptamers used for liver cancer cells

Hepatocellular carcinoma is considered one of the most common yet deadly forms of cancer. The concern of hepatocellular carcinoma lies in the late detection of tumors leading to hindrances in medical treatment to the patient. Tumor markers are employed to solve this major concern in the treatment of carcinoma. Tumor markers are those substances produced by the cancer cells in larger amounts that are found in the patient's urine, stool, blood and tissue samples. Exploiting the superior affinity and specificity of aptamers, they are been considered an ideal candidate for tumor markers and utilized as *in vitro* and *in vivo* probe nanomedicine in liver cancer therapy. Hu *et al* developed an efficient method to label hepatoma cells with aptamers and detection utilizing fluorescent silica nanoparticles. They demonstrated the efficacy of biotin-conjugated TLS11a aptamer (Bio-TLS11a) in hepatoma cells (Hu *et al* 2012). Zhou *et al* described two different types of aptamers that effectively recognized DKK1, which is a biomarker for detecting early-stage liver carcinoma. They utilized slow-off and fast-off aptamers and it was found that slow-off aptamers were suitable for ELISA assay whereas the fast-off aptamer was ideal for blotting and flow cytometry. The authors reported the quantitative data of sixty sera samples and the results revealed that a novel aptamer could be a potential candidate for *in vitro* diagnosis of hepatocellular carcinoma (Zhou *et al* 2019). Yi *et al* reported an AB3 aptamer that was functionalized comprising of a 59-base DNA oligonucleotide sequence to deliver doxorubicin to acute myeloid leukemia cancer cells.

12.5.5 Aptamers against prostate cancer cells

Next to lung cancer, prostate cancer is a commonly reported malignancy among men. With a mortality rate of 3.8% annually, the risk factors for prostate cancer include age, patient history, genetic factors, and ethnicity. It is reported that the rate of prostate cancer is higher in African-American men compared to Caucasian men. At present, diagnosis of prostate cancer involves assessing a serum prostate-specific antigen (PSA); serine protease, also called KLK3. The serine protease is secreted by prostatic epithelium cells in response to prostate cancer, old age, ejaculation and even hormonal therapy. These measurements exhibit a false positive leading to additional diagnostic tests and unnecessary treatment. Gray *et al* (2018) demonstrated the use of E3 RNA selectively that internalizes into prostate cancer cells. Further, they reported that E3-highly toxic drug conjugates are potent anti-cancer agents. Argoubi *et al* (2018) demonstrated a novel label-free electrochemical aptasensing technique for detecting prostate cancer. It exhibited the highest sensitivity, repeatability, specificity, and storage stability for PSA and was also authenticated in the spiked artificial urine and blood serum samples from a healthy male volunteer (Argoubi *et al* 2018). It is an important key to use by combining biocompatible organic macromolecules to increase system sensitivity and stability in the realm of developing immunosensors. Sun *et al* (2019) developed a dual detection fluorescence biosensor fabricated of mesoporous silica nanoparticles (MSNs) and loaded with CdTe quantum dots for the rapid detection of prostate-specific antigens. (Sun *et al* 2019) reported an ultrasensitive fluorescence assay for detecting PSA by the combined use of CdTe QDs and aptamer-PAMAM-AuNPs that demonstrated enhanced sensitivity for trace levels of antigen. A dual aptasensor was designed based on the premise of a guanine chemiluminescence reaction that was employed for the early detection of prostate cancer. The aptasensor could simultaneously quantify PSA and vascular endothelial growth factor (VEGF) in the patient's sample with reproducibility. Some applications of aptamers in the diagnosis and treatment of PCa are shown in figure 12.4.

12.5.6 Aptamers used for cervical cancer cells

As men suffer from prostate cancer, most women are prone to cervical cancer. Not only women are prone to cervical cancer, but their reproductive system may also

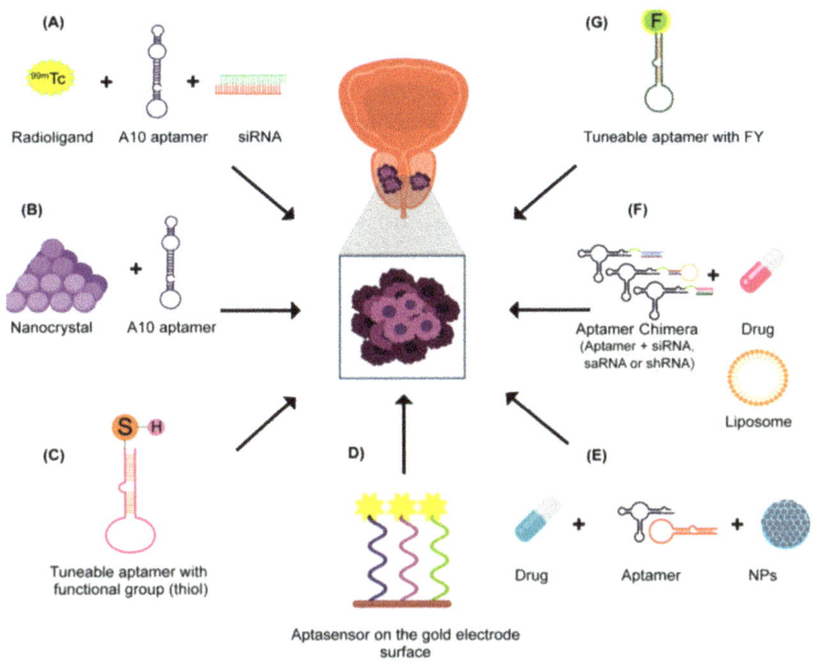

Figure 12.4. Scheme depicting some applications of aptamers in the diagnosis and treatment of PCa (Cruz-Hernández *et al* 2022).

predominantly get affected by ovarian cancer (Lengyel 2010) vaginal cancer, fallopian tube cancer, and vulvar cancer. Routinely, cervical cancer can be diagnosed and detected with cervical intraepithelial neoplasia (CIN) and Pap smear methods. (Ma *et al* 2019) produced an RNA aptamer against the HPV-16 virus, and in particular, the selected aptamers are more specific to HPV E7 oncoprotein (Toscano-Garibay *et al* 2011). Carvalho *et al* (2019) evaluated AT11-L0 G4 as a supramolecular carrier for the delivery of acridine ligands C3, C5 and C8 to HeLa cervical cancer cells.

12.6 Conclusions and future prospects of aptamers in cancer diagnosis

Small single-stranded DNA or RNA oligonucleotides known as aptamers have a three-dimensional structure that allows for target binding and selectivity. Aptamers have a special three-dimensional structure that allows them to bind to the target epitopes with a high level of specificity that bigger antibodies cannot. Because of these benefits, aptamers may one day be used for targeted delivery, cancer immunotherapy, and efficient treatment of bacterial and viral diseases. Aptamers are therefore essential for the delivery of drug-loaded nanoparticles in future personalized therapies. Additionally, after connecting to cellular receptors or other components, many aptamers aid in internalizing the cells. It may provide new opportunities for improving the drug delivery system's pharmacokinetic profile and target specificity. We now lack *in vivo* investigations, but we anticipate that the recent approval of aptamer-based medication and ongoing clinical trials will lead to new opportunities.

Aptamer technology is developing, in contrast to antibodies, which need more work to ensure their widespread adoption. Recognition of tiny molecule targets or targets that are harmful to cells should be prioritized. The application of high-throughput next-generation sequencing and reliable nucleic acid chemistry would have a significant and long-lasting impact on the aptamer field. Depending on the aptamer or the target biomarker, some minor adjustments to the current IHC protocols might be required, but in the end, aptamers can replace traditional antibodies in these applications with very little additional capital investment, resources/reagents, or staff training needed.

Successful use of aptamers includes the identification of pathogens, cancer, the detection of environmental contaminants, and stem cell markers. When a condition is acute, aptamers can be a financially viable diagnostic option for identifying viral antigens quickly after infection and for tracking illness development while receiving therapy.

Funding

This research received no external funding.

Conflicts of interest

The authors declare no conflict of interest.

References

Adachi T and Nakamura Y 2019 Aptamers: a review of their chemical properties and modifications for therapeutic application *Molecules* **24** 4229

Alipoor S D, Mortaz E, Varahram M, Movassaghi M, Kraneveld A D, Garssen J and Adcock I M 2018 The potential biomarkers and immunological effects of tumour-derived exosomes in lung cancer *Front. Immunol.* **9** 819

Argoubi W, Sánchez A, Parrado C, Raouafi N and Villalonga R 2018 Label-free electrochemical aptasensing platform based on mesoporous silica thin film for the detection of prostate-specific antigen *Sensors Actuators* B **255** 309–15

Bala J, Bhaskar A, Varshney A, Singh A K, Dey S and Yadava P 2011 *In vitro* selected RNA aptamer recognizing glutathione induces ROS-mediated apoptosis in the human breast cancer cell line MCF 7 *RNA Biology* **8** 101–11

Barfod A, Persson T and Lindh J 2009 In vitro selection of RNA aptamers against a conserved region of the *Plasmodium falciparum* erythrocyte membrane protein 1 *Parasitol. Res.* **105** 1557–66

Brockstedt U, Uzarowska A, Montpetit A, Pfau W and Labuda D 2004 *In vitro* evolution of RNA aptamers recognizing carcinogenic aromatic amines *Biochem. Biophys. Res. Commun.* **313** 1004–8

Carvalho J, Lopes-Nunes J, Lopes A C, Campello M P C, Paulo A, Queiroz J A and Cruz C 2019 Aptamer-guided acridine derivatives for cervical cancer *Org. Biomol. Chem.* **17** 2992–3002

Chou S H, Chin K H and Wang A H 2005 DNA aptamers as potential anti-HIV agents *Trends Biochem. Sci.* **30** 231–4

Cimino A, Halushka M, Illei P, Wu X, Sukumar S and Argani P 2009 Epithelial cell adhesion molecule (EpCAM) is overexpressed in breast cancer metastases *Breast Cancer Res. Treat.* **123** 701–8

Codnnell D O *et al* 1996 Calcium-dependent oligonucleotide antagonists specific for L-selectin *Proc. Natl Acad. Sci.* **93** 5883–7

Cruz-Hernández C D *et al* 2022 Aptamers as theragnostic tools in prostate cancer *Biomolecules* **12** 1056

Dai J, Carver M, Punchihewa C, Jones R A and Yang D 2007 Structure of the Hybrid-2 type intramolecular human telomeric G quadruplex in K+ solution: insights into structure polymorphism of the human telomeric sequence *Nucleic Acids Res.* **35** 4927–40

Derbyshire N, White S J, Bunka D H, Song L, Stead S, Tarbin J, Sharman M, Zhou D and Stockley P G 2012 Toggled RNA aptamers against aminoglycosides allowing facile detection of antibiotics using gold nanoparticle assays *Anal. Chem.* **84** 6595–602

Duchardt-Ferner E, Juen M, Bourgeois B, Madl T, Kreutz C, Ohlenschläger O and Wöhnert J 2020 Structure of an RNA aptamer in complex with the fluorophore tetramethylrhodamine *Nucleic Acids Res.* **48** 949–61

Ellington A D and Szostak J W 1990 In vitro selection of RNA molecules that bind specific ligands *Nature* **346** 818–22

Engelberg S, Netzer E, Assaraf Y G and Livney Y D 2019 Selective eradication of human non-small cell lung cancer cells using aptamer-decorated nanoparticles harbouring a cytotoxic drug cargo. *Cell Death Dis.* **10** 702

Ferreira C S M, Papamichael K, Guilbault G, Schwarzacher T, Gariepy J and Missailidis S 2007 DNA aptamers against the MUC1 tumour marker: design of aptamer–antibody sandwich ELISA for the early diagnosis of epithelial tumours *Anal. Bioanal. Chem.* **390** 1039–50

García-Recio E M, Pinto-Díez C, Pérez-Morgado M I, García-Hernández M, Fernández G and Martín M E *et al* 2016 Characterization of MNK1b DNA aptamers that inhibit proliferation in MDA-MB231 breast cancer cells *Mole. Ther. Nucleic Acids* **5** e275

Gijs M, Penner G, Blackler G B, Impens N R, Baatout S, Luxen A and Aerts A 2016 Improved aptamers for the diagnosis and potential treatment of HER2-positive cancer *Pharmaceuticals* **9** 29

Gray B, Kelly L, Ahrens D P, Barry A P, Kratschmer C, Levy M and Sullenger B A 2018 Tunable cytotoxic aptamer-drug conjugates for the treatment of prostate cancer *Proc. Natl Acad. Sci.* **115** 4761–6

Gronewold T M A, Baumgartner A and Hierer J *et al* 2009 Kinetic binding analysis of aptamers targeting HIV-1 proteins by a combination of a microbalance array and mass spectrometry (MAMS) *J. Proteome Res.* **8** 3568–77

Hammarström S 1999 The carcinoembryonic antigen (CEA) family: structures, suggested functions and expression in normal and malignant tissues *Semin. Cancer Biol.* **9** 67–81

Hu Y, Duan J, Zhan Q, Wang F, Lu X and Yang X D 2012 Novel MUC1 aptamer selectively delivers cytotoxic agents to cancer cells *in vitro PLoS One* **7** e31970

Huang D B, Vu D, Cassiday L A, Zimmerman J M, Maher III L J and Ghosh G 2003 Crystal structure of NF-B $(p50)_2$ complexed to a high-affinity RNA aptamer *Proc. Natl Acad. Sci.* **100** 9268–73

Hunter C, Bond J, Kuo P C, Selim M A and Levinson H 2012 The role of osteopontin and osteopontin aptamer (OPN-R3) in fibroblast activity *J. Surg. Res.* **176** 348–58

Hwang S Y, Sun H Y and Lee K H *et al* 2012 5′-Triphosphate-RNA-independent activation of RIG-I via RNA aptamer with enhanced antiviral activity *Nucleic Acids Res.* **40** 2724–33

Inamura K 2017 Lung cancer: understanding its molecular pathology and the 2015 WHO Classification *Front. Oncol.* **7** 193

Jin J, Ryu H S, Lee K B and Jang J J 2014 High expression of protein tyrosine kinase 7 significantly associates with invasiveness and poor prognosis in intrahepatic cholangiocarcinoma *PLoS One* **9** e90247

Konecny G E, Meng Y G, Untch M, Wang H J, Bauerfeind I, Epstein M, Stieber P, Vernes J M, Gutierrez J and Hong K *et al* 2004 Association between HER-2/neu and vascular endothelial growth factor expression predicts clinical outcome in primary breast cancer patients *Clin. Cancer Res.* **10** 1706–16

Lee Y J, Han S R, Kim N Y, Lee S H, Jeong J S and Lee S W 2012 An RNA aptamer that binds carcinoembryonic antigen inhibits hepatic metastasis of colon cancer cells in mice *Gastroenterology* **143** 155–65

Lee Y J, Kim I S, Park S A, Kim Y, Lee J E and Noh D Y *et al* 2013 Periostin-binding DNA aptamer inhibits breast cancer growth and metastasis *Mole. Ther.* **21** 1004–13

Lee Y J and Lee S W 2012 Regression of hepatocarcinoma cells using RNA aptamer specific to alpha-fetoprotein *Biochem. Biophys. Res. Commun.* **417** 521–7

Lee S K, Park M W, Yang E G, Yu J and Jeong S 2005 An RNA aptamer that binds to the β-catenin interaction domain of TCF-1 protein *Biochem. Biophys. Res. Commun.* **327** 294–9

Lengyel E 2010 Ovarian cancer development and metastasis *Am. J. Pathol.* **177** 1053–64

Li Z, Fu X, Huang J, Zeng P, Huang Y, Chen X and Liang C 2021 Advances in screening and development of therapeutic aptamers against cancer cells *Front. Cell Dev. Biol.* **9** 662791

Liu M, Yu X, Chen Z, Yang T, Yang D, Liu Q, Du K, Li B, Wang Z and Li S *et al* 2017 Aptamer selection and applications for breast cancer diagnostics and therapy *J. Nanobiotechnol.* **15** 81

Long S B *et al* 2008 Crystal structure of an RNA aptamer bound to thrombin *RNA (New York, N.Y.)* **14** 2504–12

Long S B, Long M B, White R R and Sullenger B A 2008 Crystal structure of an RNA aptamer bound to thrombin *RNA* **14** 2504–12

Ma X, Lakshmipriya T and Gopinath S C 2019 Recent advances in identifying biomarkers and high-affinity aptamers for gynecologic cancers diagnosis and therapy *J. Anal. Methods Chem.* **2019** 1–9

McNamara J O, Andrechek I I E R and Wang Y *et al* 2006 Cell type-specific delivery of siRNAs with aptamer-siRNA chimeras *Nat. Biotechnol.* **24** 1005–15

Ogino S and Goel A 2008 Molecular classification and correlates in colorectal cancer *J. Mol. Diagn.* **10** 13–27

Opalinska J B and Gewirtz A M 2002 Nucleic-acid therapeutics: basic principles and recent applications *Nat. Rev. Drug. Discov.* **1** 503–14

Ozalp V C, Kavruk M, Dilek O and Bayrac A T 2015 Aptamers: molecular tools for medical diagnosis *Curr. Top. Med. Chem.* **15** 1125–37

Padmanabhan K, Padmanabhan K P, Ferrara J D, Sadler J E and Tulinsky A 1993 The structure of alpha-thrombin is inhibited by a 15-mer single-stranded DNA aptamer *J. Biol. Chem.* **268** 17651–4

Patel D J, Suri A K, Jiang F, Jiang L, Fan P, Kumar R A and Nonin S 1997 Structure, recognition and adaptive binding in RNA aptamer complexes *J. Mol. Biol.* **272** 645–64

Paterni I, Granchi C, Katzenellenbogen J A and Minutolo F 2014 Estrogen receptors alpha (ER_) and beta (ER_): subtype-selective ligands and clinical potential *Steroids* **90** 13–29

Phan A T, Kuryavyi V, Ma J B, Faure A, Andreola M L and Patel D J 2005 An interlocked dimeric parallel-stranded DNA quadruplex: a potent inhibitor of HIV-1 integrase *Proc. Natl Acad. Sci. USA* **102** 634–9

Prodeus A, Abdul-Wahid A, Fischer N W, Huang E H, Cydzik M and Gariépy J 2015 Targeting the PD-1/PD-L1 immune evasion axis with DNA aptamers as a novel therapeutic strategy for the treatment of disseminated cancers *Mol. Ther. Nucleic Acids* **4** e237

Qin S, Yi M, Jiao D, Li A and Wu K 2020 Distinct roles of VEGFA and ANGPT2 in lung adenocarcinoma and squamous cell carcinoma *J. Cancer* **11** 153–67

Rentmeister A, Bill A, Wahle T, Walter J and Famulok M 2006 RNA aptamers selectively modulate protein recruitment to the cytoplasmic domain of β-secretase BACE1 *in vitro RNA* **12** 1650–60

Sae-Lim S, Soontornworajit B and Pichayanoot P 2019 Inhibition of colorectal cancer cell proliferation by regulating platelet-derived growth Factor B signaling with a DNA aptamer *Asian Pac. J. Cancer Prev. APJCP* **20** 487

Santosh B and Yadava P K 2014 Nucleic acid aptamers: research tools in disease diagnostics and therapeutics *BioMed Res. Int.* **2014** 540451

Sefah K, Meng L, Lopez-Colon D, Jimenez E and Liu C *et al* 2010 DNA Aptamers as molecular probes for colorectal cancer study *PLoS One* **5** e14269

Sengupta A, Ganguly A and Chowdhury S 2019 Promise of G-quadruplex structure binding ligands as epigenetic modifiers with anti-cancer effects *Molecules* **24** 582

Smolle E, Leithner K and Olschewski H 2020 Oncogene addiction and tumor mutational burden in non-small-cell lung cancer: clinical significance and limitations *Thorac. Cancer* **11** 205–15

Song Y, Zhu Z, An Y, Zhang W, Zhang H, Liu D, Yu C, Duan W and Yang C J 2013 Selection of DNA aptamers against epithelial cell adhesion molecule for cancer cell imaging and circulating tumor cell capture *Anal. Chem.* **85** 4141–9

Suk J S *et al* 2016 PEGylation as a strategy for improving nanoparticle-based drug and gene delivery *Adv. Drug Del. Rev.* **99** 28–51

Sun D, Luo Z, Lu J, Zhang S, Che T, Chen Z and Zhang L 2019 Electrochemical dual-aptamer-based biosensor for nonenzymatic detection of cardiac troponin I by nanohybrid electrocatalysts labeling combined with DNA nanotetrahedron structure *Biosens. Bioelectron.* **134** 49–56

Taheri M, Saragovi U, Fuks A, Makkerh J, Mort J and Stanners C P 2000 Self-recognition in the Ig superfamily: identification of precise subdomains in CEA required for intercellular adhesion *J. Biol. Chem.* **275** 26935–43

Toscano-Garibay J D, Benítez-Hess M L and Alvarez-Salas L M 2011 Isolation and characterization of an RNA aptamer for the HPV-16 E7 oncoprotein *Arch. Med. Res.* **42** 88–96

Tuerk C and Gold L 1990 Systemic evolution of ligands by exponential enrichment: RNA ligands to bacteriophage T4 DNA polymerase *Science* **249** 505–10

Ulrich H 2006 RNA aptamers: from basic science towards therapy *Handb. Exp. Pharmacol.* **173** 305–26

Ulrich H *et al* 1998 *In vitro* selection of RNA molecules that displace cocaine from the membrane-bound nicotinic acetylcholine receptor *Proc. SPIE* **95** 14051–6

Varty K, O'Brien C and Ignaszak A 2021 Breast cancer aptamers: current sensing targets, available aptamers, and their evaluation for clinical use in diagnostics *Cancers* **13** 3984

Vera-Puente O *et al* 2018 MAFG is a potential therapeutic target to restore chemosensitivity in cisplatin-resistant cancer cells by increasing reactive oxygen species *Transl. Res. J. Lab. Clin. Med.* **200** 1–17

Vinkenborg J L *et al* 2011 Aptamers for allosteric regulation *Nat. Chem. Biol.* **7** 519–27

White R, Rusconi C, Scardino E, Wolberg A, Lawson J, Hoffman M and Sullenger B 2001 Generation of species cross-reactive aptamers using 'Toggle' SELEX *Mol Ther* **4** 567–73

Xu W and Ellington A D 1996 Anti-peptide aptamers recognize amino acid sequence and bind a protein epitope *PNAS* **93** 7475–80

Xu X, Hamhouyia F, Thomas S D, Burke T J, Girvan A C, McGregor W G, Trent J O, Miller D M and Bates P J 2001 Inhibition of DNA replication and induction of S phase cell cycle arrest by Grich oligonucleotides *J. Biol. Chem.* **276** 43221–30

Yang D 2019 G-Quadruplex DNA and RNA. *G-Quadruplex Nucleic Acids: Methods and Protocols; Methods in Molecular Biology* ed D Yang and C Lin (Springer) pp 1–24

Zhou J, Li H, Li S, Zaia J and Rossi J J 2008 Novel dual inhibitory function aptamer-siRNA delivery system for HIV-1 therapy *Molecular Therapy* **16** 1481–9

Zhou Y, Li W, Tseng Y, Zhang J and Liu J 2019 Developing slow-off dickkopf-1 aptamers for early-diagnosis of hepatocellular carcinoma *Talanta* **194** 422–9

Zhou G, Wilson G, Hebbard L, Duan W, Liddle C, George J and Qiao L 2016 Aptamers: a promising chemical antibody for cancer therapy *Oncotarget* **7** 13446–63

www.ingramcontent.com/pod-product-compliance
Ingram Content Group UK Ltd.
Pitfield, Milton Keynes, MK11 3LW, UK
UKHW051858100926
8556IPUK00005B/680

9 780750 350105